T0295180

NCLEX-PN®
Prep
Seventeenth Edition

Practice Test **+** Proven Strategies

Also From Kaplan Nursing

Books

NCLEX-PN® Content Review Guide
The Basics: A Comprehensive Outline of Nursing School Content
NCLEX® Medication Review
Adult CCRN® Prep
Family Nurse Practitioner Certification Prep Plus
Dosage Calculation Workbook
Talk Like a Nurse

Online

kaptest.com/nclex-pn

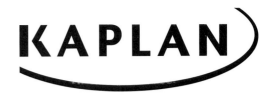

NCLEX-PN® Prep

Seventeenth Edition

Practice Test + Proven Strategies

Published by Kaplan North America, LLC dba Kaplan Publishing
1515 West Cypress Creek Road
Fort Lauderdale, Florida 33309

10 9 8 7 6 5 4 3 2 1

ISBN-13: 978-1-5062-9611-1

Kaplan Publishing print books are available at special quantity discounts to use for sales promotions, employee premiums, or educational purposes. For more information or to purchase books, please call the Simon & Schuster special sales department at 866-506-1949.

TABLE OF CONTENTS

K   v

For Any Test Changes or Late-Breaking Developments

kaptest.com/retail-book-corrections-and-updates

The material in this book is current at the time of publication. However, the National Council of State Boards of Nursing may have instituted changes in the test after this book was published. Be sure to carefully read the materials you receive when you register for the test. If there are any important late-breaking developments—or any changes or corrections to the Kaplan test preparation materials in this book—we will post that information online at **kaptest.com/retail-book-corrections-and-updates**.

ABOUT THE AUTHORS

Barbara J. Irwin, MSN, RN

Barbara Irwin is emeritus Executive Director of Nursing at Kaplan Test Prep. She supervised development of the Kaplan courses for preparation for the NCLEX-RN® and NCLEX-PN® exams for U.S. nursing students and international nurses, as well as integrated testing programs implemented by nursing schools. Irwin developed the Decision Tree, a framework of innovative test-taking strategies that help students achieve success on these high-stakes tests. Her seminars about how to effectively study to achieve deep learning have guided thousands of students nurses. Her seminars to nursing faculty have shared important insights about the NCLEX-RN® and NCLEX-PN® examinations and how to overcome the challenge of non-self-efficacious nursing students. Irwin received a bachelor of science in nursing from the University of Oklahoma and a master of science degree in nursing and nursing education from Kaplan University. Her professional background includes experience as a nursing educator and director of a home health agency.

Patricia A. Yock, BSN, RN

Patricia Yock is a nursing educator and consultant in Boulder, Colorado. She received a bachelor of science in nursing from Loyola University in Chicago. Her professional experience includes clinical nursing in varied settings from postsurgical care to comprehensive inpatient rehabilitation, and nursing education in diploma and practical nursing programs. Yock is certified in rehabilitation nursing and served as the nursing director for inpatient rehabilitation and transitional care units.

Judith A. Burckhardt, PhD, MSN, RN

Dr. Judith Burckhardt is former Dean of the Nursing and Health Programs for Kaplan Higher Education Campuses, Vice President of the Kaplan School of Nursing, and head of the Nursing division at Kaplan Test Preparation. Under Dr. Burckhardt's leadership, Kaplan introduced new methods of program provision, including online delivery. She is currently Dean of Nursing Programs at American Sentinel University. Dr. Burckhardt received a bachelor of science in nursing from Loyola University in Chicago, a master's degree in education from Washington University in St. Louis, a master of science in nursing degree from Kaplan University, and a doctorate in educational administration from the University of Nebraska at Lincoln.

Kaplan thanks the following nursing professionals for their contributions to this book:

Barbara Arnoldussen, RN, MBA, CPHQ
Jean Blank, MSN, RN
Susan Compton, MSN, RN
Cindy Finesilver, MSN, RN
Mary Fischer, MSN, CNM, RN
Joseph Ryan Goble, MSN, RN, CEN, CPEN
Pamela Guillaume, MSN, RN
Janice Hoffman, PhD, RN, ANEF
Cheryl Martin, PhD, RNC-E, WHNP-E
Patricia Porta, MSN, RN
Rebecca Potter, PhD, MSIDT, MSN/ED, RN
Marlene Redemske, MSN, MA, RN
Marian Stewart, MSN, RN
Lindsey Unterseher, MSN, RN

HOW TO USE THIS BOOK

STEP 1: Read and Complete Parts One and Two

Parts One and Two contain a comprehensive, detailed strategy guide for each type of question on the NCLEX-PN® exam. This information will teach you how to analyze each question and use your nursing knowledge to select the correct answer choice. Practice using these strategies in the quiz at the end of each chapter in Part Two, then check your work against the detailed answer explanations provided.

BONUS: Kaplan also offers realistic NCLEX-PN practice online, free. Sign up here to access Kaplan's NCLEX-PN quizzes, question of the day, and more: **kaptest.com/ nclex-pn/free/nclex-practice**

STEP 2: Read Part Three

Part Three will help you determine the most effective methods of exam preparation for you and will guide you in the licensure process.

Chapter 12, Essentials for International Nurses, contains information on certification for graduates of foreign nursing schools, work visas, and programs that can help you prepare for the NCLEX-PN® exam. This chapter also covers nursing practice in the United States and includes practice designed to help you master NCLEX-PN® exam-type questions on the important subject of nursing communication.

STEP 3: Take the Practice Test

When you are nearing your exam date, take Kaplan's full-length practice test. It follows the NCLEX-PN® Exam Test Plan and simulates the format, content, question types, and difficulty of the actual test. This 150-question practice test will help you build your stamina for the real test and give you a good sense of your level of preparation. Detailed answer explanations follow the exam, and these can help you understand why you got off track on a particular question.

STEP 4: Register for the Exam

When you are prepared to take the NCLEX-PN® exam, contact your state/provincial/ territorial Board of Nursing to initiate the registration process. All the steps you'll need to follow are contained in Chapter 10, The Licensure Process.

Practice Makes Perfect

GO ONLINE

www.kaptest.com/nclex-pn/practice/nclex-pn-qbank

Looking for even more practice? Up your game with **Kaplan's NCLEX-PN® Qbank.**

- Over 1,100 test-like NCLEX questions

- Customizable: quiz yourself by category, incorrect questions, and more

- Comprehensive explanations for every answer option, correct and incorrect

- Topic refreshers

- Detailed performance feedback to measure your progress

Learn more at: **kaptest.com/nclex-pn/practice/nclex-pn-qbank**

[PART ONE]

NCLEX-PN® EXAM OVERVIEW

CHAPTER 1

OVERVIEW OF THE NCLEX-PN® EXAM

The NCLEX-PN® exam is, among other things, an endurance test, like a marathon. If you don't prepare properly or approach it with confidence and rigor, you'll quickly lose your composure. Here is a sample, test-like question:

> A client had a permanent pacemaker implanted one year ago. The client returns to the outpatient clinic for suspected pacemaker battery failure. It is **most** important for the LPN/LVN to assess which of these?
>
> 1. Abdominal pain, nausea, and vomiting.
> 2. Wheezing on exertion, cyanosis, and orthopnea.
> 3. Palpitations, shortness of breath, and dizziness.
> 4. Chest pain, headache, and diaphoresis.

As you can see, the style and content of the NCLEX-PN® exam is unique. It's not like any other exam you've ever taken, even in nursing school!

The content in this book was prepared by the experts on Kaplan's Nursing team, the world's largest provider of test prep courses for the NCLEX-PN® exam. By using Kaplan's proven methods and strategies, you will be able to take control of the exam, just as you have taken control of your nursing education and other preparations for your career in this incredibly challenging and rewarding field. The first step is to learn everything you can about the exam.

What Is the NCLEX-PN® Exam?

NCLEX-PN® stands for *National Council Licensure Examination For Practical Nurses*. The NCLEX-PN® examination is administered by the National Council of State Boards of Nursing (NCSBN), whose members include the boards of nursing in each of the 50 states in the United States, the District of Columbia, and four U.S. territories: American Samoa, Guam, the Northern Mariana Islands, and the Virgin Islands. These boards have a mandate to protect the public from unsafe and ineffective nursing care, and each board has been given responsibility to regulate the practice of nursing in its respective state. In fact, the NCLEX-PN® exam is often referred to as "the Boards" or "State Boards."

The NCLEX-PN® exam has only one purpose: to determine if it is safe for you to begin practice as an entry-level practical/vocational nurse.

Why Must You Take the NCLEX-PN® Exam?

The NCLEX-PN® exam is prepared by the NCSBN. Each state requires that you pass this exam to obtain a license to practice as a practical/vocational nurse. The designation *licensed practical/vocational nurse* or *LPN/LVN* indicates that you have proven to your state board of nursing or regulatory body that you can deliver safe and effective nursing care.

The NCLEX-PN® exam is a test of minimum competency and is based on the knowledge and behaviors that are needed for the entry-level practice of practical/vocational nursing. This exam tests not only your knowledge, but also your ability to make competent nursing decisions. Specifically, the National Council uses the NCLEX-PN® to verify that you have the cognitive skills and clinical judgment to do the following:

- Recognize concerning cues
- Analyze the significance or implications of the cues
- Identify the topic or the priority concern
- Generate solutions that enable you to plan or assist in the planning of your client's care
- Implement the care you have planned
- Evaluate whether the nursing interventions you took improved the client's condition

What Is Entry-Level Practice of Practical/Vocational Nursing?

In order to define *entry-level* practice of practical/vocational nursing, NCSBN conducts a job-analysis study every three years to determine what entry-level nurses do on the job. The kinds of questions they investigate include: In which clinical settings does the beginning practical/vocational nurse work? What types of care do beginning practical/vocational nurses provide to their clients? What are their primary duties and responsibilities? Based on the results of this study, NCSBN adjusts the content and level of difficulty of the test to accurately reflect what is happening in the workplace.

What the NCLEX-PN® Exam Is *NOT*

The exam is not a test of achievement or intelligence. It is not designed for nurses who have years of experience. The questions do not involve high-tech clinical nursing or equipment. It is not predictive of your eventual success in the career of nursing. You will not be tested on all the content that you were taught in practical/vocational nursing school.

What Is a CAT?

CAT stands for *Computer Adaptive Test*. Each test is assembled interactively based on the accuracy of the candidate's response to the questions. This ensures that the questions you are answering are not "too hard" or "too easy" for your skill level. Your first question will be relatively easy; that is, below the level of minimum competency. If you answer that question correctly, the computer selects a slightly more difficult question. If you answer the first question incorrectly, the computer selects a slightly easier question (Figure 1.1). By continuing to do this as you answer questions, the computer is able to calculate your level of competence.

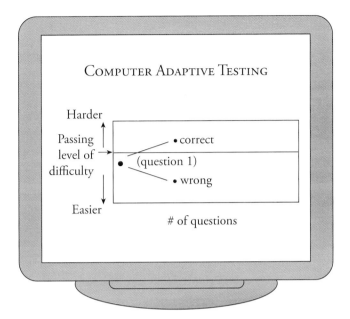

Figure 1.1

In a CAT, the questions are adapted to your level of ability. The computer selects questions that represent all areas of nursing, as defined by the NCLEX-PN® test plan and by the level of item difficulty. Each question is self-contained, so that all of the information you need to answer a question is presented on the computer screen.

Taking the Exam

There is no time limit for each individual question. You have a maximum of five hours to complete the exam, but that includes the beginning tutorial, an optional 10-minute break after the first 2 hours of testing, and an optional break after an additional 90 minutes of testing. (Time that you spend in optional breaks, however, is counted as a part of your 5 hours of total testing time.) Everyone answers a minimum of 85 questions to a maximum of 150 questions. Regardless of the number of questions you answer, you are given 15 questions that are experimental. These questions, which are indistinguishable from the other questions on the test, are being tested for future use in NCLEX-PN® exams, and your answers do not count for or against you.

Your test ends when one of the following occurs:

- You have demonstrated minimum competency and answered the minimum number of questions (85) (Figure 1.2).
- You have demonstrated a lack of minimum competency and answered the minimum number of questions (85) (Figure 1.3).
- You have answered the maximum number of questions (150).
- You have used the maximum time allowed (five hours).

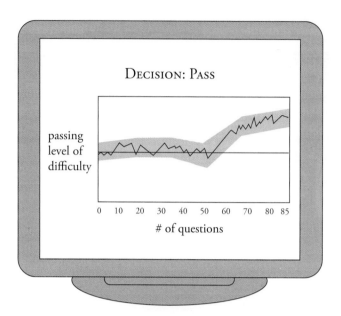

Figure 1.2

Remember, every question counts. There is no warm-up time, so it is important for you to be ready to answer questions correctly from the very beginning. Concentration is also key. You need to give your best to each question because you do not know which one will put you over the top.

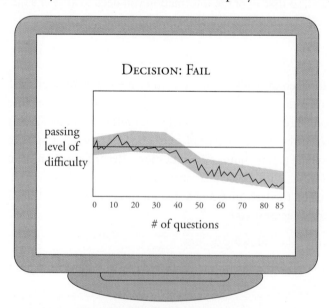

Figure 1.3

Structure of the NCLEX-PN® Exam

Whether you complete the exam in 85 questions (the minimum number) or 150 questions (the maximum), you will see a mix of standalone questions and case study question sets.

Standalone Questions

Standalone questions can be answered on their own, without considering any other question on the exam. These items may be text-based, or they may include a chart/exhibit in place of some of the text. The most common type of standalone question is also the most familiar type: text-based, four-option multiple choice question.

Some standalone questions will be case-based items and start by introducing a client, the client's diagnosis or symptoms upon admission, and the client's medical record. Depending on the context, you may be required to analyze vital signs, physical assessment findings, and/or health care provider orders. Foundational nursing knowledge is a prerequisite for answering case-based questions, but sound clinical judgment is of equal importance.

In case-based questions, different categories of information may be visible under different "tabs" of the medical record, as shown in the following illustrations.

The nurse is caring for a 38-year-old client newly admitted to the medical-surgical floor with fatigue and dehydration.

Nurse's Notes	Vital Signs

The client has a history of diabetes mellitus and has been insulin dependent for over 20 years. The client has undergone hemodialysis for the last 4 years for end-stage kidney failure. The client's skin is warm and dry to touch with poor skin turgor, and the mucous membranes are dry. The client reports feeling nauseated for several days and has not been eating or drinking. The client also reports several episodes of diarrhea. Labs have been drawn, but results are not available yet.

Figure 1.4 First Tab of a Case-Based Question

The nurse is caring for a 38-year-old client newly admitted to the medical-surgical floor with fatigue and dehydration.

Nurse's Notes	Vital Signs

Vital Sign	Result
Blood Pressure	120/82 mmHg
Pulse	118
Respirations	12
Temperature	100.8° F (38.2° C)

Figure 1.5 Second Tab of a Case-Based Question

Case Study Question Sets

You will also see case-based questions in six-item sets. Like the standalone case-based questions, these case study question sets start by introducing a client case, passage, or vignette. In the six-item sets, however, you must apply information obtained in earlier questions to help answer later questions in the set.

Each "tab" of the medical record will show an aspect of the same client case, for example:

- Nurse's notes
- History and physical
- Laboratory or diagnostic results
- Flow sheets
- Admission notes or progress notes
- Intake and output
- Medications

Additional, "unfolding" tabs of the medical record may be added as you progress through the six questions in the set. Whenever a new tab of data is provided (such as laboratory results), the information in that tab will be available for the current question and for all subsequent questions in the set. Once you have navigated to a subsequent question in a six-item set, you cannot go back to previous questions in the set to alter your responses. However, you can "course correct" based on newly added information as you answer the remaining questions in the set.

The six questions within a set are counted as six different items. If question number 11 starts the set, the next question you see after the set ends will be question number 17.

Navigation

Case-based questions take the form of a split screen. In each case study question set, the case remains static on the left-hand side of the screen, while the right-hand side of the screen changes as you answer the individual questions. Within each set of six questions, you may also see a succession of different item types; for instance, the first question in a set might be a Highlight item, the second question a Matrix item, the third a Cloze item, and so on. (You will learn more about question types on the NCLEX-PN® exam in chapter 3.)

You can determine whether a case study is a standalone question or part of a question set by looking at the boldface text in the upper left-hand corner of the screen:

- **Case Study Screen 1 of 1** indicates a standalone question.
- **Case Study Screen 1 of 6** (or **Case Study Screen 2 of 6**, etc.) indicates a question in a six-item set.

Following is a series of examples illustrating how an unfolding case study will look. Only three sample screens are shown in this example. On the NCLEX-PN® exam, however, case study question sets will always have six items.

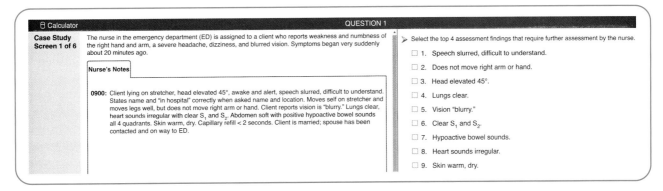

Figure 1.6 Screen 1 of 6 in an Unfolding Case Study

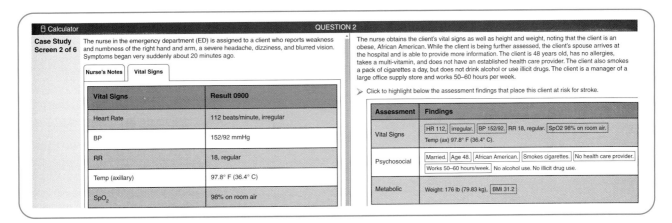

Figure 1.7 Screen 2 of 6 in an Unfolding Case Study

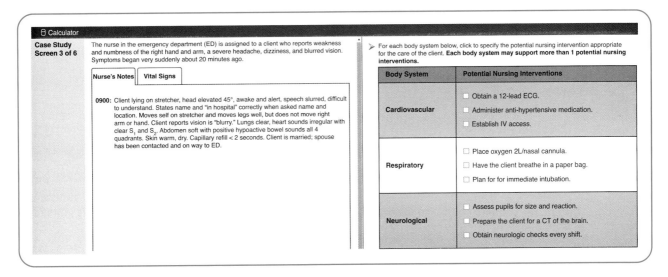

Figure 1.8 Screen 3 of 6 in an Unfolding Case Study

Structure of a Minimum Length Exam

The minimum length NCLEX-PN® exam is 85 questions. Within these first 85 questions, every test taker will receive three scored six-item question sets (18 scored questions) and 52 scored standalone items, for a total of 70 scored items. The other 15 questions are unscored, experimental items.

The scored case study question sets will be randomly selected and evenly distributed among the 70 scored questions, with the first set appearing in the first third, the second set in the middle third, and the third set in the final third (see Figure 1.9). All exam candidates will see case study question sets in the same region of the exam, but the sets will not appear in the same place for everyone. For example, you might receive the first set after the sixth item while another test taker receives the first set after the tenth item.

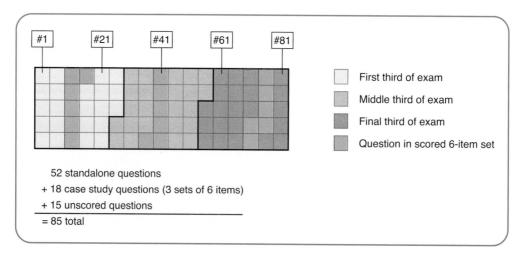

Figure 1.9 Example of a Minimum Length Exam

You may see as many as five case study question sets (30 items) on your NCLEX-PN® exam, but only three sets (18 items) will be scored. Any additional question sets you see will be part of the 15 unscored items randomly distributed in the first 85 questions. Looking at Figure 1.9, you can't tell which of the 85 items are unscored. The same is true when you are taking the exam. *You will not know* which items are scored for your NCLEX exam and which items are experimental.

Questions After the Minimum Length

If a stopping rule is not triggered after the minimum length of 85 questions, the exam will continue until either the computer reaches a pass/fail decision, you have answered 150 questions, or you have reached the maximum testing time of 5 hours. All remaining items will be scored. At this point, the computer will select only standalone questions.

- Case-based standalone items make up approximately 10% of the remaining questions.
- Non-case-based standalone items (such as "select all that apply" and four-option multiple choice questions) make up approximately 90% of the remaining questions.

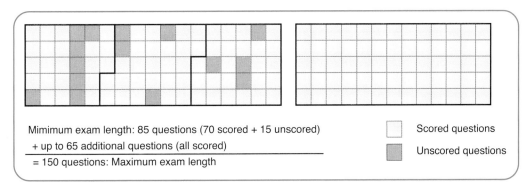

Mimimum exam length: 85 questions (70 scored + 15 unscored)

+ up to 65 additional questions (all scored)

= 150 questions: Maximum exam length

Scored questions

Unscored questions

Figure 1.10 Example of a Maximum Length Exam

When you are taking the NCLEX-PN® exam, try not to be concerned with the length of your test. In fact, you should plan on testing for 5 hours and seeing 150 questions. You are still in the game as long as the computer continues to give you test questions, so focus on answering them to the best of your ability. If you are still getting questions, it means the computer has not made a decision on your ability level and you can still pass the NCLEX!

NCLEX-PN® Exam Scoring

In past versions of the NCLEX-PN®, no partial credit was given. If the correct answers to a question were answer choices (1), (2), and (4), for example, exam candidates had to select those three answers—and *only* those answers—as correct in order to receive credit for the question. Since 2023, however, NCSBN awards partial credit. Three different scoring methodologies are used:

- 0/1 Scoring Rule
- +/– Scoring Rule
- Rationale Scoring Rule

Let's look at how the NCLEX-PN® exam applies these scoring approaches.

0/1 Scoring Rule

The 0/1 Scoring Rule is the rule that you are probably most familiar with from nursing school. This is the classic approach used to score four-option Multiple Choice questions:

- Earn 1 point for correct response.
- Earn 0 points for incorrect response.

For an item that is worth more than 1 point, the sum of all correct responses is the total score. The illustration shows an example of how a multi-point Matrix Multiple Choice item would be scored using the 0/1 Scoring Rule.

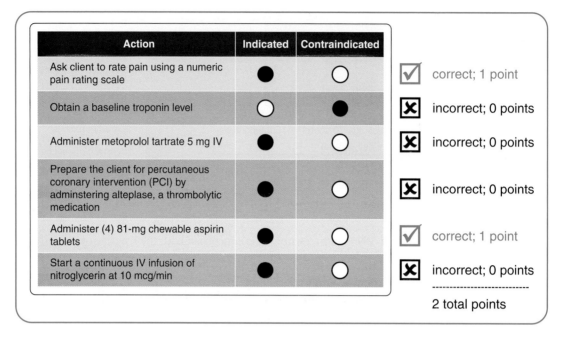

Action	Indicated	Contraindicated		
Ask client to rate pain using a numeric pain rating scale	●	○	☑	correct; 1 point
Obtain a baseline troponin level	○	●	☒	incorrect; 0 points
Administer metoprolol tartrate 5 mg IV	●	○	☒	incorrect; 0 points
Prepare the client for percutaneous coronary intervention (PCI) by adminstering alteplase, a thrombolytic medication	●	○	☒	incorrect; 0 points
Administer (4) 81-mg chewable aspirin tablets	●	○	☑	correct; 1 point
Start a continuous IV infusion of nitroglycerin at 10 mcg/min	●	○	☒	incorrect; 0 points

2 total points

Figure 1.11 0/1 Scoring Rule Applied to a Matrix Item

+/− Scoring Rule

The +/− Scoring Rule awards a higher score when you identify and select information that is more pertinent. You probably remember "Select all that apply" (or SATA) questions from nursing school. You may have dreaded them too. The good news is that you can receive partial credit on the NCLEX exam for SATA questions! The +/− Scoring Rule works like this:

- Earn 1 point for each correct selection.
- Forfeit 1 point for each incorrect selection.

While the +/− Scoring Rule subtracts points for incorrect answers, there are no negative scores. The minimum score per item is zero.

The illustration shows an example of how a multi-point item would be scored using the +/− Scoring Rule. In this example, the test-taker has selected all four correct answer options, and has also selected two incorrect options. This would result in a score of 2 out of a possible 4 points for this question.

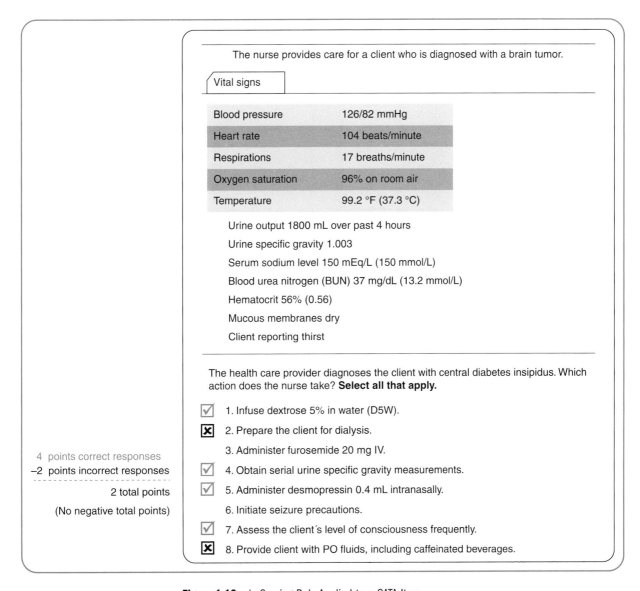

The nurse provides care for a client who is diagnosed with a brain tumor.

Vital signs

Blood pressure	126/82 mmHg
Heart rate	104 beats/minute
Respirations	17 breaths/minute
Oxygen saturation	96% on room air
Temperature	99.2 °F (37.3 °C)

Urine output 1800 mL over past 4 hours

Urine specific gravity 1.003

Serum sodium level 150 mEq/L (150 mmol/L)

Blood urea nitrogen (BUN) 37 mg/dL (13.2 mmol/L)

Hematocrit 56% (0.56)

Mucous membranes dry

Client reporting thirst

The health care provider diagnoses the client with central diabetes insipidus. Which action does the nurse take? **Select all that apply.**

☑ 1. Infuse dextrose 5% in water (D5W).

☒ 2. Prepare the client for dialysis.

3. Administer furosemide 20 mg IV.

☑ 4. Obtain serial urine specific gravity measurements.

☑ 5. Administer desmopressin 0.4 mL intranasally.

6. Initiate seizure precautions.

☑ 7. Assess the client's level of consciousness frequently.

☒ 8. Provide client with PO fluids, including caffeinated beverages.

4 points correct responses
−2 points incorrect responses
2 total points
(No negative total points)

Figure 1.12 +/− Scoring Rule Applied to a SATA Item

Rationale Scoring Rule

Finally, the Rationale Scoring Rule awards points when both elements of a linked pair of concepts are correct. This scoring method tests concepts that require justification through a rationale—that is, situations in which a nurse must perform action X because of circumstance Y. Under the Rationale Scoring Rule:

- Earn 1 point when both X and Y are correct.

- Earn 0 points when any element of the answer selection is incorrect.

The Rationale Scoring Rule requires an understanding of paired information. The illustration shows an example of how a Cloze item would be scored using the Rationale Scoring Rule. Though the test taker has correctly selected "loss of visual fields or blindness" in this example, 0 points are earned because the other element of the paired information is incorrect.

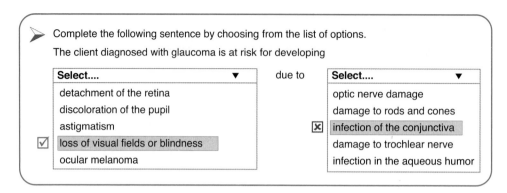

Complete the following sentence by choosing from the list of options.

The client diagnosed with glaucoma is at risk for developing

Select.... ▼		due to	Select.... ▼
detachment of the retina			optic nerve damage
discoloration of the pupil			damage to rods and cones
astigmatism	☒		infection of the conjunctiva
☑ loss of visual fields or blindness			damage to trochlear nerve
ocular melanoma			infection in the aqueous humor

Figure 1.13 Rationale Scoring Rule Applied to a Cloze Item

Having a general familiarity with the scoring rules will help you avoid surprises. On the NCLEX exam, however, you should not try to calculate the number of points you may receive based on your responses. Similarly, you should not dwell on the difficulty level of the questions that the CAT has selected. Neither is a good use of your time. Instead, you should focus solely on making safe nursing judgments.

Content of the NCLEX-PN® Exam

The NCLEX-PN® exam is not divided into separate content areas. It tests integrated nursing content. Many nursing programs are based on the medical model. Students take separate medical, surgical, pediatric, psychiatric, and obstetric classes. On the NCLEX-PN® exam, all content is integrated.

Look at the following question.

> A client with type 1 diabetes returns to the recovery room one hour after an uneventful delivery of a 9 lb, 8 oz (4,309 g), newborn. The nurse would expect which change in the client's blood glucose level?
>
> 1. From 220 to 180 mg/dL (12.21 to 10 mmol/L).
> 2. From 110 to 80 mg/dL (6.1 to 4.4 mmol/L).
> 3. From 90 to 120 mg/dL (5 to 6.7 mmol/L).
> 4. From 100 to 140 mg/dL (5.6 to 7.8 mmol/L).

Is this an obstetrical question or a medical/surgical question? In order to select the correct answer, (2), you must consider the pathophysiology of diabetes along with the principles of labor and delivery. This is an example of an integrated question.

The NCLEX-PN® Exam Test Plan

The NCLEX-PN® exam is organized according to the framework "Client Needs." For the purposes of the NCLEX-PN® examination, a client is identified as the individual, family, or group, which includes significant others. There are four major categories of client needs; two of the major categories are further divided for a total of six subcategories. This information is distributed by NCSBN, the developer of the NCLEX-PN® exam.

Client Need #1: Safe and Effective Care Environment

The first subcategory for this client need is **Coordinated Care**, which accounts for **18–24** percent of the questions on the exam. Nursing actions that are covered in this subcategory include:

- Advance directives
- Advocacy
- Client care assignments
- Client rights
- Collaboration with interdisciplinary team
- Concepts of management and supervision
- Confidentiality/information security
- Continuity of care
- Establishing priorities
- Ethical practice
- Informed consent
- Information technology
- Legal responsibilities
- Performance improvement (quality improvement)
- Referral process
- Resource management

Here is an example of a question from the Coordinated Care subcategory:

> The LPN/LVN knows that an assignment to which client would be appropriate?
>
> 1. A client with emphysema scheduled for discharge.
> 2. A client in traction for treatment of a fractured femur.
> 3. A client with low back pain scheduled for a myelogram.
> 4. A client newly diagnosed with type 1 diabetes.

The correct answer is (2). This client is in stable condition and can be cared for by an LPN/LVN.

Here is another example of a Coordinated Care question:

> After receiving hand-off of care report from the RN, which client should the LPN/LVN see **first**?
>
> 1. A client refusing to take sucralfate before mealtime.
> 2. A client with left-sided weakness asking for assistance to the commode.
> 3. A client reporting chills who is scheduled for a cholecystectomy.
> 4. A client with a nasogastric tube who had a bowel resection yesterday.

The correct answer is (3). This is the least stable client.

The second subcategory for this client need is **Safety and Infection Control**, which accounts for **10–16** percent of the questions on the exam. Nursing actions that are covered in this subcategory include:

- Accident/error/injury prevention
- Emergency response plan
- Ergonomic principles
- Handling hazardous and infectious materials
- Home safety
- Reporting of incident/event/irregular occurrence/variance
- Restraints and safety devices
- Safe use of equipment
- Security plan
- Standard precautions/transmission-based precautions/surgical asepsis

Here is an example of a question from the Safety and Infection Control subcategory:

> The primary health care provider prescribes amoxicillin 150 mg PO in oral suspension every 8 hours for a 3-year-old client. The LPN/LVN enters the client's room to administer the medication and discovers that the client does not have an identification bracelet. Which action should the LPN/LVN take?
>
> 1. Ask the parents to state their child's name.
> 2. Ask the child to say the first and last name.
> 3. Have a coworker identify the child before giving the medication.
> 4. Hold the medication until an identification bracelet can be obtained.

The correct answer is (1). This action will allow the nurse to correctly identify the child and enable the nurse to give the medication on time.

Client Need #2: Health Promotion and Maintenance

This client need accounts for **6–12** percent of the questions on the exam. Nursing actions that are covered in this category include:

- Aging process
- Ante/intra/postpartum and newborn care
- Data collection techniques
- Developmental stages and transitions
- Health promotion/disease prevention
- High-risk behaviors
- Lifestyle choices
- Self-care

It is important to understand that not everyone described in the questions will be sick, hospitalized, or in a long-term care facility. Some clients may be in a clinic or home-care setting. Some clients may not be sick at all. Wellness is an important concept on the NCLEX-PN® exam. It is necessary for a safe and effective practical/vocational nurse to know how to promote health and prevent disease.

The following is an example of a question from the Health Promotion and Maintenance category:

> The LPN/LVN in the outpatient clinic notes that the blood pressure for a client is 190/100 mmHg. The LPN/LVN should take which action?
>
> 1. Report the blood pressure reading to the RN.
> 2. Wait 20 minutes and retake the blood pressure.
> 3. Use a different cuff and retake the blood pressure.
> 4. Position the client supine with feet elevated.

The correct answer is (1). The LPN/LVN is responsible for data collection and should report findings that are abnormal to the supervising RN. Immediate action should be taken, so (2) is incorrect. It is unnecessary to recheck the blood pressure using other equipment (3) or to position the client supine with feet elevated (4).

Client Need #3: Psychosocial Integrity

This client need accounts for **9–15** percent of the questions on the exam. Nursing actions that are covered in this category include:

- Abuse/neglect
- Behavioral management
- Chemical and other dependencies
- Coping mechanisms
- Crisis intervention
- Cultural awareness
- End-of-life concepts

- Grief and loss
- Mental health concepts
- Religious and spiritual influences on health
- Sensory/perceptual alterations
- Stress management
- Support systems
- Therapeutic communication
- Therapeutic environment

This is an example of a question from the Psychosocial Integrity category:

> A client comes to the nurses' station and inquires about going to the cafeteria to get something to eat. The client becomes verbally abusive when told personal privileges do not include going to the cafeteria. Which approach by the LPN/LVN would be **most** effective?
>
> 1. Tell the client to speak softly to avoid disturbing the other clients.
> 2. Ask what the client wants from the cafeteria and have it delivered to the client's room.
> 3. Calmly but firmly escort the client back to the client's room.
> 4. Assign the unlicensed assistive personnel (UAP) to accompany the client to the cafeteria.

The correct answer is (3). The nurse should not reinforce abusive behavior. Clients need consistent and clearly defined expectations and limits.

Client Need #4: Physiological Integrity

The first subcategory for this client need is **Basic Care and Comfort**, which accounts for **7–13** percent of the questions on the exam. Nursing actions that are covered in this subcategory include:

- Assistive devices
- Elimination
- Mobility/immobility
- Non-pharmacological comfort interventions
- Nutrition and oral hydration
- Personal hygiene
- Rest and sleep

The following question is representative of the Basic Care and Comfort subcategory:

> The primary health care provider is applying a cast to an infant for treatment of talipes equinovarus. Which instruction is **most** essential for the LPN/LVN to give to the child's parents regarding care?
>
> 1. Offer age-appropriate toys.
> 2. Visit clinic frequently for cast adjustments.
> 3. Give an analgesic as needed.
> 4. Check circulation in the casted extremity.

The correct answer is (4). A possible complication that can occur after cast application is impaired circulation. All of these answer choices might be included in family teaching, but checking the child's circulation is the highest priority.

The second subcategory for this client need is **Pharmacological Therapies**, which makes up for **10–16** percent of the questions on the exam. Nursing actions that are covered in this subcategory include:

- Adverse effects/contraindications/side effects/interactions
- Dosage calculations
- Expected actions/outcomes
- Medication administration
- Pharmacological pain management

Because the brand name or trade name of drugs may vary, you should expect to see the use of generic medication names only on the NCLEX-PN® exam.

Try this question from the Pharmacological Therapies subcategory:

> The LPN/LVN notes the client is allergic to an ordered medication. Which is the correct action by the LPN/LVN?
>
> 1. Administer the medication as the primary health care provider ordered it.
> 2. Administer the medication and closely observe the client.
> 3. Call the pharmacist to verify potential allergic responses.
> 4. Call the primary health care provider and report the medication allergy.

The correct answer is (4). The LPN/LVN must notify the primary health care provider regarding the client's allergy to revise the medication order.

The third subcategory for this client need is **Reduction of Risk Potential**, which accounts for **9–15** percent of the questions on the exam. Nursing actions that are covered in this subcategory include:

- Changes/abnormalities in vital signs
- Diagnostic tests
- Laboratory values
- Potential for alterations in body systems
- Potential for complications of diagnostic tests/treatments/procedures
- Potential for complications from surgical procedures and health alterations
- Therapeutic procedures

This is a an example of a question from the Reduction of Risk Potential subcategory:

> Parents bring a school-age client with a history of type 1 diabetes and several days of illness to the emergency department (ED). Which laboratory test result would the LPN/LVN expect if the client is experiencing diabetic ketoacidosis (DKA)?
>
> 1. Serum glucose 140 mg/dL (7.8 mmol/L).
> 2. Serum creatine 5.2 mg/dL (460 µmol/L).
> 3. Blood pH 7.28.
> 4. Hematocrit 38%.

The correct answer is (3). Normal blood pH is 7.35–7.45. A blood pH of 7.28 indicates DKA.

The fourth subcategory for this client need is **Physiological Adaptation**, which accounts for **7–13** percent of exam questions. Nursing actions that are covered in this subcategory include:

- Alterations in body systems
- Basic pathophysiology
- Fluid and electrolyte imbalances
- Medical emergencies
- Radiation therapy
- Unexpected response to therapies

The following is an example of a Physiological Adaptation question:

> The LPN/LVN is delivering external cardiac compressions to a client during cardiopulmonary resuscitation (CPR). Which action by the LPN/LVN is **best**?
>
> 1. Maintain a position close to the client's side with the nurse's knees apart.
> 2. Position hands on the lower half of the sternum during compressions.
> 3. Lean on chest between compressions to prevent full chest wall recoil.
> 4. Check for a return of the client's pulse after every 8 breaths by the nurse.

The correct answer is (2). The nurse's hands should be positioned on the lower half of the client's sternum during compressions with elbows locked, arms straight, and shoulders positioned directly over the hands. The nurse should avoid leaning on the chest between compressions to allow for full chest wall recoil.

The Nursing Process

Several processes are integrated throughout the NCLEX-PN® exam. The most important of these is *the nursing process.*

For the practical/vocational nurse, the nursing process involves *data collection, planning, implementation,* and *evaluation* of nursing care. You will help the registered nurse, or other qualified health professional, formulate a plan of nursing care for clients in a variety of settings. As a graduate practical/vocational nurse, you are very familiar with each step of the nursing process and how to assist in writing a care plan using this process. Knowledge of the nursing process is essential to the performance of safe and effective care. It is also essential to answering questions correctly on the NCLEX-PN® exam.

Now we are going to review the steps of the nursing process and show you how each step is incorporated into test questions. The nursing process is a way of thinking. Using it will help you select correct answers.

Data collection. Data collection is the process of establishing and verifying a database of information about the client. This permits you to collaborate in the identification of actual and/or potential health problems. The practical/vocational nurse obtains subjective data (information given to you by the client that can't be observed or measured by others) and objective data (information that is observable and measurable by others). This data is collected by interviewing and observing the client and/or significant others, reviewing the health history, performing a physical assessment, gathering lab results, and interacting with the registered nurse and members of the health care team.

An example of a data collection test question is:

> The LPN/LVN is obtaining a health history from a client admitted with acute glomerulonephritis. Which history finding is significant for the diagnosis of acute glomerulonephritis?
>
> 1. Personal history of sore throat 10 days ago.
> 2. Family history of chronic glomerulonephritis.
> 3. Personal history of renal calculus 2 years ago.
> 4. Personal history of renal trauma several years ago.

The correct answer is (1). Acute glomerulonephritis, an immunologic disorder that affects the kidneys, can be caused by group A Streptococcus. It usually occurs about 10 days after strep throat or scarlet fever and about 21 days after a group A Streptococcus skin infection.

Planning. During the planning phase of the nursing process, the nursing care plan is formulated collaboratively with the registered nurse. Steps in planning include:

- Assigning priorities to nursing diagnosis
- Specifying goals
- Identifying interventions
- Specifying expected outcomes
- Documenting the nursing care plan

Goals are anticipated responses and client behaviors that result from nursing care. Nursing goals are client-centered and measurable, and they have an established time frame. *Expected outcomes* are the interim steps needed to reach a goal and the resolution of a nursing diagnosis. There will be multiple expected outcomes for each goal. Expected outcomes guide the practical/vocational nurse in planning interventions.

This is an example of a planning question:

> A client reporting nausea, vomiting, and severe right upper quadrant pain is admitted to the medical/surgical unit. The client's temperature is 101.3° F (38.5° C) and an abdominal x-ray reveals an enlarged gallbladder. The client is scheduled for surgery. Which action should the LPN/LVN take **first**?
>
> 1. Assess the client's need for dietary teaching.
> 2. Evaluate the client's fluid and electrolyte status.
> 3. Examine the client's health history for allergies to antibiotics.
> 4. Determine whether the client has signed consent for surgery.

The correct answer is (2). Hypokalemia and hypomagnesemia commonly occur after repeated vomiting.

Implementation. Implementation is the term used to describe the actions that you take in the care of your clients. Implementation includes:

- Assisting in the performance of activities of daily living (ADLs)
- Implementing the educational plan for the client and family
- Giving care to clients

It is important for you to remember that nursing interventions may be:

- *Independent* actions that do not require supervision by others. These nursing interventions are usually not within the scope of practice for practical/vocational nurses. However, the LPN/LVN can follow established care plans, standards of care, and established protocols.
- *Dependent* actions based on the written orders of a physician.
- *Interdependent* actions shared with the registered nurse or other members of the health team.

The NCLEX-PN® exam includes questions that involve all three types of nursing interventions.

Here is an example of an implementation question:

> A client is being treated in the burn unit for second- and third-degree burns over 45% of the body. The primary health care provider prescribes silver sulfadiazine cream application. Which method is **best** for the LPN/LVN to apply this medication?
>
> 1. Sterile dressings soaked in saline.
> 2. Sterile tongue depressor.
> 3. Sterile gloved hand.
> 4. Sterile cotton-tipped applicator.

The correct answer is (3). A sterile, gloved hand will cause the least trauma to tissues and will decrease the chances of breaking blisters.

Evaluation. Evaluation measures the client's response to nursing interventions and indicates the client's progress toward achieving the goals established in the care plan. You compare the observed results with expected outcomes in collaboration with the registered nurse.

This is an evaluation question:

> When caring for a client diagnosed with anorexia nervosa, which observation indicates to the LPN/LVN that the client's condition is improving?
>
> 1. The client eats all food on the meal tray.
> 2. The client asks friends to bring special foods.
> 3. The client weighs self daily.
> 4. The client has gained weight.

The correct response is (4). The client's weight is the most objective outcome measure in the evaluation of this client's problem.

Integrated Processes

Several other important processes are integrated throughout the NCLEX-PN® exam. They are:

Caring. As you take the NCLEX-PN® exam, remember that the test is about caring for people, not working with high-tech equipment or analyzing lab results.

Communication and Documentation. For this exam, you are required to understand and utilize therapeutic communication skills with all professional contacts, including clients, their families, and other members of the health care team. Charting or documenting your care and the client's response is both a legal requirement and an essential method of communication in nursing. On this exam you may be asked to identify appropriate documentation of a client behavior or nursing action.

Teaching/Learning Principles. Nursing frequently involves sharing information with clients and families so optimal functioning can be achieved. You may see questions concerning teaching a client about diet and/or medications.

Knowledge Is Power

The more knowledgeable you are about the NCLEX-PN® exam, the more effective your study will be. As you prepare for the exam, keep the content of the test in mind. Thinking like the test maker will enhance your chance of success on the exam.

Are you still thinking about the question involving the pacemaker battery from the beginning of the chapter? What do you think the correct answer is?

A client had a permanent pacemaker implanted one year ago. The client returns to the outpatient clinic for suspected pacemaker battery failure. It is **most** important for the LPN/LVN to assess for which of these?

1. Abdominal pain, nausea, and vomiting.
2. Wheezing on exertion, cyanosis, and orthopnea.
3. Palpitations, shortness of breath, and dizziness.
4. Chest pain, headache, and diaphoresis.

The correct answer is (3). Palpitations, shortness of breath, dizziness, lightheadedness, syncope, irregular heart rate, and tachycardia or bradycardia may occur with pacemaker battery failure.

Gastrointestinal symptoms (1) are not found with pacemaker malfunction. The items listed in (2) are not symptoms of pacemaker failure. And although chest pain may occur with decreased output (4), chest pain is suggestive of angina. Headache and diaphoresis are not seen with pacemaker failure.

[CHAPTER 2]

GENERAL TEST STRATEGIES

As a nursing student, you are used to taking multiple choice tests. In fact, you've taken so many tests by the time you graduate from nursing school, you probably believe that there won't be any more surprises on any nursing test, including the NCLEX-PN® exam.

But if you've ever talked to graduate practical/vocational nurses about their experiences taking the NCLEX-PN® exam, they probably told you that the test wasn't like *any* nursing test they had ever taken. How can that be? How can the NCLEX-PN® exam seem like a practical/vocational nursing school test but be so different? The reason is that the NCLEX-PN® exam is a standardized test that analyzes a different set of behaviors from those tested in nursing school.

Standardized Exams

Many of you have some experience with standardized exams. You may have been required to take the SAT or ACT to get into nursing school. Remember taking that exam? Was your experience positive or negative?

All standardized exams share the same characteristics:

- Tests are written by content specialists and test-construction experts.
- The content of the exam is researched and planned.
- The questions are designed according to test construction methodology (all answer choices are about the same length, the verb tenses all agree, etc.).
- All the questions are tested before use on the actual exam.

The NCLEX-PN® exam is similar to other standardized exams in some ways yet different in others:

- The NCLEX-PN® exam is written by nurse specialists who are experts in a content area of nursing.
- All content is selected to allow the beginning practical/vocational nurse to prove minimum competency on all areas of the test plan.
- Minimum-competency questions are most frequently asked at the application level, not the recognition or recall level. All the responses to a question are similar in length and subject matter, and are grammatically correct.
- All test items have been extensively tested by NCSBN. The questions are valid; all correct responses are documented in two different sources.

What does this mean for you?

- NCSBN has defined what is minimum-competency, entry-level nursing.
- Questions and answers will be written in such a way that you cannot, in most cases, predict or recognize the correct answer.
- NCSBN is knowledgeable about strategies regarding length of answers, grammar, and so on. It makes sure that you can't use these strategies in order to select correct answers. English majors have no advantage!
- The answer choices have been extensively tested. The people who write the test questions make the incorrect answer choices look attractive to the unwary test taker.

What Behaviors Does the NCLEX-PN® Exam Test?

The NCLEX-PN® exam does *not* just test your nursing knowledge: It assumes that you have a body of knowledge and you understand the material because you have graduated from nursing school. So what does the NCLEX-PN® exam test? The NCLEX-PN® exam primarily tests your nursing decisions. It tests your ability to think critically and solve problems.

Critical Thinking

What does the term *critical thinking* mean? Critical thinking is problem solving that involves thinking creatively. It requires that the practical/vocational nurse:

- Observe.
- Decide what is important.
- Look for patterns and relationships.
- Identify normal and abnormal.
- Identify the problem.
- Transfer knowledge from one situation to another.
- Apply knowledge.
- Evaluate according to criteria established.

You successfully solve problems every day in the clinical area. You are probably comfortable with this concept when actually caring for clients. Although you've had lots of practice critically thinking in the clinical area, you may have had less practice critically thinking your way through test questions. Why is that?

During nursing school, you take exams developed by nursing instructors to test a specific body of content. Many of these questions are at the knowledge level. This involves recognition and recall of ideas or material that you read in your nursing textbooks and discussed in class. This is the most basic level of testing. Figure 2.1 illustrates the different levels of questions on nursing exams.

The following is an example of a knowledge-based question you might have seen in nursing school.

Which of the following is a complication that occurs during the first 24 hours after a percutaneous liver biopsy?

1. Nausea and vomiting.
2. Constipation.
3. Hemorrhage.
4. Pain at the biopsy site.

The question restated is, "What is a common complication of a liver biopsy?" You may or may not remember the answer. So, as you look at the answer choices, you hope to see an item that looks familiar. You do see something that looks familiar: "Hemorrhage." You select the correct answer based on recall or recognition. The NCLEX-PN® exam rarely asks questions at the recall/recognition level.

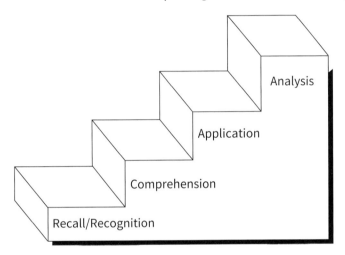

Figure 2.1 Levels of Questions in Nursing Tests

In nursing school, you are also given test questions written at the comprehension level. These questions require you to understand the meaning of the material. Let's look at this same question written at the comprehension level.

The LPN/LVN understands that hemorrhage is a complication of a liver biopsy due to which of the following reasons?

1. There are several large blood vessels near the liver.
2. The liver cells are bathed with a mixture of venous and arterial blood.
3. The test is performed on clients with elevated enzymes.
4. The procedure requires a large piece of tissue to be removed.

The question restated is, "Why does hemorrhage occur after a liver biopsy?" In order to answer this question, the nurse must understand that the liver is a highly vascular organ. The portal vein and the hepatic artery join in the liver to form the sinusoids that bathe the liver in a mixture of venous and arterial blood.

The NCLEX-PN® exam asks few minimum-competency questions at the comprehension level. It assumes you know and understand the facts you learned in practical/vocational nursing school.

Minimum-competency NCLEX-PN® exam questions are written at the application and/or analysis level. Remember, the NCLEX-PN® exam tests your ability to make safe judgments about client care. Your ability to solve problems is not tested with questions at the recall/recognition or comprehension level.

Let's look at this same question written at the application level.

> Which symptom observed by the LPN/LVN during the first 24 hours after a percutaneous liver biopsy would indicate a complication from the procedure?
>
> 1. Anorexia, nausea, and vomiting.
> 2. Abdominal distention and discomfort.
> 3. P 112 beats/minute, BP 86/60 mmHg.
> 4. Redness and pain at the biopsy site.

Can you select an answer based on recall or recognition? No. Let's analyze the question and answer choices.

The question is: What is a complication of a liver biopsy? In order to begin to analyze this question, you must *know* that hemorrhage is the major complication. However, it's not listed as an answer. Can you find hemorrhage in one of the answer choices?

ANSWERS:

(1) "Anorexia, nausea, and vomiting." Does this indicate that the client is hemorrhaging? No, these are not symptoms of hemorrhage.

(2) "Abdominal distention and discomfort." Does this indicate that the client is hemorrhaging? Perhaps. Abdominal distention could indicate internal bleeding.

(3) "P 112 beats/minute, BP 86/60 mmHg." Does this indicate that the client is hemorrhaging? Yes. An increased pulse and a decreased blood pressure indicate shock. Shock is a result of hemorrhage.

(4) "Redness and pain at the biopsy site." Does this indicate the client is hemorrhaging? No. Pain and some redness at the biopsy site may occur as a normal result of the procedure.

Ask yourself, "Which is the best indicator of hemorrhage?" Abdominal distention or a change in vital signs? Abdominal distention can be caused by liver disease. The correct answer is (3).

This question tests you at the application level. You were not able to answer the question by recalling or recognizing the word *hemorrhage*. You had to take information you learned (hemorrhage is the major complication of a liver biopsy) and select the answer that best indicates hemorrhage. Application involves taking the facts that you know and using them to make a nursing judgment. You must be able to answer questions at the application level in order to prove your competence on the NCLEX-PN® exam.

Let's look at a question that is written at the analysis level.

> The LPN/LVN is caring for a client receiving haloperidol 2 mg PO bid. The LPN/LVN assists the client to choose which menu?
>
> 1. 6 oz (168 g) roast beef, baked potato, salad with dressing, dill pickle, baked apple pie, and milk.
> 2. 3 oz (84 g) baked chicken, green beans, steamed rice, 1 slice of bread, banana, and milk.
> 3. 6 oz (168 g) burger on a bun, french fries, apple, chocolate chip cookie, and milk to drink 30 minutes after mealtime.
> 4. 3 oz (84 g) baked fish, slice of bread, broccoli, ice cream, and pineapple juice to drink 60 minutes after mealtime.

Many students panic when they read this question because they can't immediately recall any diet restriction required by a client taking haloperidol. Because students can't recall the information, they assume that they didn't learn enough information. Analysis questions are often written so that a familiar piece of information is put in an unfamiliar setting. Let's think about this question.

What type of diet do you choose for a client receiving haloperidol? In order to begin analyzing this question, you must first recall that haloperidol is an antipsychotic medication used to treat psychotic disorders. There are *no* diet restrictions for clients taking haloperidol. Because there are no diet restrictions, you must problem-solve to determine what this question is *really* asking. Based on the answer choices, it is obviously a diet question. What kind of diet should you choose for this client? Because you have been given no other information, there is only one type of diet that can be considered: a regular balanced diet. This is an example of taking the familiar (a regular balanced diet) and putting it into the unfamiliar (a client receiving haloperidol). In this question, the critical thinking is deciding what this question is *really* asking.

QUESTION: "What is the most balanced regular diet?"

ANSWERS:

(1) "6 oz (168 g) roast beef, baked potato, salad with dressing, dill pickle, baked apple pie, and milk." Is this a balanced diet? Yes, it certainly has possibilities.

(2) "3 oz (84 g) baked chicken, green beans, steamed rice, 1 slice of bread, banana, and milk." Is this a balanced diet? Yes, this is also a good answer because it contains foods from each of the food groups.

(3) "6 oz (168 g) burger on a bun, french fries, apple, chocolate chip cookie, and milk to drink 30 minutes after mealtime." Is this a balanced diet? No. This diet is high in fat and does not contain all of the food groups. Eliminate this answer.

(4) "3 oz (84 g) baked fish, slice of bread, broccoli, ice cream, and pineapple juice to drink 60 minutes after mealtime." Does this sound like a balanced diet? The choice of foods isn't bad, but why would the intake of fluids be delayed? This sounds like a menu to prevent dumping syndrome. Eliminate this answer.

Which is the better answer choice: (1) or (2)? Dill pickles are high in sodium, so the correct answer is (2).

Choosing the menu that best represents a balanced diet is not a difficult question to answer. The challenge lies in determining that a balanced diet is the topic of the question. Note that answer choices (1) and (2) are very similar. Because the NCLEX-PN® exam is testing your discretion, you will be making decisions between answer choices that are very close in meaning. Don't expect obvious answer choices.

These questions highlight the difference between the knowledge/comprehension-based questions that you may have seen in nursing school, and the application/analysis-based questions that you will see on the NCLEX-PN® exam.

Strategies That Don't Work on the NCLEX-PN® Exam

Whether you realize it or not, you developed a set of strategies in nursing school to answer teacher-generated test questions that are written at the knowledge/comprehension level. These strategies include:

- "Cramming" in hundreds of facts about disease processes and nursing care
- Recognizing and recalling facts rather than understanding the pathophysiology and the needs of a client with an illness
- Knowing who wrote the question and what is important to that instructor
- Predicting answers based on what you remember or who wrote the test question
- Selecting the response that is a different length compared to the other choices
- Selecting the answer choice that is grammatically correct
- When in doubt, choosing answer choice (C)

These strategies will not work on the NCLEX-PN® exam. Remember, the NCLEX-PN® exam is testing your ability to make safe, competent decisions.

Becoming a Better Test Taker

The first step to becoming a better test taker is to assess and identify the following:

- The kind of test taker you are
- The kind of learner you are

Successful NCLEX-PN® Exam Test Takers

- Have a good understanding of nursing content.
- Have the ability to tackle each test question with a lot of confidence because they assume that they can figure out the right answer.
- Don't give up if they are unsure of the answer. They are not afraid to think about the question, and the possible choices, in order to select the correct answer.

- Possess the know-how to correctly identify the question.
- Stay focused on the topic of the question.

Unsuccessful NCLEX-PN® Exam Test Takers

- Assume that they either know or don't know the answer to the question.
- Memorize facts to answer questions by recall or recognition.
- Read the question, read the answers, re-read the question, and pick an answer.
- Choose answer choices based on a hunch or a feeling instead of thinking carefully.
- Answer questions based on personal experience rather than nursing theory.
- Give up too soon, because they aren't willing to think hard about questions and answers.
- Don't stay focused on the topic of the question.

If you are a successful test taker, congratulations! This book will reinforce your test taking skills. If you have many of the characteristics of an unsuccessful test taker, don't despair! You can change. If you follow the strategies in this book, you will become a successful test taker.

What Kind of Learner Are You?

It is important for you to identify whether you think predominantly in images or words. Why? This will assist you in developing a study plan that is specific for your learning style. Read the following statement:

A nurse walks into a room and finds the client lying on the floor.

As you read those words, did you hear yourself reading the words? Or did you see a nurse walking into a room, and see the client lying on the floor? If you heard yourself reading the sentence, you think in words. If you formed a mental image (saw a picture), you think in images.

Students who think in images sometimes have a difficult time answering nursing test questions. These students say things like:

"I have to study harder than the other students."
"I have to look up the same information over and over again."
"Once I see the procedure (or client), I don't have any difficulty understanding or remembering the content."
"I have trouble understanding procedures from reading the book. I have to see the procedure to understand it."
"I have trouble answering test questions about clients or procedures I've never seen."

Why is that? For some people, imagery is necessary to understand ideas and concepts. If this is true for you, you need to visualize information that you are learning. As you prepare for the NCLEX-PN® exam, try to form mental images of terminology, procedures, and diseases. For example, if you're reviewing information about traction but you have never seen traction, it would be ideal for you to see a client in traction. If that isn't possible, find a picture of traction and rig up a traction setup with whatever material you have available. As you read about traction, use the photo or model to visualize care of the client. If you can visualize the theory that you are trying to learn, it will make recall and understanding of concepts much easier for you.

It is also important that you visualize test questions. As you read the question and possible answer choices, picture yourself going through each suggested action. This will increase your chances of selecting correct answer choices.

Let's look at a test question that requires imagery.

> An adolescent sustains a left femur fracture during a sledding accident. The health care provider reduces the fracture and applies a cast. The client is taught how to use crutches for ambulating without bearing weight on the left leg. The LPN/LVN expects the client to learn which crutch-walking gait?
>
> 1. Two-point gait.
> 2. Three-point gait.
> 3. Four-point gait.
> 4. Swing-through gait.

Don't panic if you can't remember crutch-walking gaits. Instead, visualize!

STEP 1. "See" a person (or yourself) walking normally. First the right leg and left arm are extended, and then the left leg and right arm are extended.

STEP 2. Put crutches in your hands. Now walk. Each foot and each crutch is a point.

STEP 3. "See" a person (or yourself) with a full cast on the left leg, with the foot never touching the ground.

STEP 4. Visualize the answers.

(1) Two-point gait. One leg and one crutch would be touching the ground at the same time. Sounds like normal walking. Eliminate this choice because the client is non-weight-bearing.

(2) Three-point gait. Both crutches and one foot are on the ground. This would be appropriate for a non-weight-bearing client.

(3) Four-point gait. This would require both legs and crutches to touch the ground. However, in this question the client is non-weight-bearing. Eliminate this option.

(4) Swing-through gait. This gait means advancing both crutches, then both legs, and requires weight-bearing. The gait is not as stable as the other gaits. Eliminate this option: the client in this question is non-weight-bearing.

The correct answer is (2).

Even if you are unsure of crutch walking gaits, imagining and thinking through the answer choices will enable you to select the correct answer.

PART TWO

NCLEX-PN®
STRATEGIES AND
PRACTICE

CHAPTER 3

COMPUTER ADAPTIVE TEST STRATEGIES

NCLEX-PN® Exam Question types

NCSBN has developed a variety of question types designed to assess your nursing knowledge and critical thinking ability. Some are most likely familiar to you already. Some are new to the NCLEX-PN® as of 2023. Broadly speaking, the exam is composed of multiple choice questions with four options and alternate format question types—that is, questions that take a form other than four-option, text-based multiple choice.

Take a moment to review this list of all the question types and subtypes that you may encounter on the exam.

(1) **Multiple Choice**

(2) **Multiple Response**
   - Multiple Response Select All That Apply (SATA)
   - Multiple Response Grouping
   - Multiple Response Select N

(3) **Highlight**
   - Highlight Table
   - Highlight Text

(4) **Hot Spot**

(5) **Fill-in-the-Blank**

(6) **Drag-and-Drop**
   - Drag-and-Drop Ordered Response
   - Cloze Drag-and-Drop
   - Drag-and-Drop Rationale

(7) **Dropdown**
   - Cloze Dropdown
   - Cloze Dropdown Rationale
   - Dropdown Table

(8) **Matrix**
   - Matrix Multiple Choice
   - Matrix Multiple Response

(9) **Bowtie**

(10) **Trend**

After reading this list, you may be thinking, "That's a lot of question types, and I've never even heard of some of them!" Don't panic. The following sections contain strategies that will help you correctly answer alternate format questions and four-option, text-based, multiple choice questions. We will identify each question type in the following sections and walk you through how to tackle them. Let's get started.

Multiple Choice Test Questions

Multiple choice questions with four answer options may take the form of a text-based question or may include an exhibit/chart or graphics in place of some of the text. Each of the four options will be preceded by an empty circle. To select an option as correct, you will click on that empty circle to fill it in. While you can click to a different circle to change your answer before confirming it as your selection, the computer will allow you to fill in *only one* of these circles, or "radio buttons," at any time.

No matter the form, you need to understand the components of a multiple choice NCLEX-PN® question to effectively apply the strategies discussed in this book. They are as follows:

- The *stem* of the question. The stem includes the situation that describes the client, their problems or health care needs, and other relevant information. It also includes a question or an incomplete statement. This is the question that you must answer.
- Three incorrect answers, referred to here as *distracters*.
- The correct answer.

The three distracters will probably sound logical to you. They may even be based on information provided in the stem, but they don't really answer the question. Other incorrect answers may be actions that are common nursing practice but not ideal nursing practice.

The correct answer is the only choice that is recognized as correct by the NCLEX-PN® exam, so you need to learn to select it. Remember that most answer choices are written on the application level, so you will not be able to select answers based on recognition or recall. You must understand the *whys* of nursing care in order to select the correct response.

Read the following exam-style question. In addition to selecting an answer, identify the components of this question.

> The LPN/LVN is planning care for a 4-year-old client who has been sexually abused by the parent. Play therapy is scheduled. The LPN/LVN knows that the **primary** goal of play therapy for a 4-year-old client is which of these?
>
> 1. Provide the opportunity to express anger and hostility by playing with dolls.
> 2. Promote communication because the client may lack capacity to verbally express perceptions.
> 3. Assess whether the client function at an age-appropriate developmental level.
> 4. Reveal the type of abuse experienced through direct observation of the client at play.

The Components

- The stem:
    - 4-year-old client
    - Sexually abused by the father
    - Play therapy is scheduled
    - What is the primary goal of play therapy for a 4-year-old client?
- The answer choices:
    (1) Provide the opportunity to express anger and hostility. Play therapy will allow children to express anger and hostility if that's what they want to communicate. Some students select this answer because they focus on the treatment of sexual abuse mentioned in the situation. This is a distracter.

    (2) Promote communication. Play is the universal language of children. The purpose of play therapy is to give children the opportunity to communicate using their own "language." This is the correct answer.

    (3) Assess developmental level. The nurse might be able to assess whether a child is functioning at an age-appropriate level, but this is not the primary purpose of play therapy. This is a distracter.

    (4) Find out what type of abuse the client has experienced. The child might communicate the type of abuse experienced if that is what the child chooses to communicate. The nurse should focus on the purpose of play therapy, not the type of abuse. This is a distracter.

Let's try another question.

> A client is being treated for heart failure with diuretic therapy. Which finding **best** indicates to the LPN/LVN that the client's condition is improving?
>
> 1. The client's weight has remained stable since admission.
> 2. The client's systolic blood pressure has decreased.
> 3. There are fewer crackles heard when auscultating the client's lungs.
> 4. The client's urinary output is 1,500 mL per day.

The Components

- The stem:
    - Heart failure
    - Treatment is diuretic therapy
    - How do you know the client's condition is improving?
- The answer choices:
    (1) Weight has remained stable. The client's weight should decrease with diuretic therapy. Weight addresses issues involved with diuretic therapy. However, it is not the best indication of improvement in a client with heart failure. This is a distracter.

(2) The systolic blood pressure has decreased. Decreased blood pressure may be the result of diuretic therapy, but it could also be due to other causes (change of position, calm rather than an excited state, etc.). This is not the best indication of an improvement in a client with heart failure. This is a distracter.

(3) There are fewer crackles. A client with heart failure has crackles due to pulmonary edema. Diuretics are given to promote excretion of sodium and water through the kidneys. Decreased crackles would indicate that the pulmonary edema is improving. This is the correct answer.

(4) Urinary output of 1,500 mL in 24 hours. This is within normal limits. Although a normal output addresses diuretic therapy, it is not the best indication of improvement of heart failure. This is a distracter.

Alternate Format Test Questions

If a question is not a four-option multiple choice item, it is known as an *alternate format question*. As outlined earlier, the NCLEX-PN® exam uses several different alternate format question types. These may appear either as standalone questions or as questions in a six-item case study question set. Let's look at each alternate format question type and the strategies that will help you correctly answer these questions.

Multiple Response

Like multiple choice questions, Multiple Response alternate format questions present a list of options for you to evaluate. Unlike traditional multiple choice questions, where there is a single best answer choice, more than one option may be correct. In a Multiple Response item, you must identify and select *all of the correct answer options*.

The NCLEX-PN® exam includes three varieties of Multiple Response questions:

- Multiple Response Select All That Apply (SATA)
- Multiple Response Grouping
- Multiple Response Select N

Take a look at the following Multiple Response question.

> The LPN/LVN is caring for a client diagnosed with a right-sided stroke with dysphagia. Which action by the LPN/LVN reflects appropriate care for the client? **(Select all that apply.)**
>
> ☐ 1. The LPN/LVN assesses the client's ability to swallow.
>
> ☐ 2. The LPN/LVN positions the client with the head of bed elevated 25 degrees.
>
> ☐ 3. The LPN/LVN offers the client scrambled eggs.
>
> ☐ 4. The LPN/LVN instructs the client to place food on the left side of the mouth.
>
> ☐ 5. The LPN/LVN turns off the television.

You will know that the question is a "Select all that apply" (SATA) alternate format question because it gives you the instruction **"Select all that apply"** after the question stem and before the answer choices. You will see that there are more than four possible answer choices; usually five or six are provided, and up to ten are possible. Instead of the radio buttons you see with multiple choice, four-option, text-based questions, there is a box in front of each answer choice.

To answer this type of question, determine which of the answer choices provided are correct. To receive full credit for a **Multiple Response SATA** question, you must select *all* of the answer choices that apply, not just the best response. Left-click on the box in front of each answer choice that you think is correct. A small check mark will appear in the box indicating that you have selected that answer. If you change your mind about a particular answer choice, simply click on the box again. The check mark will disappear and the answer choice will no longer be selected.

How should you approach this type of question? What *does not* work is to compare and contrast the individual answer choices. In a Multiple Response SATA question, any number of answer choices may be correct. Instead, consider each answer choice a True/False question. Reword this question to ask, "What is appropriate care for a client with a right-sided stroke who has dysphagia?" Dysphagia means the client is having difficulty swallowing; if the stroke involves the right hemisphere, the client's left side is affected.

Let's look at the answers. The strategy is to change each answer choice into a statement, and then determine if the statement is true or false.

(1) "I should assess the client's ability to swallow." Is this true for a client with dysphagia? Yes. This is a correct response because the nurse needs to make sure that the client can swallow food before providing anything to eat. The results of the evaluation will also determine whether the nurse should offer the client clear liquids or thickened liquids. Some clients will require thickened liquids while others will not. Select this answer choice.

(2) "I should position the client with the head of bed elevated 25 degrees." Is this the correct position for a client with dysphagia? No. The client should be sitting upright in a chair or with the head of the bed elevated at least 30 degrees. Eliminate this answer choice.

(3) "I should offer the client scrambled eggs." Is this an appropriate food for a client with dysphagia? Yes. Soft or semi-soft foods are more easily tolerated than a regular diet. Select this answer choice.

(4) "I should instruct the client to place food on the left side of the mouth." Is this what should be done? If the client has a right-sided stroke, that means the left side of the client's body is affected. The food should be placed on the unaffected side—the right side of the mouth for this client. Eliminate this answer.

(5) "I should turn off the television." What are they getting at with this statement? Many clients are easily distracted after a stroke. If the client has dysphagia, you don't want the client to aspirate while being distracted by the television. It is best to turn off the TV during meals. Select this answer choice.

So, which answers should be checked as correct? For this question, choices (1), (3), and (5) are correct. Left-click on the box in front of each of these answer choices to select them. When you have selected all the responses you believe to be correct, click on the NEXT (N) button in the bottom left of the screen or press the Enter key on the keyboard to lock in your answer and go on to the next question. Remember, once you click on the NEXT (N) button or press the Enter key, you have entered your answer to the question and you cannot return to the question.

The LPN/LVN is caring for a client diagnosed with a right-sided stroke with dysphagia. Which action by the LPN/LVN reflects appropriate care for the client? **(Select all that apply.)**

- [✓] 1. The LPN/LVN assesses the client's ability to swallow.
- [ ] 2. The LPN/LVN positions the client with the head of bed elevated 25 degrees.
- [✓] 3. The LPN/LVN offers the client scrambled eggs.
- [ ] 4. The LPN/LVN instructs the client to place food on the left side of the mouth.
- [✓] 5. The LPN/LVN turns off the client's television.

A variation of the Multiple Response item type is **Multiple Response Grouping**. In this question type, you will again see a box in front of each answer option, and you will be prompted to select all of the correct answers. However, the options are arranged in groupings within a table. The figure gives an example of a Multiple Response Grouping question.

> For each body system below, click to specify the potential nursing intervention appropriate for the care of the client. **Each body system may support more than 1 potential nursing interventions.**

Body System	Potential Nursing Interventions
Cardiovascular	[ ] Obtain a 12-lead ECG. [ ] Administer anti-hypertensive medication. [ ] Establish IV access.
Respiratory	[ ] Place oxygen 2L/nasal cannula. [ ] Have the client breathe in a paper bag. [ ] Plan for immediate intubation.
Neurological	[ ] Assess pupils for size and reaction. [ ] Prepare the client for a CT of the brain. [ ] Obtain neurologic checks every shift.

Figure 3.1 Example of Multiple Response Grouping Question

As in a Multiple Response SATA question, the strategy is to reword each answer option as a True/False question and consider it individually. In the first row of the figure, for example, you would reword the first option as "Is obtaining a 12-lead ECG an appropriate cardiovascular intervention for this client?", the second option as "Is administering anti-hypertensive medication an appropriate nursing intervention for this client?", and so on.

The last variation of the Multiple Response item type is **Multiple Response Select N**, in which the question tells you the correct number of responses to choose, for example:

- "Which 3 findings are most concerning?"
- "Which 3 findings require follow-up?"

Read the question stem carefully. If the question stem directs you to choose three answers, choose *exactly three answers*—and no fewer—before proceeding to the next question. Again, reword each answer option as a True/False question and consider it individually.

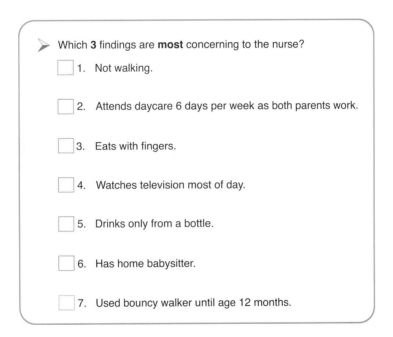

Figure 3.2 Example of Multiple Response Select N Question

Highlight

This type of alternate format question asks you to identify relevant text within a passage. For example, a Highlight question may ask you to select concerning or priority findings that require follow-up by the nurse or health care provider or, alternatively, to select client findings that indicate an improvement in condition. Highlight questions may take either of two forms: a table or a paragraph.

The figure shows an example of a **Highlight Table** question.

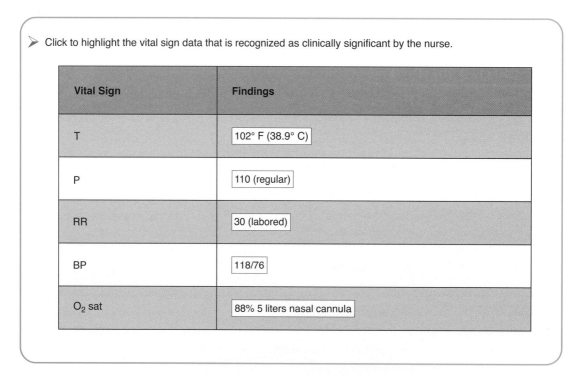

➤ Click to highlight the vital sign data that is recognized as clinically significant by the nurse.

Vital Sign	Findings
T	102° F (38.9° C)
P	110 (regular)
RR	30 (labored)
BP	118/76
O₂ sat	88% 5 liters nasal cannula

Figure 3.3 Example of Highlight Table Question

Highlighting is achieved by selecting "tokenized text"—that is, preselected phrases or words that can be highlighted in response to an exam question. The tokenized text may be a mix of "keys" (correct answers) and distracters (incorrect answers).

Highlighting tokenized text on the NCLEX-RN exam is much like physically marking a book with a highlighter pen. Hover the cursor over tokenized text and click once to highlight the text. Hovering the cursor over the tokenized text and clicking again would remove the highlighting.

To answer a Highlight question, analyze each piece of tokenized text individually. As in a Multiple Response SATA question, the strategy is to change each answer choice into a statement, then determine if the statement is correct/incorrect, right/wrong, true/false, significant/insignificant, priority/non-priority, indicated/contraindicated, expected/unexpected, and so on.

Here is how you would begin to answer the Highlight question in the example:

(1) T 102° F (38.9° C). Is this finding significant? Yes, it is outside the normal range. Hover the cursor over the tokenized text and left-click.

(2) P 110 (regular). Is this finding significant? Yes, it is outside the normal range. Hover the cursor over the tokenized text and left-click.

(3) RR 30 (labored). Is this finding significant? Yes, respiratory rate is high, and labored breathing is significant. Hover the cursor over the tokenized text and left-click.

Continue with this method of questioning for each remaining assessment finding. Then enter your answer by clicking on the NEXT (N) button or pressing the Enter key.

➢ Click to highlight the vital sign data that is recognized as clinically significant by the nurse.

Vital Sign	Findings
T	102° F (38.9° C)
P	110 (regular)
RR	30 (labored)
BP	118/76
O$_2$ sat	88% 5 liters nasal cannula

Figure 3.4 Example of Highlight Table Question, Marked

In a **Highlight Text** question, the tokenized text is located in a sentence or text-based paragraph.

- Hover the cursor over tokenized text and click once to mark an answer choice as correct.
- Hover the cursor over tokenized text and click again to remove the highlighting.

Approach it in the same way as in a table. The figure shows an example of a Highlight Text alternate format question.

> ➤ Click to highlight the information in the Nurse's Notes that concerns the nurse at this time.

Client was brought to the urgent care clinic by spouse due to abdominal pain. The client states, "I have been having pain on and off for several days, but today the pain was very severe." The client has a history of atrial fibrillation, myocardial infarction, hypertension, and hyperlipidemia. The client also reports a 40-pound (18 kg) weight loss over the last three months. Vital Signs: T 99.9° F (37.7° C), P 76, RR 20, BP 148/90, pulse oximetry reading 95% on room air. Upon assessment the client's breathing is unlabored, and lungs are clear bilaterally. Pain intermittent, located in the epigastric area and often radiates to the right shoulder, rated "7" on 1-10 pain scale. Abdomen slightly distended, and firm to palpation. Client is alert and oriented to person, place, and time. Currently taking digoxin, metoprolol, and atorvastatin.

Figure 3.5 Example of Highlight Text Question

Hot Spot

This type of alternate format question asks you to identify a location on a graphic or table. It is important to understand that this is not a test of your fine motor skills. Hot Spot questions are designed to evaluate your knowledge of nursing content, anatomy, and physiology and pathophysiology.

Let's take a look at a question that involves a hot spot.

The LPN/LVN is palpating peripheral pulses on an adult client. Identify the appropriate area in which the LPN/LVN would expect to palpate a client's dorsalis pedis pulse.

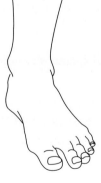

The question asks you to identify where you would palpate one of the two commonly assessed peripheral pulses found in the foot. The strategy you should use is to locate anatomical landmarks. You need to know that the dorsalis pedis pulse is located on the top (dorsum) of the client's foot. It is found between the first and second metatarsal bones (between the great and first toes) over the dorsalis pedis artery.

Move the cursor to the location you think is correct. Then, left-click the mouse. Check to make sure that you have selected the location you wanted. Then enter your answer by clicking on the NEXT (N) button or pressing the Enter key. If you click between the second and third toes, for example, the location would be inaccurate for the dorsalis pedis pulse and the question would be counted as incorrect. Just do your best and use the anatomical landmarks to get your bearings and select the location.

Here's the answer to this Hot Spot question.

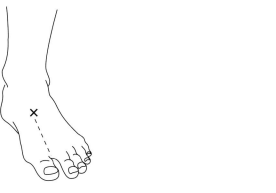

The LPN/LVN is palpating peripheral pulses on an adult client. Identify the appropriate area in which the LPN/LVN would expect to palpate a client's dorsalis pedis pulse.

Fill-in-the-Blank

This type of alternate format question asks you to fill in the blank with a number based on a calculation.

The following is an example of a **Fill-in-the-Blank** question.

> The LPN/LVN is caring for a client who has a primary health care provider order for strict intake and output. The client drinks 12 oz of lemon-lime soda and 1/2 cup of grape juice between breakfast and lunch, and voids 200 mL of urine. Calculate and record the client's oral intake in milliliters for this period.
>
> _____ mL

To answer this question, calculate the client's intake from the information provided. **Note: Pay close attention to the unit of measure you need for your final answer.** In this situation, you are asked for the client's intake in milliliters, not cups or ounces.

You can use the drop-down calculator provided on the computer to do the math. The button that displays the calculator is on the bottom of the right side of the computer screen. Use your mouse to click on the numbers or functions you want. Remember, the slash (/) is used for division.

First, convert cups into ounces. One cup of fluid = 8 oz. Then convert ounces into milliliters. One ounce = 30 mL.

The client's intake is:

> 12 oz lemon-lime soda = 360 mL
> 1/2 cup grape juice = 4 oz = 120 mL

Move the cursor inside the text box, and left-click on the mouse. Type in the correct intake using the number keys on the keyboard. The correct answer is 480. Do not put "mL" or any other unit of measure after the number. *Only the number* goes into the box. Rules for rounding are typically provided with the question.

The LPN/LVN is caring for a client who has a primary health care provider order for strict intake and output. The client drinks 12 oz of lemon-lime soda and 1/2 cup of grape juice between breakfast and lunch, and voids 200 mL of urine. Calculate and record the client's oral intake in milliliters for this period.

<u>480</u>_____ mL

Drag-and-Drop

Drag-and-Drop alternate format questions ask you to arrange answers in the correct order or to supply missing information to complete a passage of text. The NCSBN defines three Drag-and-Drop varieties.

- Drag-and-Drop Ordered Response
- Cloze Drag-and-Drop
- Drag-and-Drop Rationale

Drag-and-Drop Ordered Response questions direct you to place answers in a specific order.

Take a look at the following question.

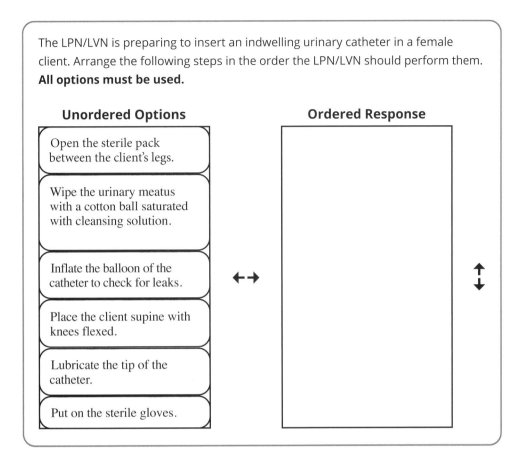

The strategy to use when answering this kind of question is to visualize: Picture yourself performing the procedure. First, prepare the client. Next, prepare the equipment in the correct order, using sterile technique. Open the sterile insertion kit. Then, put on the sterile gloves. Next, inflate the balloon of the catheter to check for leaks. (NOTE: This step may vary per facility policy and manufacturer guidelines. Silicone catheter balloons should not be pre-inflated.) Lubricate the tip of the catheter. After preparing the equipment, prepare the client for the insertion of the catheter. The last step from those provided is to cleanse the periurethral area using swabsticks or cotton balls saturated with cleansing solution.

To place the options in the correct order, click on an option and drag it to the box on the right. You can also move an answer from the left column to the right column by highlighting the option and clicking the arrow key that points to the column on the right. You may also rearrange the order of the options in the right column using the arrow keys pointing up and down.

Here's the answer to this question.

The nurse is preparing to insert an indwelling urinary catheter in a female client. Arrange the following steps in the order the LPN/LVN should perform them. **All options must be used.**

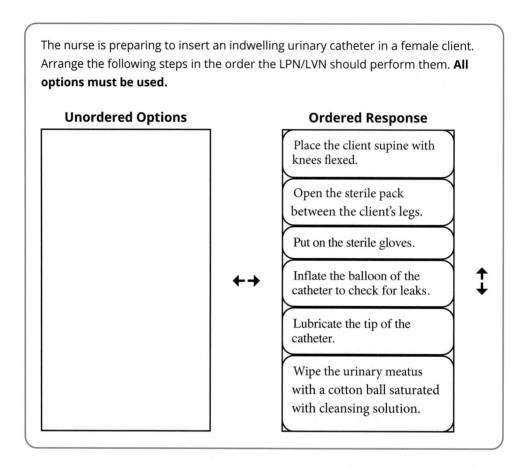

Unordered Options

Ordered Response

- Place the client supine with knees flexed.
- Open the sterile pack between the client's legs.
- Put on the sterile gloves.
- Inflate the balloon of the catheter to check for leaks.
- Lubricate the tip of the catheter.
- Wipe the urinary meatus with a cotton ball saturated with cleansing solution.

A variation is **Cloze Drag-and-Drop**, in which you choose a word or words from an answer well to complete a sentence. (The word *cloze* is derived from "closure.") With the cursor, drag "tokens" (answer choices) from the answer well to complete the sentence. If you mistakenly drag an incorrect token into the sentence, you can remove it by either returning it to the answer well or dragging the correct token from the answer well to replace the incorrect token.

The figure shows an example of a Cloze Drag-and-Drop alternate format question.

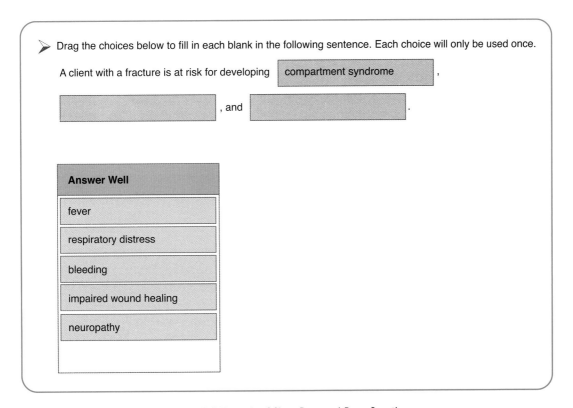

Figure 3.6 Example of Cloze Drag-and-Drop Question

Another variation is **Drag-and-Drop Rationale**. Again, you use the cursor to drag tokens from the answer well to complete a sentence. In this question type, however, the word or words you choose complete a *rationale-based* sentence. A Drag-and-Drop Rationale question requires you to recognize a cause-and-effect relationship.

Take a look at the following question.

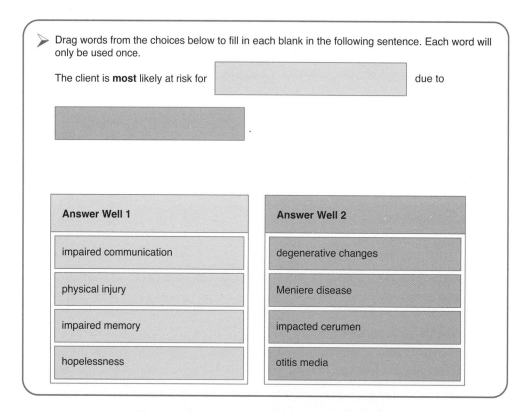

Figure 3.7 Example of Drag-and-Drop Rationale Question

You will know that an item is a rationale-based question because it includes the words "due to" or "as evidenced by."

To complete the sentence, drag a color-coded token from each answer well and drop it into the blank in the sentence with the corresponding color. Note that a token "dropped" into a noncorresponding blank will be rejected and automatically returned to its answer well.

Drag-and-Drop Rationale questions on the NCLEX-PN® exam come in two forms:

- A single dyad has one cause and one effect. (The sample question is an example of a single dyad.)
- A single triad has one cause and two effects.

How should you approach this question? The strategy you should use is to identify the client's priority problem based on cues in the case study. Starting with the first answer well, consider each answer choice: Is it related to the priority problem or potential condition you identified for this client? If the answer is yes, select the answer option. Identifying the priority problem or potential condition in the first answer well is essential to earning any credit on the item.

After choosing your answers from the answer wells, pause to consider each of your selections. Ask yourself:

- "Do the answers I chose make sense?"
- "Have I selected answers based on my foundational nursing knowledge?"
- "Have I selected answers based on the client's priority problem/condition?"

If you can answer "Yes," you have selected the best choices to answer the Drag-and-Drop Rationale item.

Dropdown

Dropdown alternate format questions ask you to select a word or phrase from a dropdown menu to complete a passage of text or table. There are three Dropdown varieties.

- Cloze Dropdown
- Cloze Dropdown Rationale
- Dropdown Table

The **Cloze Dropdown** question type asks you to complete a sentence by choosing a word or words from a dropdown list.

Take a look at the following question.

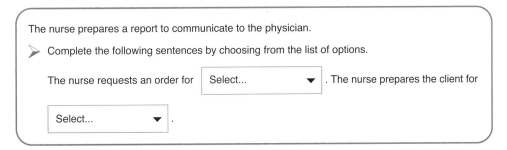

Figure 3.8 Example of Cloze Dropdown Question

To populate the answer choices, place the cursor on the first dropdown, labeled with the instruction "Select" beside an inverted triangle, and left-click. Typically, three to five answer choices are provided in each dropdown.

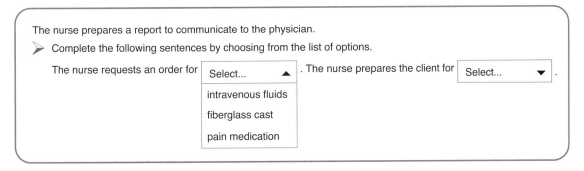

Figure 3.9 Example of Cloze Dropdown Options

The first step to answer a Cloze Dropdown question is to identify the client's priority problem based on cues in the case study. Next, consider each answer choice in the first dropdown menu.

- Does the answer choice help validate or address the priority problem or potential condition you identified for this client?
- Will the action in the answer choice help the client "right here, right now"?

If not, eliminate that answer choice. Repeat this process with each answer choice in each dropdown menu. After choosing your answers, pause to consider each of your selections. Ask yourself:

- "Does this choice make sense?"
- "Have I selected answers based on my foundational nursing knowledge?"

If you can answer "Yes," you have selected the best choices to answer the Cloze Dropdown item.

A variation of the dropdown question type is **Cloze Dropdown Rationale**, in which you complete a rationale-based sentence. Like Drag-and-Drop Rationale, this question type requires you to recognize a cause-and-effect relationship. In Cloze Dropdown Rationale questions, however, you select answers to complete the sentence from dropdown menus rather than answer wells. As in any rationale-based question, the sentence will include the words "due to" or "as evidenced by."

Look at the following Cloze Dropdown Rationale question.

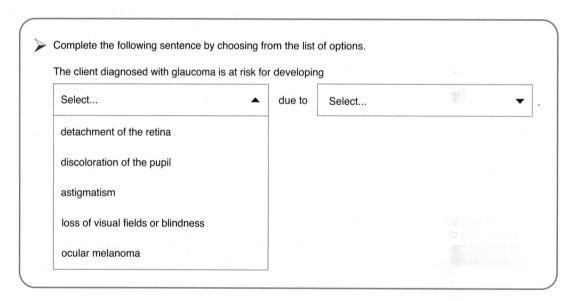

Figure 3.10 Example of Cloze Dropdown Rationale Question, First Dropdown

To answer a Cloze Dropdown Rationale question, identify the client's priority problem based on cues in the case study. Then, starting with the first dropdown, consider each answer choice: Is it related to the priority problem or potential condition you identified for this client? If not, eliminate that answer choice. Identifying the priority problem or potential condition in the first dropdown is essential to earning any credit on the item.

Repeat this process with each answer choice in each dropdown. After choosing your answers, pause to consider each of your selections. Ask yourself:

- "Do the answers I chose make sense?"
- "Have I selected answers based on my foundational nursing knowledge?"
- "Have I selected answers based on the client's priority problem/condition?"

If you can answer "Yes," you have selected the best choices to answer the Cloze Dropdown Rationale question.

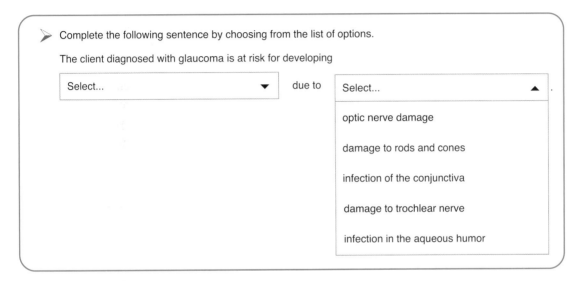

Figure 3.11 Example of Cloze Dropdown Rationale Question, Second Dropdown

Another dropdown variation is **Dropdown Table**, in which you select from a series of dropdowns incorporated into a chart. As in the other dropdown question types, you select only one answer choice per dropdown.

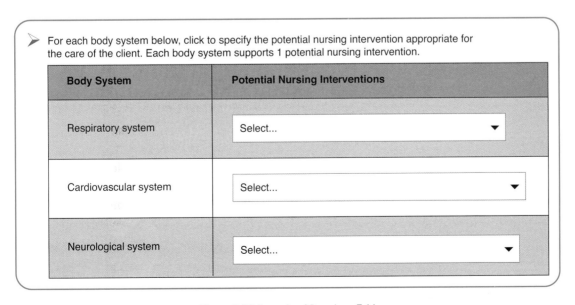

Figure 3.12 Example of Dropdown Table

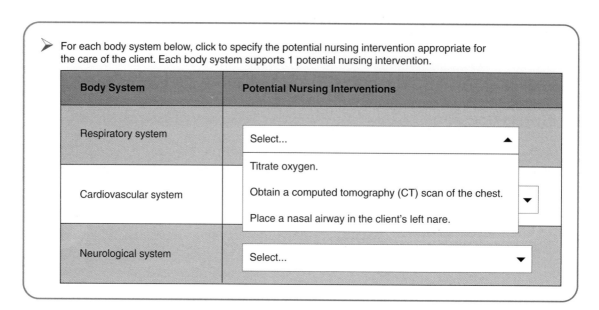

> For each body system below, click to specify the potential nursing intervention appropriate for the care of the client. Each body system supports 1 potential nursing intervention.

Body System	Potential Nursing Interventions
Respiratory system	Select... ▲
Cardiovascular system	Titrate oxygen. / Obtain a computed tomography (CT) scan of the chest. / Place a nasal airway in the client's left nare. ▼
Neurological system	Select... ▼

Figure 3.13 Example of Dropdown Table, First Dropdown

The strategy you should use in a Dropdown Table question is to reword each answer option as a True/False question and consider it individually. In the first row of the figure, for example, you would reword the first option as "Is titrating oxygen an appropriate respiratory intervention for this client?", the second option as "Is obtaining a CT scan of the chest an appropriate respiratory intervention for this client?", and so on.

After choosing your answers, pause to consider each of your selections. Ask yourself:

- "Do the answers I chose make sense?"
- "Have I selected answers based on my foundational nursing knowledge?"

If you can answer "Yes," you have selected the best choices to answer the Dropdown Table question.

Matrix

Matrix alternate format questions present answer options arranged in a table and prompt you to select an answer or answers from each row. There are two varieties, Matrix Multiple Choice and Matrix Multiple Response.

In the **Matrix Multiple Choice** question type, there is only one correct answer per row, which you will select from a set of radio buttons. The question will prompt you to evaluate each item of a series against the same set of answer options. For instance, you would decide for each item in a series:

- Is the intervention indicated or contraindicated?
- Is the intervention priority or nonpriority?
- Does the client response indicate that teaching is effective or ineffective?

Look at the following Matrix Multiple Choice question.

On day 3 of the client's hospitalization, the nurse assesses the client and documents care. The nurse provides additional discharge teaching.

➤ For each client statement, click to indicate if the client understands discharge teaching or requires **further** education.

Statement	Understands	Further education
"If my blood glucose is below 60 mg/dL (3.33 mmol/L), I should drink 4 ounces of fruit juice or cola."	○	○
"Fifteen minutes after I eat or drink something to correct hypoglycemia, I should recheck my blood glucose."	○	○
"If my blood glucose remains low after I eat or drink something, I should come to the emergency department (ED)."	○	○
"I should keep hard candies with me at all times."	○	○
"It is very important for me to eat as soon as I have injected my regular insulin dose."	○	○

Figure 3.14 Example of Matrix Multiple Choice Question

The strategy you should use to answer a Matrix Multiple Choice question is the same as for SATA questions. Change each answer choice into a statement, and then determine if the statement is correct. Let's look at the answers.

- "If my blood glucose is below 60 mg/dL (3.33 mmol/L), I should drink 4 ounces of fruit juice or cola." Does this statement indicate client understanding? Yes, this statement indicates understanding of the "15–15" rule. Select "Understands" for this row.

- "Fifteen minutes after I eat or drink something to correct hypoglycemia, I should recheck my blood glucose." Does this statement indicate client understanding? Yes, this statement indicates understanding of the "15–15" rule. Select "Understands" for this row.

- "If my blood glucose remains low after I eat or drink something, I should come to the emergency department (ED)." Does this statement indicate client understanding? No. As the immediate next step, the client should follow the "15–15" rule and ingest an additional 15 grams of carbohydrates. Select "Further education" for this row.

- "I should keep hard candies with me at all times." Does this statement indicate client understanding? Yes, this statement indicates understanding of the "15–15" rule. Select "Understands" for this row.

- "It is very important for me to eat as soon as I have injected my regular insulin dose." Does this statement indicate client understanding? Yes. Having injected regular insulin, the client needs to take in a bolus of food so that there is glucose in the bloodstream when the peak action of insulin occurs. Select "Understands" for this row.

Matrix Multiple Response questions may prompt you to correlate a set of client symptoms or nursing assessment findings with a medical problem. In this question type, there is *potentially more than one correct answer* per row. Instead of radio buttons, you will see a box for each answer option. Left-click in the box to select the option. Remember, you may select more than one option per row.

It is important to note that each column in a Matrix Multiple Response question must have at least one option selected. Otherwise, you will be unable to progress to the next question.

Here is a sample Matrix Multiple Response question.

> For each assessment finding below, click to specify whether the finding is consistent with the disease process of pneumonia, heart failure, or sepsis. Each finding may support more than one disease process. **Each column must have at least 1 response option selected.**

Assessment Finding	Pneumonia	Heart failure	Sepsis
Shortness of breath.	☐	☐	☐
BP 94/62 mmHg.	☐	☐	☐
1+ edema to lower extremities.	☐	☐	☐
Temperature 101.4° F (38.8° C).	☐	☐	☐
Coarse crackles to lung bases.	☐	☐	☐

Figure 3.15 Example of Matrix Multiple Response Question

Let's look at the answer options for the first two rows of the table. The strategy for this type of question is, once again, to change each answer choice into a statement, and then determine if the statement is true or false based on your foundational nursing knowledge.

- "Shortness of breath is expected with pneumonia." Yes, this is a true statement. Select this answer choice.
- "Shortness of breath is expected with heart failure." True. Select this answer choice.
- "Shortness of breath is expected with sepsis." True. Select this answer choice.
- "Hypotension is expected with pneumonia." No, this statement is false. Eliminate this answer.
- "Hypotension is expected with heart failure." Perhaps, if the client has a reduced ejection fraction rate. Refer to information in the case to determine whether the client has a reduced ejection fraction.
- "Hypotension is expected with sepsis." True. Select this answer choice.

Continue with this method for each remaining assessment finding.

Bowtie

This is a standalone, case-based alternate format question type in which you "drag and drop" answer choices into a bowtie-shaped diagram. The **Bowtie** question type requires you to make multiple clinical decisions that range from recognizing concerning cues to evaluating client outcomes.

Take a look at the following Bowtie question.

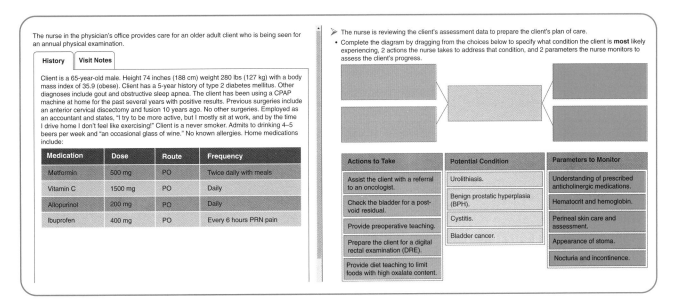

Figure 3.16 Example of Bowtie Question and Case Study

The answer choices in a Bowtie item are laid out in an uneven table with five options in the left column, four in the middle column, and five in the right column. In each Bowtie item, two options are correct in the left and right columns, and one answer is correct in the middle column.

The color-coded columns of these answer wells correspond with the targets above each column. For example, tokens from the "Actions to Take" column can only be dragged to a corresponding-colored "Actions to Take" target location directly above it. As with other drag-and-drop question types, a token dropped into a non corresponding blank will be rejected and automatically returned to its answer well.

To remove a token that you have mistakenly dragged into the diagram, you can either return it to its answer well or drag the desired token to the target to replace the discarded token. Note that paired options, such as the two options chosen for "Actions to Take" and "Parameters to Monitor" in the example, are interchangeable and do not need to be in a specific order in the diagram.

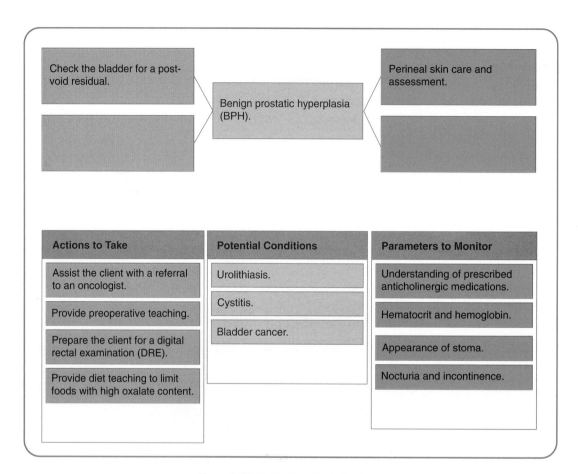

Figure 3.17 Bowtie Question in Progress

To answer a Bowtie question, start with the middle of the diagram.

- First, identify the Potential Condition you believe the client is experiencing, and place it in the middle target. You should derive the Potential Condition by recognizing cues in the case record and analyzing their significance based on your foundational nursing knowledge.

- Next, select the two Actions to Take based on the Potential Condition you have identified, and place them (in either order) in the left-hand targets of the diagram.

- Finally, select the two Parameters to Monitor based on the Potential Condition you have identified, and place them (in either order) in the right-hand targets of the diagram.

The Potential Condition that you select will help you determine which Actions to Take are appropriate and which Parameters to Monitor are necessary. Use the *if/then* principle as you consider these: "If the potential condition is most likely _____, then the actions the nurse will take are _____ and _____, and the parameters to monitor are _____ and _____."

Trend

This standalone, case-based alternate format question type also requires clinical decision-making skills and clinical judgment. The name of the question, **Trend**, is representative of what you will be asked to do: recognize and interpret a pattern of changes over a period of time. Some trends may be desired and therapeutic, such as a decline in blood glucose readings after starting an antidiabetic medication. Other trends may be harmful, such as steady increases in blood pressure readings after increasing sodium intake in the diet.

Different "tabs" in the medical record provide different categories of information gathered over a period of time, such as:

- Nurse's Notes
- Laboratory Results
- Diagnostic Results
- Vital Signs
- Intake and Output

The time evolution could occur over minutes, hours, days, and so on. For example, a Trend question might provide a "Nurse's Notes" tab documenting a client's vital signs throughout the shift, and then ask you to interpret the vital signs and make a clinical decision regarding care of the client. Trend items can feature any item response type except Bowtie, so you could see a Trend question in the form of Cloze, Matrix, Highlight, Multiple Response, or four-option multiple choice.

Following is an example of a Trend question.

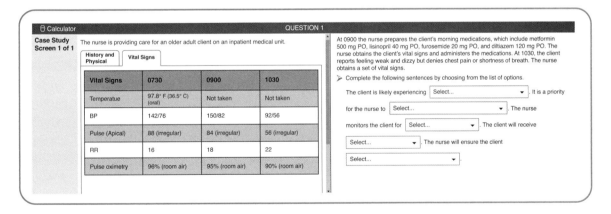

Figure 3.18 Example of Trend Question

Each time you receive a set of trended data, analyze it and consider whether the trend is therapeutic or nontherapeutic for the client's condition. Making that determination sets the stage for you to respond successfully to the trended data.

Critical Thinking Strategies

- The NCLEX-PN® exam is not a test about recognizing facts.
- You must be able to correctly identify what the question is asking.
- Do not focus on background information that is not needed to answer the question.
- The NCLEX-PN® exam focuses on thinking through a problem or situation.

Now that you are more knowledgeable about the components of a multiple choice test question and the structure of the various alternate format question types, let's talk about specific strategies that you can use to problem-solve your way to correct answers on the NCLEX-PN® exam.

Remember, the NCLEX-PN® exam tests your ability to think critically. Critical thinking for the practical/vocational nurse involves:

- Observation (recognizing cues)
- Applying knowledge and deciding what is important (analyzing cues and prioritizing)
- Looking for patterns and relationships (trends)
- Identifying the problem (based on cue recognition)
- Transferring knowledge from one situation to another
- Discriminating between possible choices and/or courses of action
- Evaluating according to criteria established

Are you feeling overwhelmed as you read these words? Don't be! We are going teach you a step-by-step method to choose the appropriate path. The Kaplan Nursing team has developed a Decision Tree that shows you how to approach every NCLEX-PN® exam question. In this book, these strategies appear as 9 critical thinking paths.

There are some strategies that you must follow on *every* NCLEX-PN® exam test question. You must *always* figure out what the question is asking, and you must *always* eliminate answer choices.

Choosing the right answer often involves choosing the best of several answers that have correct information. This may entail your correct analysis and interpretation of what the question is really asking. So let's talk about how to figure out what the question is asking.

Reword the Question

The first step to correctly answering NCLEX-PN® exam questions is to find out what each question is *really* asking.

STEP 1. Read each question carefully from the first word to the last word. Do not skim over the words or read them too quickly.

STEP 2. Look for hints in the wording of the question stem. The adjectives *most, first, best, primary,* and *initial* indicate that you must establish priorities. The phrase *further teaching is necessary* indicates that the answer will contain incorrect information. The phrase *client understands the teaching* indicates that the answer will be correct information.

STEP 3. Reword the question stem in your own words so that it can be answered with a *yes* or a *no,* or with a specific bit of information. Begin your questions with *what, when,* or *why.* We will refer to this reworded version as THE REWORDED QUESTION in the examples that follow.

STEP 4. If you can't complete step 3, read the answer choices for clues.

Let's practice rewording a question.

> A preschool-age child is brought to the emergency department (ED) by the parents for treatment of a femur fracture. When asked how the injury occurred, the parents state that the child fell from the sofa. On examination, the LPN/LVN finds old and new lesions on the child's buttocks. Which statement **most** appropriately reflects how the LPN/LVN should document these findings?
>
> 1.
> 2.
> 3.
> 4.

We omitted the answer choices to make you focus on the question stem this time. The answer choices will be provided and discussed later in this chapter.

STEP 1. Read the question stem carefully.

STEP 2. Pay attention to the adjectives. *Most appropriately* tells you that you need to select the best answer.

STEP 3. Reword the question stem in your own words. In this case, it is, "What is the best documentation for this situation?"

STEP 4. Because you were able to reword the question, the fourth step is unnecessary. You didn't need to read the answer choices for clues.

We have all missed questions on a test because we didn't read accurately. The following question illustrates this point.

> A client is admitted to the hospital for treatment of active tuberculosis (TB). The LPN/LVN reinforces teaching about TB. Which statement by the client indicates to the LPN/LVN that further teaching is necessary?
>
> 1.
> 2.
> 3.
> 4.

Again, just the question stem is given to encourage you to focus on rewording the question. We will discuss the answer choices for this question later in this chapter.

STEP 1. Read the question stem carefully.

STEP 2. Look for hints. Pay particular attention to the statement "further teaching is necessary." You are looking for negative information.

STEP 3. Reword the question stem in your own words. In this case, it is, "What is incorrect information about TB?"

STEP 4. Because you were able to reword the question, the fourth step is unnecessary. You didn't need to read the answer choices for clues to determine what the question is asking.

Try rewording this test question.

> A client admitted to the hospital in premature labor has been treated successfully. The client is to receive a regimen of betamethasone. Which statement by the client indicates to the LPN/LVN that the client understands the teaching about the medication?
>
> 1.
> 2.
> 3.
> 4.

Again, just the question stem is given to encourage you to focus on rewording the question. We will discuss the answer choices for this question later in this chapter.

STEP 1. Read the question stem carefully.

STEP 2. Look for hints. Pay attention to the words *client understands*. You are looking for true information.

STEP 3. Reword the question stem. This question is asking, "What is true about betametasone?"

STEP 4. Because you were able to reword this question, the fourth step is unnecessary. You didn't need to obtain clues about what the question is asking from the answer choices.

Eliminate Incorrect Answer Choices

Now that you've mastered rewording the question, let's examine how to select the correct answer.

Remember the characteristics of unsuccessful test takers? One of their major problems is that they do not thoughtfully consider each answer choice. They react to questions using feelings and hunches. Unsuccessful test takers look for a specific answer choice. The following strategy will enable you to consider each answer choice in a thoughtful way.

STEP 1. Do not look at any of the answer choices except answer choice (1).

STEP 2. Read answer choice (1). Then repeat THE REWORDED QUESTION after reading the answer choice. Ask yourself, "Does this answer THE REWORDED QUESTION?" If you know the answer choice is wrong, eliminate it. If you aren't sure, leave the answer choice in for consideration.

STEP 3. Repeat the above process with each remaining answer choice.

STEP 4. Note which answer choices remain.

STEP 5. Reread the question to make sure you have correctly identified THE REWORDED QUESTION.

STEP 6. Ask yourself, "Which answer choice best answers the question?" That is your answer.

Let's practice the elimination strategy using the same questions.

> A preschool-age child is brought to the emergency department (ED) by the parents for treatment of a femur fracture. When asked how the injury occurred, the parents state that the child fell from the sofa. On examination, the LPN/LVN finds old and new lesions on the child's buttocks. Which statement most appropriately reflects how the LPN/LVN should document these findings?
>
> 1. "Six lesions in various stages of healing noted on buttocks."
> 2. "Multiple lesions on buttocks due to child abuse."
> 3. "Lesions noted on buttocks from unknown causes."
> 4. "Several lesions noted on buttocks caused by cigarettes."

THE REWORDED QUESTION: "What is good documenting?"

STEP 1. Do not look at any of the answer choices except for answer choice (1). Thoughtfully consider each answer choice individually.

STEP 2. Read answer choice (1). Does it answer the question, "What is good documenting for this situation?"

(1) "Six lesions in various stages of healing noted on buttocks." Is this good documenting? Maybe. Leave it in for consideration.

STEP 3. Repeat the process with each remaining answer choice.

(2) "Multiple lesions on buttocks due to child abuse." Is this good documenting? No, because the LPN/LVN is making a judgment about the cause of the lesions.

(3) "Lesions noted on buttocks from unknown causes." Is this good documenting? Maybe. Leave it in for consideration.

(4) "Several lesions noted on buttocks caused by cigarettes." Is this good documenting? No. The question does not include information about how the burns occurred.

STEP 4. Answer choices (1) and (3) remain.

STEP 5. Reread the question to make sure you have correctly identified THE REWORDED QUESTION. This question asks you to identify good documenting.

STEP 6. Which is better documenting? "Six lesions in various stages of healing noted on buttocks," or "Lesions noted on buttock from unknown causes"? Good documenting is accurate, objective, concise, and complete. It must reflect the client's current status. The correct answer is (1).

Some students will select answer (3), thinking, "How can I be sure about the stages of healing?" But the purpose of this question is to test your ability to select good documenting. Select the answer choice that shows you are a safe and effective nurse. Remember, questions on the NCLEX-PN® exam are not designed to trick you. Stay focused on the question.

Let's select the correct answer for the second question.

> A client admitted to the hospital for treatment of active tuberculosis (TB). The LPN/LVN reinforces teaching about TB. Which statement by the client indicates to the LPN/LVN that further teaching is necessary?
>
> 1. "I will have to take medication for 6 months."
> 2. "I should cover my nose and mouth when coughing or sneezing."
> 3. "I will remain in isolation for at least 6 weeks."
> 4. "I will always have a positive skin test for TB."

THE REWORDED QUESTION: What is incorrect information about TB?

STEP 1. Do not look at any of the answer choices except answer choice (1).

STEP 2. Read answer choice (1). Does it answer THE REWORDED QUESTION, "What is incorrect (or wrong) information about TB?"

(1) "I will have to take medication for 6 months." Is this wrong information? No, it is a true statement. The client will need to take a medication, such as isonicotinyl hydrazine (INH), for 6 months or longer. Eliminate this choice.

STEP 3. Repeat the process with each remaining answer choice.

(2) "I should cover my nose and mouth when coughing or sneezing." Is this wrong information about TB? No, this is a true statement. TB is transmitted by droplet contamination. Eliminate it.

(3) "I will remain in isolation for at least 6 weeks." Is this wrong information about TB? Maybe. Leave it in for consideration.

(4) "I will always have a positive skin test for TB." Is this a wrong statement about TB? No, this is true. A positive skin test indicates that the client has developed antibodies to the tuberculosis bacillus. Eliminate this choice.

STEP 4. Only answer choice (3) remains.

STEP 5. Reread the question to make sure you have correctly identified THE REWORDED QUESTION. The question is, "What is incorrect information about TB?"

STEP 6. The correct answer is (3). You "know" this is the correct answer because you've eliminated the other three answer choices. The client does not need to be isolated for 6 weeks. The client's activities will be restricted for about 2–3 weeks after medication therapy is initiated.

A couple of things to remember when using this strategy:

- Eliminate only what you know is wrong. However, once you eliminate an answer choice, do not retrieve it for consideration. You may be tempted to do this if you do not feel comfortable with the one answer choice that is left. Resist the impulse!
- Stay focused on THE REWORDED QUESTION. How many of you have missed a question that asked for negative information because you selected the answer choice that contained correct information?

Here's another question.

> A client admitted to the hospital in premature labor has been treated successfully. The client is to receive a regimen of betamethasone. Which statement by the client indicates to the LPN/LVN that the client understands the teaching about the medication?
>
> 1. "As long as I receive my medication, I won't deliver prematurely."
> 2. "It is important that I count the fetal movements for one hour, twice a day."
> 3. "I have insomnia and a rapid heart beat while on this medication."
> 4. "Bed rest is necessary in order for the medication to work properly."

THE REWORDED QUESTION: What is true about antenatal betamethasone?

STEP 1. Do not look at any of the answer choices except answer choice (1).

STEP 2. Read answer choice (1). Does it answer the question, "What is true about betamethasone?"

(1) "As long as I receive my medication, I won't deliver prematurely." Is this true about betamethasone? No. Betamethasone will help fetal lung maturation in case the client delivers prematurely, but it doesn't prevent premature delivery. Eliminate it.

STEP 3. Repeat the process with each remaining answer choice.

(2) "It is important that I count the fetal movements for one hour, twice a day." Is this true about betamethasone? Maybe. Clients are told to be aware of fetal movement. Keep it as a possibility.

(3) "I may have insomnia and a rapid heart beat while on this medication." Is this true of betamethasone? Yes. Betamethasone is a corticosteroid. Side effects include insomnia, increased maternal heart rate, and hypertension. Leave this choice in for consideration.

(4) "Bed rest is necessary for the medication to work properly." Is this true about betamethasone? No. Betamethasone will work whether the client is on bedrest or not. Eliminate it.

STEP 4. Note that only answer choices (2) and (3) remain.

STEP 5. Reread the question to make sure you have correctly identified THE REWORDED QUESTION. The rewarded question is, "What is true about betamethasone?"

STEP 6. Which choice best answers the question, (2) or (3)? If you are focused on the question, you will select (3). Some students focus on the background information (pregnancy). This question has nothing to do with pregnancy. If you chose (2), you fell for a distracter.

Remember: Focus on the question, and not the background information. If you can answer the question—"What is true about betamethasone?"—without considering the background information (pregnancy), do it. Many students answer a question incorrectly because they don't focus on THE REWORDED QUESTION. Don't fall for the distracters.

At this point you're probably thinking, "Will I have enough time to finish the test using these strategies?" or "How will I ever remember how to answer questions using these steps?" Yes, you will have time to finish the test. Unsuccessful test takers spend time agonizing over test questions. By using these strategies, you will be using your time productively. You will remember the steps because you are going to practice, practice, practice with test questions. You will not be able to absorb this strategy by osmosis; the process must be practiced repeatedly.

Don't Predict Answers

On the NCLEX-PN® exam, you are asked to select the best answer from the four choices that you are given. Many times, the "ideal" answer choice is not there. Don't sit and moan because the answer that you think should be there isn't provided. Remember:

- Identify THE REWORDED QUESTION.
- Select the best answer *from the choices given.*

Look at this question.

> The LPN/LVN is explaining the procedure for clean-catch urine specimen collection for culture and sensitivity to a male client. Which explanation by the LPN/LVN would be **most** accurate?
>
> 1. "The urinary meatus is cleansed with an iodine solution and then a urinary drainage catheter is inserted to obtain urine."
> 2. "You will be asked to empty your bladder one-half hour before the test; you will then be asked to void into a container."
> 3. "Before voiding, the urinary meatus is cleansed with an iodine solution and urine is voided into a sterile container; the container must not touch the penis."
> 4. "You must void a few drops of urine, then stop; then void the remaining urine into a clean container, which should be immediately covered."

STEP 1. Read the question stem.

STEP 2. Focus on the adjectives. "*Most accurate*" tells you that more than one answer may seem correct.

STEP 3. Reword the question stem. What is true about a clean-catch urine specimen for culture and sensitivity?

STEP 4. Read each answer choice and ask yourself, "Is this true about a clean-catch urine specimen for culture and sensitivity?"

(1) "The urinary meatus is cleansed with an iodine solution and then a urinary drainage catheter is inserted to obtain urine." This choice describes how to obtain a catheterized urine specimen. Urine isn't usually collected by catheterization due to the increased risk of infection. This answer does not answer the question about a clean-catch urine specimen. Eliminate.

(2) "You will be asked to empty your bladder one-half hour before the test; you will then be asked to void into a container." This describes a double-voided specimen. This action is usually done when testing urine for glucose and ketones. It is not relevant to a clean-catch urine specimen. Eliminate.

(3) "Before voiding, the urinary meatus is cleansed with an iodine solution and urine is voided into a sterile container; the container must not touch the penis." This is true of a clean-catch urine specimen for culture and sensitivity. The urinary meatus is cleansed, a sterile container is used, and the penis must not touch the container. Leave this answer in for consideration.

(4) "You must void a few drops of urine, then stop; then void the remaining urine into a clean container, which should be immediately covered." This does describe a clean-catch urine specimen. The client does void a few drops of urine, stops, and then continues voiding into the container. There is only one problem. For a culture and sensitivity, the container must be sterile. Eliminate.

The correct answer is (3). Many students will select answer choice (4) because they see the expected words: "Void a few drops, stop, continue voiding." Be careful. This question is a good example of why scanning for expected words could get you into trouble. You may see expected words in an answer choice that is not correct.

Okay. You've practiced how to identify the topic of the question and how to eliminate answer choices. You know that predicting answers does not work on the NCLEX-PN® exam. You are well on your way to correctly answering NCLEX-PN® exam test questions. Unfortunately, this is just the starting point. Let's talk about specific paths and how you can correctly decide which paths to use on the NCLEX-PN® exam. Remember, the correct answer is at the end of the path!

Recognize Expected Outcomes

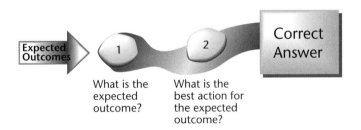

You spent much of your time in practical/vocational nursing school learning about what might go wrong with clients and their care. This makes sense; after all, nurses need to deal with problems and illnesses. Many test questions that your practical/vocational nursing school faculty wrote focused on what was wrong with clients and their care. In order to prove minimum competence, the beginning practical/vocational nurse must demonstrate the ability to make appropriate nursing judgments.

Competent nursing judgments include recognizing both expected and unexpected behaviors, so it is important for you to recognize expected outcomes on the NCLEX-PN® exam. Expected outcomes are the behaviors and changes you think are going to occur as a result of nursing care. These outcomes allow the nurse to evaluate whether goals have been met.

Look at the following question.

> The LPN/LVN is checking the morning's serum electrolyte results for a client. The LPN/LVN notes that the client's sodium is 142 mEq/L (142 mmol/L), potassium is 4.4 mEq/L (4.4 mmol/L), and chloride is 102 mEq/L (102 mmol/L). Which should the nurse do **first**?
>
> 1. Encourage the client to drink additional fluids.
> 2. Notify the primary health care provider of electrolyte results.
> 3. Record electrolyte results in the client's medical record.
> 4. Withhold the client's potassium supplement.

If this question were included on one of your fundamentals tests, you would assume that a problem was being described. You would choose an answer that involved "fixing" the problem. Let's look at this question.

THE REWORDED QUESTION: What should you do with a client with these electrolyte results?

STEP 1. Recognize normal. Interpret the serum electrolyte results. All are within normal limits.

STEP 2. Decide how you should use this information. Because the values are all normal, let's reword the question again using this information.

Now THE REWORDED QUESTION is: What should you do for a client with normal serum electrolytes?

ANSWERS:

(1) Encourage the client to drink additional fluids. Although good fluid intake is usually recommended, this is not a priority because the serum electrolytes are within normal limits. Eliminate.

(2) Notify the physician of the client's electrolyte results. This is unnecessary because the serum electrolytes are normal. Most physicians request notification only for abnormal test results. Eliminate.

(3) Record the electrolyte results in the client's chart. This action should be done because the electrolyte results are normal.

(4) Withhold the client's morning potassium supplement. The client's K^+ is within normal limits, which suggests that the potassium supplement has helped maintain this serum level. There is no indication with the information you have been given that this would be necessary or prudent. Eliminate.

The correct answer is (3). The electrolytes are within normal limits. Some students select answer choice (1) because they think there's something they missed, or it must be a trick question. The "trick" is deciding whether the information that you are given is normal or abnormal, and then answering the question accordingly.

Try this question.

> A client reporting chest pressure is brought to the emergency department (ED). Vital signs include blood pressure 150/90 mmHg, pulse 88 beats/minute, respirations 20 breaths/minute. The LPN/LVN administers nitroglycerin 0.4 mg sublingually as ordered. After five minutes, the client's vital signs include blood pressure 100/60 Hg, pulse 96 beats/minute, respirations 20 breaths/minute. Which action should the LPN/LVN take next?
>
> 1. Notify the primary health care provider of hypotension.
> 2. Place the client in semi-Fowler position and administer oxygen at 4 L/minute.
> 3. Administer a second dose of nitroglycerin 0.4 mg sublingually, as ordered.
> 4. Document vital signs and continue to monitor the client.

THE REWORDED QUESTION: What should you do for this client?

To answer this question you need to know what these vital signs indicate.

STEP 1. Recognize normal. Nitroglycerin is a potent vasodilator with anti-anginal, anti-ischemic, and antihypertensive actions. It increases blood flow through the coronary arteries. Side effects include orthostatic hypotension, tachycardia, dizziness, and palpitations. Decreased blood pressure, increased pulse rate, and stable respiratory rate after administration of a potent vasodilator is normal and expected.

STEP 2. Decide how you should use this information. The question should be reworded as, "What should you do for a client who has responded as expected to a dose of nitroglycerin?"

ANSWERS:

(1) "Notify the primary health care provider of hypotension." The blood pressure has decreased due to vasodilation. Decreased blood pressure is expected. Eliminate.

(2) "Place the client in semi-Fowler position and administer oxygen at 4 L/minute." Respiratory rate is stable and there is no indication of respiratory distress. Eliminate.

(3) "Administer a second dose of nitroglycerin 0.4 mg sublingually, as ordered." The nurse should assess the client for chest pain first, and administer a second dose of the medication only if the client continues to report chest pain. Eliminate.

(4) "Document the vital signs and continue to closely monitor the client." This is the correct choice. You identified it by recognizing the client's response as normal, thus eliminating the other three answer choices.

The correct answer is (4). You would expect a client's blood pressure to decrease after administration of nitroglycerin. The key to this question is understanding how the medication works and correctly identifying the expected outcome.

Read Answer Choices to Obtain Clues

Because the NCLEX-PN® exam tests your critical thinking, the topic of the questions may be unstated. You may see a question that concerns a disease process or procedure with which you are unfamiliar. Most test takers who are "clueless" about a question will read the question and answer choices over and over again. They do this because they hope that:

- They will remember seeing the topic in their notes or on a textbook page.
- The light will dawn and they will remember something about the topic.
- They believe there is some clue in the question that will point them toward the correct answer.

What usually happens? Absolutely nothing! The student then randomly selects an answer choice. When you randomly select an answer, you have one chance in four of getting it right. You can better those odds, and here's how: when you encounter a question that deals with unfamiliar nursing content, look for clues in the answer choices instead of in the question stem.

If you find yourself "clueless" after you carefully read a question, follow these steps:

STEP 1. Resist the impulse to read and reread the question. Read the question only once. Identify the topic of the question. It is often unstated.

STEP 2. Read the answer choices, not to select the correct answer, but to figure out, "What is the topic of the question?" or "What should I be thinking?" You are looking for clues from the answer choices.

STEP 3. After reading the answer choices, reword the question using the clues that you have obtained. Then use the strategies previously discussed to answer the question you have formulated.

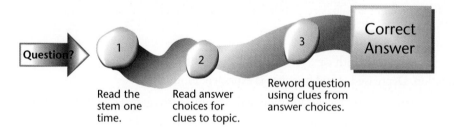

Let's try this strategy with a question.

> A client with type 1 diabetes contacts the home care LPN/LVN to report nausea and abdominal pain. What should the LPN/LVN advise the client to do?
>
> 1. "Hold your regular dose of insulin."
> 2. "Check your blood glucose level every 3 to 4 hours."
> 3. "Increase consumption of foods containing simple sugars."
> 4. "Increase your activity level."

STEP 1. Read the stem of the question. Can you identify the topic of the question? No, you can't. The LPN/LVN is telling the client to do something, but about what topic? The topic is unstated in the question.

STEP 2. Read the answer choices to obtain clues about the topic of the question. What topic are they prompting you to think about? Each answer choice deals with ways to maintain a normal blood glucose.

STEP 3. Reword the question. "What does the LPN/LVN tell the client about 'sick day rules'?"

ANSWERS:

(1) "Hold your regular dose of insulin." This is an implementation that would increase the blood glucose level. The LPN/LVN should collect data first. Eliminate.

(2) "Check your blood glucose level every 3 to 4 hours." This is data collection. Before you can advise the client, you must identify whether the client is hypoglycemic or hyperglycemic. Keep this answer for consideration.

(3) "Increase your consumption of foods containing simple sugars." This is an implementation and would increase the client's blood glucose level. The LPN/LVN should collect data first. Eliminate.

(4) "Increase your activity level." This is an implementation that would decrease the client's blood glucose level. The LPN/LVN should collect data first. Eliminate.

The nurse should always collect data before implementing nursing care. The correct answer is (2).

No matter how much you prepare for the NCLEX-PN® exam, there may be topics you see on your test with which you are unfamiliar. Reading the answer choices for clues will increase your chances of selecting a correct answer. Remember, you do have a body of knowledge. You just have to be calm and access this knowledge.

Read this question.

> A client is being treated for Addison disease. The primary health care provider orders cortisone 25 mg PO daily. The LPN/LVN should explain to the client that a dosage adjustment may be required in which situation?
>
> 1. Dosage is increased when the blood glucose level increases.
> 2. Dosage is decreased when dietary intake is increased.
> 3. Dosage is decreased when infection stimulates endogenous steroid secretion.
> 4. Dosage is increased relative to an increase in the level of stress.

Not sure what Addison disease is? Not sure how to adjust the dose of cortisone?

STEP 1. Read the question once. Resist the impulse to reread the question.

STEP 2. Read the answer choices. What should you be thinking? The question concerns cortisone. If the client is receiving cortisone, Addison disease must be something that requires cortisone, a hormone from the adrenal glands. You notice that dosages are both increased and decreased.

STEP 3. Reword the question using clues from the answer choices: "What is true about adjusting corti-sone dosage?" Consider each answer choice. Does it answer THE REWORDED QUESTION?

(1) "Dosage is increased when the blood glucose level increases." Is this true about cortisone? No. This sounds like insulin. Eliminate.

(2) "Dosage is decreased when dietary intake is increased." Is this true about cortisone? No. Cortisone requirements are not related to diet. Eliminate.

(3) "Dosage is decreased when infection stimulates endogenous steroid secretion." Endogenous means "within the client." If the client is receiving cortisone for Addison's disease, the client must have adrenal insufficiency. Therefore, infection can't stimulate steroid secretion. Eliminate.

The correct answer is (4) because it is the only choice remaining. Even if you are not confident that cortisone is increased during periods of stress, you can conclude that this is the correct answer because the other choices have been eliminated.

If you're not sure about the topic of the question, read the answer choices for clues.

Let's look at another critical thinking path.

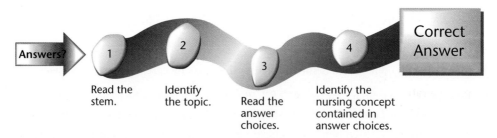

In some questions, the NCLEX-PN® exam asks you to figure out the topic of the question. In other questions, you are required to use critical thinking skills to figure out what the answer choices *really* mean. The NCLEX-PN® exam can take a concept with which you are very familiar and make it difficult to recognize. The following question illustrates this point.

> A client with a history of heart failure visits the clinic. The client states, "I have not been feeling like my old self for about 2 weeks." It would be **most** important for the LPN/LVN to ask which question?
>
> 1. "Do your ankles swell at the end of the day?"
> 2. "How do you position yourself for sleep?"
> 3. "How do you feel after you eat dinner?"
> 4. "Do you have chest pain when you inhale?"

It is not difficult to identify the topic of this question, "What is a priority for a client with heart failure?" Many students get tripped up on this question by not thinking through the answers as carefully as they should. In some questions, you have to figure out the topic of the question. In this question, you have to figure out what the answer choices mean.

STEP 1. Read the stem of the question.

STEP 2. Reword the question in your own words.

STEP 3. Read the answer choices.

STEP 4. Think: "What nursing concept should I identify in the answer choices?"

THE REWORDED QUESTION: What is a priority for a client with heart failure?

ANSWERS:

(1)   "Do your ankles swell at the end of the day?" Why would you ask a client this question? Because edema is a symptom of right-sided heart failure. Is right-sided failure your priority? No, left-sided failure takes priority because it affects the lungs. Eliminate this answer.

(2)   "How do you position yourself for sleep?" Why would you ask a client this question? If the client sleeps flat in bed, breathing is not compromised. If the client sleeps in a recliner, the client experiences orthopnea, a symptom of left-sided failure. This would be a priority. Keep this answer for consideration.

(3)   "How do you feel after you eat dinner?" Why would you ask a client this question? Bloating after meals is a symptom of right-sided failure. This is not as important as breathing problems. Eliminate this answer.

(4)   "Do you have chest pain when you inhale?" Why would you ask a client this question? It does indicate a breathing problem. The student who reacts rather than thinks may select this answer. Pain on inspiration may indicate irritation of the parietal pleura of the lung, which is not associated with heart failure. Eliminate this answer.

The correct answer is (2). In order to select this answer, you must recognize that "Where do you sleep at night?" represents orthopnea. The NCLEX-PN® exam can take important concepts such as this and "hide" the concept in some fairly simple behaviors.

Let's try another question where you have to figure out what the answer choices really mean.

> The LPN/LVN is caring for a client immediately after a paracentesis. It is **most**
> important for the LPN/LVN to ask which question?
>
> 1.   "Do your clothes feel tight?"
> 2.   "Do you need to void?"
> 3.   "Are you feeling dizzy?"
> 4.   "Do you have any pain?"

STEP 1. Read the stem of the question.

STEP 2. Reword the question in your own words.

STEP 3. Read the answer choices.

STEP 4. Think: "What nursing concept should I identify in the answer choices?"

THE REWORDED QUESTION: What is the highest priority for a client after a paracentesis?

ANSWERS:

(1) "Do your clothes feel tight?" Why would you ask a client this question? Clothes should fit looser because the abdominal girth has decreased after fluid has been removed with a paracentesis. This is an expected outcome. Eliminate.

(2) "Do you need to void?" Why would you ask a client this question? It is imperative to empty the bladder prior to the procedure, not after the procedure. There is no compelling reason to ask the client this question. Eliminate.

(3) "Are you feeling dizzy?" What makes a client dizzy? One of the causes is a decrease in cerebral perfusion due to a fall in blood pressure. Could this client have a decreased blood pressure? Yes. Hypotension and hypovolemic shock are complications of a paracentesis due to removal of a large volume of fluid. Keep this answer for consideration.

(4) "Do you have any pain?" You ask this question to assess pain level. This client may have discomfort where the paracentesis was performed, but this is an expected outcome. Eliminate.

The correct answer is (3).

Strategy Recap

These questions illustrate why knowing nursing content is not enough to answer application/analysis-level questions. You must be able to effectively use the information you learned in practical/vocational nursing school to answer NCLEX-PN® exam-style test questions.

Review the strategies that you learned in this chapter:

- Reword the question.
- Eliminate answer choices you know to be incorrect.
- Don't predict answers.
- Recognize expected outcomes.
- Read answer choices to obtain clues.

Chapter Quiz

1. The LPN/LVN is reinforcing teaching for a client after a right mastectomy and axillary lymph node dissection. Which statement by the client requires further intervention by the LPN/LVN? **(Select all that apply).**

    1. "I will wear gloves and long sleeves whenever I go out and work in my garden."
    2. "The risk for arm swelling will decrease one year after my treatment is completed."
    3. "I will sleep with my right arm elevated on a small flat pillow from now on."
    4. "If my right arm begins to feel heavy, I should contact my primary health care provider."
    5. "It will be necessary for me to wear a compression bandage for the rest of my life."

2. The LPN/LVN is preparing to reinforce instructions for a client about the use of an incentive spirometer. Arrange the following steps in the order the client should perform them. **All options must be used.**

    1. Seal lips around the mouthpiece.
    2. Assume high Fowler position.
    3. Exhale slowly and cough.
    4. Hold breath for 3 to 5 seconds.
    5. Inhale slowly and deeply.

3. The LPN/LVN is preparing to infuse 1 L of normal saline solution at a rate of 125 mL/hr. The drop factor for the intravenous tubing is 15 drops per mL. What is the drip rate per minute? Round to the nearest whole number.

    _____ gtt/minute

4. The LPN/LVN is preparing to administer an intramuscular injection to a 6-month-old client. Identify the area where the injection should be given.

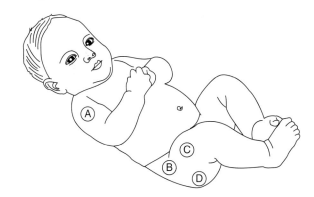

    1. A.
    2. B.
    3. C.
    4. D.

Refer to the Case Study to answer the next six questions.

The LPN/LVN is caring for a middle-aged adult client in a rural hospital.

Admission Notes	Nurse's Notes

The client is admitted for evaluation of symptoms characterized primarily by a cough of 3 months duration with productive sputum, night sweats, loss of 5% body weight, extreme fatigue, and general decline in health. The client was diagnosed 4 years ago with human immunodeficiency virus (HIV) infection. The client tested positive for latent tuberculosis infection (LTBI) at the time of the HIV diagnosis but did not complete the recommended treatment. Various social and personal factors have also negatively impacted the client's adherence to antiretroviral therapy (ART) for HIV infection. The client volunteers at an HIV/AIDS support clinic and a homeless shelter. The client cannot remember when last screened for tuberculosis (TB) disease.

Social History: The client does not have stable employment and currently lives in temporary housing. Over the past several years, the client has experienced homelessness and lived in numerous overcrowded housing and community homeless shelters. The client reports a 25 pack-year history of cigarette smoking and has an uncertain history of substance use disorder (SUD).

Pending diagnostic studies:
Tuberculosis (TB) blood test.
Chest x-ray.
Sputum for acid fast bacilli (AFB) smear and culture.

History	Nurse's Notes

Vital Signs	Results
BP	118/78 mmHg
Heart rate	106, irregular
Respiratory rate	26, regular
Temperature (oral)	99.6° F (37.5° C)
Body Mass Index (BMI)	19 kg/m^2, normal weight

Assessment	Client Finding
General	Frail appearing Lethargic
Integument	Skin intact, pale, warm, and dry Dry mucous membranes Decreased turgor
Cardiovascular	S1 and S2 auscultated, regular rhythm, no murmurs Capillary refill less than 2 seconds 2+ radial pulses, equal
Respiratory	Crackles in bilateral lung bases Productive cough with discolored sputum No dyspnea or chest pain
Abdomen	Soft, flat, nontender Normoactive bowel sounds x 4 quadrants
Musculoskeletal	Moves all extremities Full range of motion of all joints, no pain or tenderness Muscle strength 4/5 bilaterally

5. The LPN/LVN reviews the admission notes and the nurse's notes.

Highlight below findings that are concerning to the LPN/LVN.

Documentation	Findings
Admission Notes	Night sweats Weight loss Untreated latent tuberculosis infection (LTBI) HIV infected
Cardiovascular	Heart rate 106, regular 2 + radial pulses
Respiratory	Crackles bilateral lung bases Productive cough of three (3) months duration Respiratory rate 26 Pulse oximetry 95% on room air

6. Complete the following sentence by choosing from the list of options.

The LPN/LVN recognizes that the client's symptoms may be related to [Select from list 1] that is associated with risk factors of [Select from list 2] and [Select from list 3].

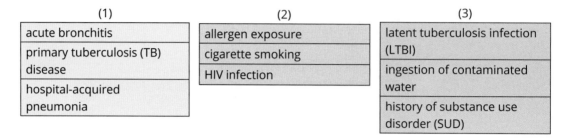

(1)
acute bronchitis
primary tuberculosis (TB) disease
hospital-acquired pneumonia

(2)
allergen exposure
cigarette smoking
HIV infection

(3)
latent tuberculosis infection (LTBI)
ingestion of contaminated water
history of substance use disorder (SUD)

7. The client's AFB smear strongly indicates a diagnosis of TB. The health care team begins treatment while awaiting the finalization of sputum cultures.

Which transmission precaution does the LPN/LVN use when caring for the client?

1. Contact precautions.

2. Droplet precautions.

3. Airborne precautions.

4. Protective environment precautions.

8. The LPN/LVN and the RN develop the plan of care. Select **3** goals which are appropriate to include in the plan.

1. Reduce transmission of TB.

2. Educate about radiation therapy.

3. Improve pulmonary function.

4. Promote therapy adherence.

5. Decrease the risk for dysrhythmias.

6. Monitor immunotherapy treatment.

9. The LPN/LVN implements care related to infection control using standard precautions and airborne precautions. For each potential intervention below, specify whether the intervention is appropriate or not appropriate care.

Potential Nursing Intervention	Appropriate	Not Appropriate
Place the client in a single room with negative pressure airflow.	○	○
Put on shoe and hair coverings before entering room.	○	○
Wear a proper fitting high-efficiency particulate air (HEPA) mask (e.g., N95 respirator).	○	○
Keep the door to the client's room closed.	○	○
Wear a surgical face mask when within 3 to 6 feet of the client.	○	○
Reinforce effective cough etiquette.	○	○
Allow the client to leave the isolation room if wearing an isolation gown.	○	○

10. The client's condition improves and the client is discharged. The RN provides discharge teaching about reducing transmission of TB in the community.

The LPN/LVN recognizes which client statement indicates understanding about the discharge teaching? **(Select all that apply.)**

1. "I will keep my clinic visits so that I can get my phlegm checked for TB to know how I'm doing."
2. "It's so good that I don't need to worry my close friends about getting screened for TB now that I'm on my meds."
3. "A public health nurse may need to visit and check that I am taking my medicine correctly."
4. "I like to be outdoors by myself and won't mind not being around lots of people or riding the public bus."
5. "Once I feel pretty good, I can begin cutting back on my medicine."
6. "Taking my medicine is the best way to keep from spreading TB to my friends."

11. The LPN/LVN is caring for a client diagnosed with Parkinson disease. The LPN/LVN observes that the client has tremors of the hands and slurred speech. The family reports that the client appears depressed. What is the **priority** of care for this client?

1. Place a clock and calendar within the client's view in room.

2. Encourage the client to perform range-of-motion exercises.

3. Ask the family about the client's favorite television shows.

4. Assist client to sit on the edge of the bed before ambulation.

12. The client is waiting to be picked up by family members after a cystogram. The LPN/LVN is reinforcing teaching about the client's home care for the first 48 hours. Which instruction is appropriate for the LPN/LVN to include? **(Select all that apply.)**

1. Decrease water and other fluid intake.

2. Avoid consuming alcoholic beverages.

3. Seek medical attention for a slight burning sensation when voiding.

4. Seek medical attention for the appearance of blood in the urine.

5. Apply heat to the lower abdomen to relieve pain and muscle spasm.

6. Report fever, chills, or increased pulse to the primary health care provider.

13. The LPN/LVN is caring for the client who has just undergone surgery for an inflamed appendix. The surgeon made a traditional incision directly over the organ removed. Identify the area where the LPN/LVN would check for bleeding and infection.

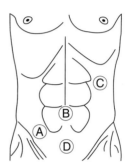

1. A.
2. B.
3. C.
4. D.

Refer to the Case Study to answer the next question.

The LPN/LVN in the community clinic is caring for a young adult client.

| History and Physical | Vital Signs |

Client presents in the clinic for follow up care for acute human immunodeficiency virus (HIV) type-1 infection. One month ago, the client was evaluated for sore throat, fever, transient nausea and diarrhea, fatigue, night sweats, and swollen lymph nodes. Subsequent HIV antigen/antibody assays and nucleic acid test results were positive for HIV-1. The client's most recent CD4 T-cell lymphocyte count is 400 cells/mm^3 (low) and HIV RNA assay (viral load) is high. Initiating antiretroviral therapy (ART) has been recommended and discussed with the client. The client has expressed concern about committing to treatment, and states, "I feel well now and know I should take the treatment. But, I'm overwhelmed about how I'm going to manage it all."

Physical Exam: Pleasant and conversational, appropriately groomed. Appears slightly anxious, speaking rapidly. Alert, oriented x 4. Skin pale, warm, and dry. Slightly enlarged axillary lymph nodes. Lungs clear bilaterally, breathing non-labored, dry cough. S1 and S2 auscultated, regular rhythm, no murmurs, 2$^+$ radial pulses. Abdomen soft, rounded, positive bowel sounds x 4. Moves all extremities, no lower leg edema. Slight joint tenderness in knees and shoulders, full range of motion.

Social History: The client has had inconsistent access to care and poor coordination of care. Uncertain history of substance abuse. Lives alone, with prior erratic living arrangements and job security. Low health literacy and questionable social support.

| History and Physical | Vital Signs |

Vital Signs	Results
BP	128/72 mmHg
Pulse	74, regular
Respiratory rate	16, regular
Temperature (oral)	98.9° F (37.16° C)
Pulse oximetry	97% on room air
Body Mass Index (BMI)	23 kg/m^2, normal

14. The LPN/LVN is reviewing the client's history and physical and provides care.

Complete the diagram by dragging from the choices below to specify the priority concern, 2 actions the LPN/LVN takes to address that concern, and 2 parameters the LPN/LVN monitors to assess the client's progress.

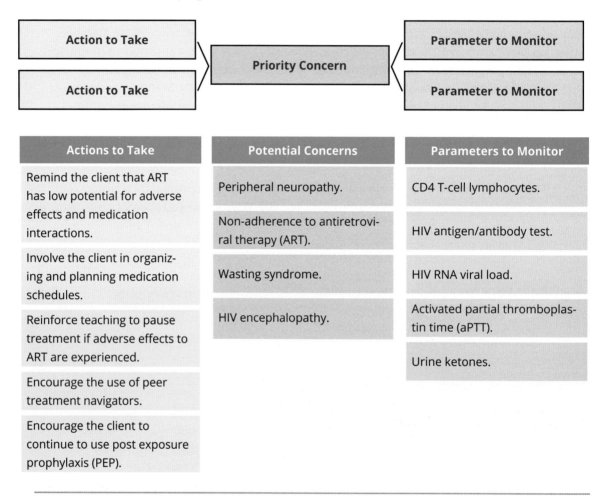

Actions to Take	Potential Concerns	Parameters to Monitor
Remind the client that ART has low potential for adverse effects and medication interactions.	Peripheral neuropathy.	CD4 T-cell lymphocytes.
Involve the client in organizing and planning medication schedules.	Non-adherence to antiretroviral therapy (ART).	HIV antigen/antibody test.
Reinforce teaching to pause treatment if adverse effects to ART are experienced.	Wasting syndrome.	HIV RNA viral load.
Encourage the use of peer treatment navigators.	HIV encephalopathy.	Activated partial thromboplastin time (aPTT).
Encourage the client to continue to use post exposure prophylaxis (PEP).		Urine ketones.

---

15. The LPN/LVN is explaining how to estimate sodium intake to a client prescribed the DASH diet. The DASH diet limits daily sodium intake to 1,500 mg, which must account for sodium in food and added to food. A quarter-teaspoon of salt contains 500 mg of sodium. What is the maximum total amount of salt that the client could ingest per day, in teaspoons?

_____ teaspoons

Chapter Quiz Answers and Explanations

1. The answer is 2, 3, and 5

The LPN/LVN is reinforcing teaching for a client after a right mastectomy and axillary lymph node dissection. Which statement by the client requires further intervention by the LPN/LVN? **(Select all that apply.)**

Strategy: First, identify the topic of the question. If unable to identify the topic after reading the question, read the answers for clues. All answers relate to prevention of lymphedema. Note that the client had a right mastectomy. When a question includes a reference to left or right, that is often important for identifying the correct answer.

Then, rephrase each answer choice as a "yes/no" question that asks "Will this action by the client prevent lymphedema?" Be careful! The question asks which statements *require further intervention* by the LPN/LVN. You are looking for incorrect statements.

Category: Evaluation/Physiological Integrity/Reduction of Risk Potential

(1) Will wearing gloves and long sleeves while gardening prevent lymphedema? Yes. Any injury to the right arm, including insect bites or scrapes, may become infected and cause lymphedema. This is a correct action. Eliminate.

(2) CORRECT: Will the risk of lymphedema decrease one year after the mastectomy procedure? No. The risk for lymphedema remains for the rest of the client's life. This statement is not true. Select this answer.

(3) CORRECT: Will arm elevation on a small flat pillow decrease the risk of lymphedema? No. The arm should be elevated above the level of the heart at night. It is an incorrect action. Select this answer.

(4) Arm heaviness is a sign of lymphedema development. Client instruction includes notifying primary health care provider if the involved arm feels heavy, has decreased muscle function, or has numbness and tingling. This is a correct action. Eliminate.

(5) CORRECT: Is the use of a compression bandage needed for the rest of the client's life? No. Compression bandages may be used if the client develops acute lymphedema. Compression bandages are not routinely used after mastectomy and lymph node dissection. Select this answer.

2. The answer is 2, 1, 5, 4, 3

The LPN/LVN is preparing to reinforce instructions for a client about the use of an incentive spirometer. Arrange the following steps in the order the client should perform them. **All options must be used.**

Strategy: Picture the client using the incentive spirometer. What is the purpose of incentive spirometry? To open the alveoli and lower airway passages and increase oxygenation. What position enables the client to inhale deeply to promote lung expansion? The upright position (2).

Now think about the steps used for incentive spirometry. Before the client inhales through the mouthpiece, there must be a tight seal (1). To make the volume indicator move, the client must inhale slowly and deeply (5). To achieve maximum expansion of the lungs, the client should hold the inhalation for 3 to 5 seconds (4). The last step is slow exhalation (3), which will continue to promote expansion of the lower airways.

Category: Planning/Physiological Integrity/Reduction of Risk Potential

(2) Assume high Fowler position.

(1) Seal lips around the mouthpiece.

(5) Inhale slowly and deeply.

(4) Hold breath for 3 to 5 seconds.

(3) Exhale slowly and cough.

3. The answer is 31

The LPN/LVN is preparing to infuse 1 L of normal saline solution at a rate of 125 mL/hr. The drop factor for the intravenous tubing is 15 drops per mL. What is the drip rate per minute? Round to the nearest whole number.

Strategy: Apply the conversion equations, being careful to avoid calculation errors. Only the numerical drip rate should be recorded. Note that specific rounding instructions are given.

Category: Planning/Physiological Integrity/Pharmacological Therapies

The formula is:

$$\frac{\text{mL/hr} \times \text{drop factor}}{\text{time in minutes}}$$

For this problem, you need to convert the hour to 60 minutes:

$$\frac{125 \text{ mL/hr} \times 15 \text{ gtt/min}}{60 \text{ min}} = \frac{1875}{60}$$
$$= 31.25 \text{ gtt /min}$$

Round to the nearest whole number. The correct answer is 31.

4. The answer is 3

The LPN/LVN is preparing to administer an intramuscular injection to a 6-month-old client. Identify the area where the injection should be given.

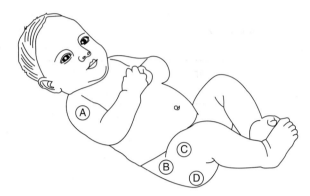

Strategy: To answer this hot spot question, recall the age of the client (6 months old) and the preferred site for intramuscular injections in infants (the vastus lateralis muscle in the thigh). Then think about the anatomical landmarks necessary to locate the correct site.

Category: Implementation/Physiological Integrity/Pharmacological Therapies

(1) A: The deltoid muscle is not the correct location.

(2) B: The hip is not the correct location.

(3) CORRECT: Location C is correct. For infants, IM injection should be given in the middle third of the anterior thigh, between the midline anterior thigh and the midline lateral thigh. To identify the IM injection site, locate the greater trochanter, then the knee joint; divide the area between the trochanter and the knee joint into thirds and note the middle third; then locate the area between the midline anterior thigh and the midline of the outer aspect of the thigh.

(4) D: The buttock is not the correct location.

5. See explanation for answers

Documentation	Findings
Admission Notes	Night sweats Weight loss Untreated latent tuberculosis infection (LTBI) HIV infected
Cardiovascular	Heart rate 106, regular 2 + radial pulses
Respiratory	Crackles bilateral lung bases Productive cough of three (3) months duration Respiratory rate 26 Pulse oximetry 95% on room air

Admission Notes: The LPN/LVN recognizes abnormal findings of **night sweats** and **weight loss**. The LPN/LVN is concerned that the client's **untreated latent tuberculosis infection (LTBI)** and **HIV co-infection** are strong risk factors for progressing to tuberculosis (TB) disease.

Cardiovascular: Tachycardia (i.e., **heart rate of 106**) is concerning. INCORRECT OPTION: The LPN/LVN is not concerned with the client's 2 + radial pulses because this is a normal adult assessment finding.

Respiratory: Concerning, abnormal findings include the client's **crackles in bilateral lung bases**, **productive cough of three (3) months duration**, and **respiratory rate of 26**. INCORRECT OPTION: The LPN/LVN is not concerned with the client's pulse oximetry of 95% on room air because this is a normal adult assessment finding.

6. See explanation for answers

CORRECT OPTION: The LPN/LVN recognizes that the client's symptoms may be related to **primary tuberculosis (TB) disease**. Productive cough, night sweats, fever, weight loss, and abnormal lung sounds are present in clients who have active TB. INCORRECT OPTIONS: Acute bronchitis is characterized by inflammation of the bronchi, resulting in a common symptom of cough that may be accompanied by headache, malaise, fever, and dyspnea. It is an illness that is usually self-limiting and may last up to three weeks. A pneumonia that develops after 48 hours of admission in a non-intubated client and not present at the time of admission is known as hospital-acquired pneumonia. The client presented with respiratory symptoms at the time of admission.

CORRECT OPTION: Immunosuppression from varying causes, cancer, and long-term corticosteroid use increases the risk for the development of TB. **Clients living with HIV have a high risk for developing TB.** INCORRECT OPTIONS: Allergen exposure is not associated with the development of TB. Cigarette smoking is a risk factor for different lower respiratory disorders, including lung cancer and chronic obstructive pulmonary disease. Risk factors for TB include immunocompromised status, immigration from or recent travel to countries with a high prevalence of TB, institutionalization, overcrowded living conditions, and others.

CORRECT OPTION: Clients with **latent TB infection (LTBI)**, a condition when TB bacteria are inactive in the body, may develop TB disease if untreated. HIV infection is the strongest risk factor for progressing to TB disease among clients with LBTI. INCORRECT OPTIONS: Ingestion of contaminated water is a risk for other reemerging infections, but not a risk for the development of TB. A history of SUD does not increase the client's risk for the development of primary TB.

7. The answer is 3

CORRECT OPTION: **Airborne precautions** are used for diseases that are transmitted by smaller droplets and remain in the air for longer periods of time. Examples of diseases requiring airborne precautions include TB, varicella virus, and rubeola virus.

INCORRECT OPTIONS: Contact precautions are used for clients who have illnesses acquired by direct contact or by contact with items in the client environment, such as *Clostridioides difficile* and methicillin-resistant *Staphylococcus aureus* (MRSA). Droplet precautions are used to protect against illnesses that are transmitted by larger droplets expelled at close contact such as influenza virus, pertussis, pneumonia, and meningitis. Protective environment precautions are focused on clients highly vulnerable to infection, such as clients who have received an organ transplant or hematopoietic stem cell transplant (HSCT). These clients are placed in positive pressure rooms intended to keep them safe from human and environmental pathogens.

8. The answer is 1, 3, and 4

CORRECT OPTIONS: The LPN/LVN and RN include **goals to reduce transmission of TB, improve pulmonary function, and promote therapy adherence**. Reducing transmission of TB is important in the acute care setting as it is an infectious disease usually spread from person to person by small airborne droplets expelled during talking or coughing that remain in the air over longer periods of time. Improving pulmonary function is a goal related to preventing further complications from TB such as scarring and residual cavitation in the lung. Medication therapy is the cornerstone of TB treatment, and fostering adherence is essential for effective treatment.

INCORRECT OPTIONS: Radiation therapy may be used as a method of cancer treatment in which energy released from a source results in cellular DNA damage in the form of ionization; it is not a treatment method for TB disease. TB disease is not a risk factor for dysrhythmias. Monitoring immunotherapy is not a nursing goal; the standard treatment for TB is anti-tubercular medications. Immunotherapy is a cancer treatment in which the immune system is boosted or directed to defend the body and fight cancer.

9. See explanation for answers

Appropriate: The LPN/LVN appropriately implements care by **placing the client in a single room with negative pressure airflow**, or an airborne infection isolation room (AIIR). An infected client with TB expels smaller droplets that remain suspended in the air over longer distances and can be inhaled by another person. Thus, air is filtered through a high-efficiency particulate air filter so it is not returned to the inside ventilation system and instead exhausted to the outside. **A proper fitting high-efficiency particulate air (HEPA) mask (e.g., N95 respirator)** is worn by the LPN/LVN when entering the room due to its highly effective protection from small droplets. **Closing the door to the room** to control the direction of airflow is an important isolation precaution for clients with TB to prevent transmission to health care workers. Teaching the client **proper cough etiquette** (i.e., covering the nose and mouth with paper tissues during coughing or sneezing) is a part of standard precautions in clients with symptoms of respiratory infection.

Not Appropriate: **Shoe and hair coverings before entering the room are not required in airborne or standard precautions.** In illnesses such as influenza, larger droplets are expelled into the air and spread at close contact. **Droplet precautions require the LPN/LVN to wear a surgical mask when within 3 to 6 feet of the client** in these circumstances. A single room with positive pressure airflow creates a protective, contaminant free environment for clients who are highly vulnerable to infection (e.g., after hematopoietic stem cell or organ transplant). If medically necessary, the **client may leave the isolation room wearing a standard isolation mask or surgical mask**.

10. The answer is 1, 3, 4, and 6

CORRECT OPTIONS: The LPN/LVN recognizes the client's understanding of discharge teaching when the client states **keeping clinic visits to have phlegm checked for TB**. Sputum for AFB smear and culture is obtained at frequent intervals. Notifying the public health department is required, and **public health nurses provide follow up and assessment for adherence**. Additionally, while clients are infectious, exposure to close contacts should be minimized. **Spending time outdoors is encouraged, and reducing time in public areas is important.** The client's statement indicates understanding of this information. TB is communicable and **taking medications is the best means to prevent transmission**. The client's statement indicates understanding about medication adherence and its importance in controlling the spread of infection.

INCORRECT OPTIONS: The LPN/LVN recognizes that to prevent transmission of TB, close contacts of the client should be identified and screened for TB, and anyone testing positive for TB will need further evaluation. The client's statement does not indicate understanding of this information. Treatment failures occur when clients stop taking medication too soon or when taking it irregularly. The client's statement does not indicate understanding regarding adherence to the prescribed treatment regimen.

11. The answer is 4

The LPN/LVN is caring for a client diagnosed with Parkinson disease. The LPN/LVN observes that the client has tremors of the hands and slurred speech. The family reports that the client appears depressed. What is the **priority** of care for this client?

Strategy: The client has hand tremors, slurred speech, and depression, but the topic of this question is unknown. Read the answers for clues: The question asks about priority of care. Remember that physical and safety needs take priority over psychosocial needs.

Category: Implementation/Safe and Effective Care Environment/Safety and Infection Control

(1) Place a clock and calendar within the client's view in room—This is a psychosocial answer. Although clients diagnosed with Parkinson disease can have cognitive impairment, other answers relate to physical or safety needs. Eliminate.

(2) Encourage the client to perform range-of-motion exercises—This is a physical answer. Think about what you know about Parkinson disease: Clients can develop muscle rigidity, and range of motion exercises may help with that. Is it a priority of care? Keep for consideration.

(3) Ask the family about the client's favorite television shows—This is a psychosocial answer. Eliminate.

(4) CORRECT: Assist client to sit on the edge of the bed before ambulation—This is a safety answer. Clients diagnosed with Parkinson disease are at risk for orthostatic hypotension due to autonomic dysfunction. Does this answer make sense? Yes. Select this answer. The important concept in this question is safety, which is a priority over psychosocial needs.

12. The answer is 2, 5, and 6

The client is waiting to be picked up by family members after a cystogram. The LPN/LVN is reinforcing teaching about the client's home care for the first 48 hours. Which of the following instructions is appropriate for the LPN/LVN to include? **(Select all that apply).**

Strategy: For each answer choice, identify the outcome for the client.

Category: Implementation/Health Promotion and Maintenance/Self-Care

(1) Decrease water and other fluid intake—The client needs to increase, not decrease, water and other fluid intake.

(2) Avoid consuming alcoholic beverages—CORRECT: The excretion of alcoholic beverages might irritate the bladder, so it is advisable to avoid them for 2 days.

(3) Seek medical attention for a slight burning sensation when voiding—A slight burning sensation when voiding can be expected as a normal, not emergency, outcome.

(4) Seek medical attention for the appearance of blood in the urine—Minor bleeding during the first 2 days can occur without being a cause for immediate concern.

(5) CORRECT: Apply heat to the lower abdomen to relieve pain and muscle spasm—Heat can relieve the pain and muscle spasm that are normal after the cystogram.

(6) CORRECT: Report fever, chills, or increased pulse to primary health care provider—Fever, chills, or an increased pulse could signify an infection; the clinician should be notified.

13. The answer is 1

The LPN/LVN is caring for the client who has just undergone surgery for an inflamed appendix. The surgeon made a traditional incision directly over the organ removed. Identify the area where the LPN/LVN would check for bleeding and infection.

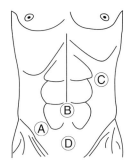

Strategy: Examine the diagram carefully. Locate the appendix. Know the client's right side from left side.

Category: Implementation/Physiological Integrity/ Physiological Adaptation

(1) CORRECT: Location A is correct. The lower right-hand side of the abdomen is directly over the organ removed.

(2) B: The umbilicus is a possible site of a laparoscopic incision, not a traditional surgical incision.

(3) C: The upper left-hand side of the abdomen is not used for either a traditional or a laparoscopic incision to remove an inflamed appendix.

(4) D: The groin is a possible site of a laparoscopic incision, not a traditional surgical incision.

14. See explanation for answers

Priority Concern	
Nonadherence to antiretroviral therapy (ART).	☑

CORRECT OPTION: The LPN/LVN's priority concern is that the **client fails to adhere to antiretroviral therapy (ART)**. When ART is taken consistently and correctly, it can significantly reduce viral loads, achieve treatment goals, and impact the emergence of medication resistance. There are multiple factors, including the adverse effects and complexity of the medication regimen, which can negatively affect adherence.

INCORRECT OPTIONS: Peripheral neuropathy can commonly occur at any stage of HIV infection or as an adverse effect of antiretroviral (ART) medications. The client is not experiencing significant pain in the hands or feet. Wasting syndrome attributed to HIV/AIDS is unintentional loss of 10% or more of ideal body mass along with weakness, fever, or diarrhea lasting more than 30 days. HIV encephalopathy is a clinical syndrome associated with decline in cognitive and behavioral function as a result of HIV. The client is not experiencing early symptoms of memory deficit, headache, and psychomotor slowing.

Actions to Take	
Involve the client in organizing and planning medication schedules.	☑
Encourage the use of peer treatment navigators.	☑

CORRECT OPTIONS: The LPN/LVN is a resource to provide assistance with treatment adherence to help reduce the client's viral load. The LPN/LVN should **involve the client in organizing and planning medication schedules**. The LPN/LVN can suggest reviewing the regimen and linking taking medications to daily activities or the use of memory aids. **A peer or paraprofessional navigator can serve as a resource to the client**; utilizing these navigators is a strategy to monitor and enhance retention in care.

INCORRECT OPTIONS: The LPN/LVN does not reinforce teaching that medication regimens have low potential for adverse effects and medication interactions. While treatment regimens may be simplified, HIV care can be very complex. The combination of medications needed for care and prevention of opportunistic infections can result in serious adverse effects and medication interactions. The LPN/LVN does not reinforce teaching to pause treatment when the client experiences adverse effects. It's important to take ART as prescribed because inadequate dosing or missing a few doses of HIV medication therapy can lead to medication resistance and delayed treatment goals. The LPN/LVN does not reinforce teaching about the use of post-exposure prophylaxis (PEP). PEP is related to reducing the risk of acquiring HIV after a potential exposure.

Parameters to Monitor	
CD4 T-cell lymphocytes.	☑
HIV RNA viral load.	☑

CORRECT OPTIONS: The LPN/LVN monitors **CD4 T-cell lymphocytes** and **HIV RNA viral load**. Viral load is a strong biologic measure of adherence. The CD4 count is a primary indicator of immune function and a strong predictor for subsequent disease. Highly effective treatment regimens can reduce HIV to undetectable levels, resulting in CD4 T-cell counts returning to normal.

INCORRECT OPTIONS: The LPN/LVN does not monitor the HIV antigen/antibody test, activated partial thromboplastin time (aPTT), or urine ketones. The HIV antigen/antibody test is used to diagnose HIV infection. It tests for both the virus, the antigen, and antibodies for HIV. The aPTT is a measure of blood coagulation ability and is commonly used to evaluate heparin therapy. Urine ketones are produced as a complication of diabetic ketoacidosis, when glucose utilization is impaired and fat is used for energy.

15. The answer is 0.75

The LPN/LVN is explaining how to estimate sodium intake to a client prescribed the DASH diet. The DASH diet limits daily sodium intake to 1,500 mg, which must account for sodium in food and added to food. A quarter-teaspoon of salt contains 500 mg of sodium. What is the maximum total amount of salt that the client could ingest per day, in teaspoons?

Strategy: Apply the conversion equation. Be careful to avoid calculation errors.

Category: Data Collection/Physiological Integrity/ Basic Care and Comfort

Each quarter-teaspoon of table salt contains 500 mg sodium, and the daily maximum is 1,500 mg:

1,500 mg ÷ 500 mg = 3

3 × ¼ teaspoon = ¾ teaspoon = 0.75 teaspoon

THE NCLEX-PN® EXAM VERSUS REAL-WORLD NURSING

Some of you are CNAs or other unlicensed assistive personnel (UAPs) completing your practical/vocational nursing studies, while others are EMTs. Some of you worked during school as student techs. All of you, however, spent time in clinical during your practical/vocational nursing education. All of this adds up to a lot of experience. Experience will help you get a job, but answering questions based on your experience can be dangerous on the NCLEX-PN® exam.

Look at the following question.

> On admission to the hospital, an elderly client is confused and appears disheveled and restless. During the client's second day on the unit, an LPN/LVN approaches the client to administer medication. The LPN/LVN is unable to identify the client because the identification band is missing. Which action by the LPN/LVN is **best**?
>
> 1. Have the roommate identify the client.
> 2. Ask the client to state the full name.
> 3. Ask another LPN/LVN to identify the client.
> 4. Look at photograph in client's medical record.

Let's see how someone using real-world experience would approach this question:

(1) "The roommate is never involved in identification of a client."

(2) "A confused client cannot be relied on for an accurate identification."

(3) "Sounds reasonable. I have seen this done in some circumstances."

(4) "A photograph? What photograph? I've never seen a photograph of a client in a medical record!"

Possible conclusions drawn by this person would include: *"OK, I've seen one LPN/LVN ask another for information so (3) must be the answer,"* or *"Well, maybe the client isn't all that confused, so I'll select (2)."*

According to nursing textbooks, asking another health care professional is not the correct way to identify a client. Many acute-care settings now include a photograph of the client in the medical record for just this type of situation. The correct answer to this question is (4). Many students reject this answer because there are rarely photographs of clients in the medical records. Real-world experience doesn't count, though; in this case, the client does have a photograph in the medical record.

The NCLEX-PN® exam is a standardized exam administered by the NCSBN. Because the NCLEX-PN® exam is a national exam, students should be aware that in some parts of the country, practical/vocational nursing is practiced slightly differently. However, to ensure that the test is reflective of national trends, questions and answers are all carefully documented. The test makers ensure that the correct answers are documented in at least two standard nursing textbooks or one textbook and one nursing journal.

When you are unsure of an answer choice, don't ask yourself, "What do they do on my floor?" but "What does the medical/surgical textbook writer Brunner say?" or "What do Potter and Perry say to do?" This test does not necessarily reflect what happens in the "real world," but is based on textbook nursing.

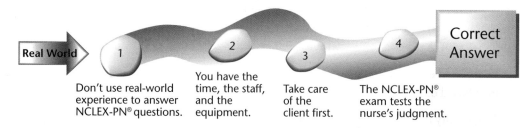

Remember the following when taking the NCLEX-PN® exam:

- You have all of the time and resources you need to provide appropriate care to your client. (Checking for bowel sounds for 5 minutes in all four quadrants, no problem!)
- You have all of the equipment you need. (Remember the bath thermometer you learned to use in the nursing lab? For the NCLEX-PN® exam, you will have one available to test the temperature of bath water.)
- There are no staffing problems on the NCLEX-PN® exam. You are caring only for the client described in the question, and that person is your only concern.
- All care given to clients is "by the book." No shortcuts are used.

Answer the following question.

> The LPN/LVN is preparing an agitated and confused client for surgery. For preoperative medication, the LPN/LVN administers morphine sulfate 5 mg IM and lorazepam 0.5 mg IM, as prescribed. The LPN/LVN should take which precaution after the preoperative medication is administered?
>
> 1. Ask the security guard to remain with the client.
> 2. Have the unlicensed assistive personnel (UAP) remain with client.
> 3. Leave the client alone until the medications take effect.
> 4. Restrain the client with the help of a coworker.

Let's look at this using real-world logic.

(1)   "Ask the security guard to stay with the client." Yes, in the real world, security is called when clients are agitated.

(2)   "Have the unlicensed assistive personnel (UAP) remain with the client." Sounds good, but what if you don't have enough staff to assign a UAP to remain with the client?

(3)   "Leave the client alone until the medications take effect." Yes, that is done in the real world for most medicated preoperative clients, but this client is agitated and confused. This is not the best answer.

(4)   "Restrain the client with the help of a coworker." Yes, this is done in the real world.

According to real-world logic, the correct answer must be (1) or (4). However, textbook theoretical nursing practice states that this client should not be left alone while in an agitated state. A member of the health care staff should remain with the client. Therefore, the correct answer is (2).

Use your real-world experience to help you visualize the client described in the test question, but select your answers based on what is found in nursing textbooks.

Your nursing faculty has been very conscientious about instructing you in the most up-to-date nursing practice. According to the National Council of State Boards of Nursing, the primary source for documenting correct answers is in nursing textbooks, and the most up-to-date practice might not always agree with the textbooks. When in doubt, always select the textbook answer!

The next question illustrates this point.

> A client is admitted to the hospital in active labor. After delivery of a healthy infant, the client decides to bottle-feed. Which statement by the client after a teaching session indicates to the LPN/LVN that the client needs further instruction?
>
> 1.   "I'll pump my breasts and use warm packs to relieve breast pain."
> 2.   "I'll wear a tight bra and apply ice packs to relieve engorgement discomfort."
> 3.   "I'll take the prescribed pain medication when I have pain or discomfort."
> 4.   "I'll take the prescribed pills to help stop the production of milk."

Let's look at these answers more closely.

(1)   Pumping the breasts will stimulate milk production. This is clearly wrong.

(2)   Wearing a tight bra and using ice packs are appropriate interventions for a nonbreastfeeding mother.

(3)   Taking a medication (mild analgesic) is an appropriate intervention for a nonbreastfeeding mother.

(4)   Medication to prevent lactation is not frequently prescribed because of potentially dangerous side effects. However, a medication may be prescribed to prevent lactation. This would be considered an appropriate intervention.

The correct answer is (1).

First Take Care of the Client, Then the Equipment

The NCLEX-PN® exam tests your ability to use critical thinking skills to make nursing judgments. It is very important that you remember to:

- Take care of the client first.
- Take care of the equipment second.

Look at the following question.

> A client who sustained a left femur fracture in a motor vehicle accident is being treated with balanced-suspension skeletal traction using a Thomas splint and a Pearson attachment. The client reports "terrible" pain in the left thigh. Which should the LPN/LVN do **first**?
>
> 1. Determine that the traction weights and ropes are aligned and hanging free.
> 2. Ask the client about the characteristics and location of the pain.
> 3. Check the Thomas splint and Pearson attachment for proper positioning.
> 4. Explain to client that pain in the affected leg is expected.

Let's review the answers:

(1) "Determine that traction weights and ropes are aligned and hanging free." This answer choice has you checking the equipment, not the client. Your first concern should be the client, not the traction. Eliminate this answer.

(2) "Ask the client about the characteristics and location of the pain." This answer choice focuses on the client first. All reports of pain should be thoroughly investigated by the LPN/LVN. Keep in this answer for consideration.

(3) "Check the Thomas splint and Pearson attachment for proper positioning." This answer choice also has you checking the equipment, not the client. Your first concern should be the client. Eliminate.

(4) "Explain to client that pain in the affected leg is expected." This is incorrect. Any reports of pain are considered abnormal, and you should investigate them thoroughly. Eliminate.

The correct answer is (2).

Laboratory Values

Answering questions about laboratory values is another example of how the real world does not work on the NCLEX-PN® exam. In practical/vocational nursing school, you learned laboratory values for specific tests and you may not have remembered them after the test. While you were in the clinical setting, the emphasis was on interpretation of laboratory values. Because most lab slips contained a listing of normal values, you were able to compare the client's results to the normal values. Questions on the NCLEX-PN® exam will not provide you with a listing of normal laboratory values.

To answer questions on the NCLEX-PN® exam, you must:

- Know normal laboratory test results.
- Correctly interpret normal or abnormal laboratory test results.

Compare the following two questions.

> A client is admitted to the hospital with influenza-like symptoms. When taking the client's history, the LPN/LVN learns that the client had been taking digoxin 0.125 mg PO daily and furosemide 40 mg PO daily for 3 years. Last month the primary health care provider changed the prescription for digoxin to 0.25 mg daily. The LPN/LVN would expect the primary health care provider to prescribe which laboratory tests?
>
> 1. Serum electrolyte and digoxin levels.
> 2. Hemoglobin level and hematocrit.
> 3. Cardiac enzymes and arterial blood gas analysis.
> 4. Blood culture and sensitivity and urinalysis.

Most of you are probably familiar with the concepts presented in this question. The primary health care provider has increased the client's digoxin dose. Furosemide is a loop diuretic that inhibits resorption of sodium and chloride; side effects include hypotension, hypokalemia, GI upset, and weakness. Hypokalemia may increase the client's risk of digitalis toxicity. Serum electrolytes and digoxin levels (1) is the correct answer.

Now look at this question.

> The LPN/LVN is caring for a client admitted with fever, vomiting, and diarrhea. The LPN/LVN sees the following nursing diagnosis on the client's care plan: "fluid volume deficit." Which of the following changes in laboratory test results would demonstrate an improvement in the client's condition?
>
> 1. Urine specific gravity, 1.015; hematocrit, 37% (0.37).
> 2. Urine specific gravity, 1.020; hematocrit, 45% (0.45).
> 3. Urine specific gravity, 1.032; hematocrit, 52% (0.52).
> 4. Urine specific gravity, 1.025; hematocrit, 35% (0.35).

To correctly answer this question, you must know:

- Normal urine specific gravity ranges 1.010–1.030 and normal hematocrit ranges 42–50% (0.42–0.50) for a male, 40–48% (0.40–0.48) for a female
- How fluid volume deficit affects hematocrit and specific gravity

Fluid volume deficit occurs when fluids and electrolytes are lost in the same proportion as they exist in the body. When a client becomes dehydrated, both the urine specific gravity and hematocrit become elevated. The correct answer is (2).

Answer this question:

> A client is hospitalized with a diagnosis of atrial fibrillation. The primary health care provider prescribes heparin 5,000 units every 12 hours to be given by subcutaneous injection and a daily partial thromboplastin time (PTT). The result of the client's most recent PTT is 55 seconds. Which action should be taken by the LPN/LVN?
>
> 1. Document the results and administer the heparin.
> 2. Withhold the heparin.
> 3. Notify the primary health care provider of the test results.
> 4. Have the test repeated.

To answer this question you need to know:

- Normal PTT ranges 20–45 seconds.
- Therapeutic range PTT for a client receiving heparin, an anticoagulant, ranges 1.5–2 times the control or normal level.
- To calculate the therapeutic range, take the lower number for the normal range for a PTT (20) and multiply it by 1.5. The result is 30. Multiply the higher number (45) by 2. The result is 90. Thus the therapeutic range ranges from 30 to 90 seconds. Therapeutic PTT ranges 30 to 90 seconds, the goal of therapy.

Evaluate the answer choices:

(1) "Document the results and administer the heparin." The client's most recent PTT is 55 seconds. This falls within the therapeutic range of 30 to 90 seconds, so the LPN/LVN should administer the medication.

(2) "Withhold the heparin." A side effect of heparin is bleeding, which can occur when PTT rises above therapeutic range. If the PTT measures greater than 90 seconds, the nurse should notify the primary health care provider.

(3) "Notify the primary health care provider of the test results." There is no reason to notify the primary health care provider, since the PTT falls within the therapeutic range.

(4) "Have the test repeated." There is no reason to have the test repeated, since it falls within normal range.

The correct answer is (1).

CHAPTER 4
THE NCLEX-PN® EXAM VERSUS REAL-WORLD NURSING

Medication Administration

An important function in providing safe and effective care to clients is the administration of medications. Because this is one of the responsibilities of a beginning LPN/LVN, questions about medications are often an important part of the NCLEX-PN® exam. The LPN/LVN who is minimally competent is knowledgeable about medications and uses the "rights" of medication administration.

In nursing school, most questions about medication followed the same pattern. You were told the client's diagnosis, the name of the medication, and then were asked a question. Even if you didn't know the information about the medication, sometimes you were able to select the correct answer by knowing the diagnosis.

The NCLEX-PN® exam does not give you any clues from the context of the question. The questions on this exam include the name of the medication, usually identifying it by generic name only. Most of the time, you will not be given the reason the client is receiving the medication.

Let's look at some medication questions.

> The primary health care provider orders furosemide and spironolactone for a client. Prior to administering the medication, the LPN/LVN determines that the client's potassium is 3.2 mEq/L (3.2 mmol/L). In addition to notifying the supervising RN, the LPN/LVN should anticipate taking which action?
>
> 1. Hold both the furosemide and spironolactone.
> 2. Administer the spironolactone only.
> 3. Administer the furosemide only.
> 4. Administer the furosemide and spironolactone.

This is a typical exam-style medication question. The question concerns the side effects and nursing implications of furosemide and spironolactone.

(1) "Hold both the furosemide and spironolactone." The potassium level falls below normal (3.5–5 mEq/L[3.5–5 mmol/L]). Furosemide is a potassium-wasting diuretic, and spironolactone is a potassium-sparing diuretic. There is no reason to hold the spironolactone because the client has a low potassium level. Eliminate this answer.

(2) "Administer the spironolactone only." The spironolactone should be administered.

(3) "Administer the furosemide only." Do not administer the furosemide because it is a potassium-wasting diuretic. The client's potassium level is already low. Eliminate.

(4) "Administer the furosemide and spironolactone." Do not administer the furosemide. Eliminate.

The correct answer is (2).

Let's try this next question.

> A client returns to the clinic 2 weeks after being started on allopurinol 200 mg PO daily. The LPN/LVN reviews information about this medication with the client. Which statement by the client indicates that the teaching was effective?
>
> 1. "I should take my medication on an empty stomach."
> 2. "I should take my medication with orange juice."
> 3. "I should increase my daily intake of protein."
> 4. "I should drink at least 8 glasses of water every day."

To answer this question you need to know information about allopurinol, an antigout agent that reduces uric acid.

(1) "I should take my medication on an empty stomach." Allopurinol is best tolerated with or immediately after meals to reduce gastrointestinal (GI) irritation. Eliminate.

(2) "I should take my medication with orange juice." Orange juice makes the urine acidic. Allopurinol is more soluble in alkaline urine. Eliminate.

(3) "I should increase my daily intake of protein." It is not necessary to increase the intake of protein when taking allopurinol. Eliminate.

(4) "I should drink at least 8 glasses of water every day." Allopurinol can cause kidney stones. The client should drink 3,000 mL/day to reduce the risk of renal calculi formation.

The correct answer is (4). You must know the side effects and nursing implications of medications for the NCLEX-PN® exam.

Notify the Primary Health Care Provider

Another behavior that commonly occurs in the real world is notifying the primary health care provider. In nursing school you were encouraged to notify your instructor of changes in your client's condition. Be very careful how you handle this on the NCLEX-PN® exam. More often than not, the answer choice that states "notify the primary health care provider," "contact the social worker," or "refer to the chaplain" is the WRONG answer. Usually there is something you need to do first before you notify them. The NCLEX-PN® exam does not want to know what the primary health care provider is going to do. The NCLEX-PN® exam wants to know what you, the LPN/LVN, will do in a given situation.

Answer this question.

> The LPN/LVN notes that there is no urine in the client's urinary drainage bag 3 hours after the bag was last emptied. Which action should the LPN/LVN take **first**?
>
> 1. Check for kinks in urinary drainage tubing.
> 2. Insert a new indwelling urinary catheter.
> 3. Irrigate existing indwelling urinary catheter.
> 4. Notify client's primary health care provider.

THE REWORDED QUESTION: What should you do *first* for this client? Have this client's kidneys stopped producing urine? Is there an obstruction in the urinary drainage system?

(1) "Check for kinks in urinary drainage tubing." If there is no urine in the urinary drainage bag, could there be an obstruction in the drainage system? Checking for kinks in the urinary drainage tubing could provide a simple explanation for your observations.

(2) "Insert a new indwelling urinary catheter." Inserting a new indwelling urinary catheter may address a possible catheter obstruction but increases the client's risk for catheter-associated urinary tract infection. Are you sure you want to do this first?

(3) "Irrigate existing indwelling urinary catheter." Irrigating the indwelling urinary catheter in hopes of dislodging a possible obstruction increases the client's risk for catheter-associated urinary tract infection. Are you sure you want to do this first?

(4) "Notify client's primary health care provider." If you notify the client's primary health care provider of "no urinary output in 3 hours" as your first action, will you be able to answer potential questions regarding the client's lack of urine output? Are you transferring your responsibility to the primary health care provider? Is there something *you* should do first?

The correct answer is (1).

Before you choose the answer choice that involves "call the primary health care provider," look at the other answer choices very carefully. Make sure that there isn't an answer that contains data collection or an action you should take before making the phone call. The test makers want to know what you would do in a situation, not what the primary health care provider would do!

Here is one more real-world question.

> The LPN/LVN is approached in the elevator by an employee from another unit. The employee states that a close friend is a client on the LPN/LVN's unit. The employee asks about the friend's condition and laboratory test results. How should the LPN/LVN respond?
>
> 1. Answer the employee's questions softly to prevent others from overhearing.
> 2. Refuse to discuss the friend's medical condition with the employee.
> 3. Refer the employee to the client's primary health care provider for information.
> 4. Tell the employee the client's normal test results.

THE REWORDED QUESTION: What should an LPN/LVN do when asked about a client by a hospital employee?

(1) Answer softly. Discussing client information in a public place breaches confidentiality. Eliminate.

(2) Refuse to discuss. This does not violate the client's right to privacy and confidentiality. Keep in consideration.

(3) Refer to the client's provider. Providing any information about a client to someone not directly involved in the client's care breaches privacy. Eliminate.

(4) Share the normal test results. Sharing any information without the client's permission breaches confidentiality. Eliminate.

The correct answer is (2).

Expect to see real-world situations on your NCLEX-PN® exam, but make sure that you do not choose real-world answers! These strategies should help you use your previous nursing experience without encountering any pitfalls.

Chapter Quiz

1. Two hours after the insertion of a Salem sump nasogastric (NG) tube, the client vomits a moderate amount of yellow-green fluid. What is the **most** appropriate action for the LPN/LVN to take?

   1. Inject 30 mL air and auscultate the left upper quadrant.
   2. Instill 20 mL carbonated beverage into the drainage tube.
   3. Inform the primary health care provider of the vomiting.
   4. Irrigate nasogastric (NG) tube with 20 mL normal saline.

2. The LPN/LVN is caring for a client after a motor vehicle accident. The LPN/LVN observes that the client is restless, anxious, and has tremors of the hands. The family reports that the client has consumed 4 to 6 beers a day for the past 8 years. What is the **priority** action for the LPN/LVN to take?

   1. Reorient client to the environment frequently.
   2. Maintain the client in a cool, darkened room.
   3. Assist the client to drink more isotonic fluids.
   4. Administer thiamine 100 mg intramuscularly.

3. The LPN/LVN is preparing to administer isoniazid 300 mg PO. Which of the following is a **priority** laboratory value to monitor before administering the medication?

   1. B-type natriuretic peptide (BNP).
   2. Aspartate aminotransferase (AST).
   3. Potassium.
   4. Vitamin B12.

Refer to the Case Study to answer the next six questions.

The LPN/LVN is providing care for an 84-year-old client in a medical surgical unit.

| Admission Notes | Nurse's Notes |

The client is a thin, frail, 84-year-old who lives alone after the spouse's death six months ago. For the past three months, the client has been experiencing frequent episodes of bloody diarrhea and abdominal pain. At the same time, the client has had an unintentional loss of 5% body weight. The client has mild memory decline but has no cognitive impairments. A colonoscopy is scheduled in the morning. The client is NPO (nothing by mouth) after midnight and is completing a bowel prep using laxatives today. Results are pending for a barium enema and computerized tomography (CT) scan.

Past History: Prostate cancer treated with hormone and radiation therapy, hypertension, coronary artery disease (CAD), and degenerative disc disease, status post discectomy. No allergies.

Vital Signs	Results at Admission
BP	118/72 mmHg
Heart rate	82, regular
Respiratory rate	20, regular
Temperature (oral)	97.4° F (36.3° C)
Pulse oximetry	96% on room air

Admission Notes | Nurse's Notes

1400: Client returns to the clinical unit after the colonoscopy procedure. Peripheral IV intact at keep vein open (KVO) rate. Site without redness or edema.

Assessment	Client Finding
General	Frail appearing. Calm affect, cooperative.
Neurological	Sleeping, rouses to voice stimuli, oriented to person and place. Needs reorienting to time and situation. Speech flow is slow but understandable. Pupils equal, round, and reactive to light (PERRL).
Integument	Skin intact, warm and dry, uneven pigmentation. Hands and feet are cool to touch. Dry lips and oral mucous membranes. Decreased skin turgor.
Cardiovascular	S1 and S2 auscultated, regular rhythm, no murmurs. Capillary refill less than 2 seconds. 1 + radial pulses, equal.
Respiratory	Vesicular breath sounds bilaterally. Non-labored breathing.
Abdomen	Soft, flat, nontender. Bowel sounds present × 4.
Musculoskeletal	Moves all extremities. No joint tenderness or deformity, full range of motion. Muscle strength, 4/5 bilaterally.

Vital Signs	Results at 1400
BP	90/60 mmHg
Heart rate	104, regular
Respiratory rate	20, regular
Temperature (oral)	97.6° F (36.4° C)
Pulse oximetry	95% on room air

4. The client returns to the clinical unit after the colonoscopy procedure. The LPN/LVN reviews the admission notes and the nurse's notes at 1400.

For each assessment below, specify the client findings that are concerning to the LPN/LVN. Each assessment may support more than 1 client finding.

Assessment	Client Finding
General	☐ Client age 84. ☐ Mild memory decline. ☐ Bowel prep with laxatives.
Neurological	☐ Needs reorienting to time and situation. ☐ Pupils equal round and reactive to light (PERRL). ☐ Speech flow is slow but understandable.
Integument	☐ Hands and feet are cool to touch. ☐ Skin intact, warm and dry, uneven pigmentation. ☐ Dry lips and oral mucous membranes.
Cardiovascular	☐ Capillary refill less than 2 seconds. ☐ 1 + radial pulses, equal. ☐ S1 and S2 auscultated, regular rhythm, no murmurs.
Vital Signs	☐ Blood pressure 90/60. ☐ Pulse oximetry 95% on room air. ☐ Heart rate 104.

Admission Notes	Nurse's Notes	Vital Signs

Vital Signs	1415	1430	1445
BP	88/60	86/58	82/56
Heart rate	110	114	120
Respiratory rate	22, regular	22, regular	22, regular
Temperature (oral)	----	97.7° F (36.5° C)	----
Pulse oximetry	94% on room air	94% on room air	94% on room air

5. The LPN/LVN monitors the client's vital signs every 15 minutes.

Complete the following sentences by choosing from the list of options.

The LPN/LVN recognizes the client is most likely experiencing [Select from list 1]. The LPN/LVN associates the client's blood pressure with the potential for [Select from list 2]. The LPN/LVN identifies the client's heart rhythm as [Select from list 3].

(1)	(2)	(3)
orthopnea	decreased tissue perfusion	normal
orthostatic hypotension	potassium loss	tachycardia
hypovolemia	atelectasis	bradycardia

6. The LPN/LVN reports the client's vital signs to the RN.

A **priority** concern for the LPN/LVN is to reduce the client's risk for developing which complication?

1. Hyperactive reflexes.
2. Heart failure.
3. Hypovolemic shock.
4. Pulmonary edema.

7. The LPN/LVN and the RN determine the plan of care for the client.

Select **4** client goals that are appropriate to plan for the client.

1. Restore vascular volume.
2. Reduce infection with antibiotics.
3. Increase the client's daily caloric intake.
4. Maintain oxygenation status.
5. Achieve normal vital signs.
6. Reduce risk for injury from falls.

8. For each nursing intervention, specify if the intervention is indicated or not indicated in the client's plan of care.

Assessment Finding	Indicated	Not Indicated
Monitor infusion of IV fluid bolus (500 mL of 0.9% normal saline) as prescribed.	○	○
Report changes in capillary refill, peripheral pulses, and skin color and temperature to RN.	○	○
Provide high-flow oxygen per Venturi mask.	○	○
Report changes in blood pressure, respirations, pulse rate, strength and rhythm to RN.	○	○
Administer epinephrine as prescribed.	○	○
Place on continuous EKG monitoring.	○	○
Have the client sit on the side of bed and dangle feet prior to standing.	○	○
Report changes in mental status to RN.	○	○
Reinforce teaching that abdominal distention and rectal bleeding are expected after a colonoscopy.	○	○

9. The RN evaluates the client at 1630 and documents a nurse's note. The LPN/LVN reviews the findings.

Which client findings indicate nursing care has been effective? Highlight correct sections.

Client is awake, oriented × 4. Speech is fluid and is understandable. Skin pale and cool. Chest expansion full and equal. Slight dyspnea at rest. Respiratory rate 24, regular. BP 108/70 mmHg. Heart rate 90, regular. 2⁺ radial pulses, equal. Pulse oximetry 96% on room air.

10. The LPN/LVN is reinforcing instructions for a client taking clopidogrel 75 mg PO daily. Which statement by the client indicates understanding of the reinforced instructions?

    1. "It will be necessary for me to have frequent blood tests done now."
    2. "I will need to discontinue the garlic tablets I take to control cholesterol."
    3. "I can continue to take several ibuprofen a day for my low back pain."
    4. "I will need to make sure I take a daily multivitamin tablet now."

11. The LPN/LVN is preparing a primigravid client for a primary health care provider examination. Laboratory test results are available. Which fasting serum glucose level result would indicate that gestational diabetes is likely?

    1. Serum glucose level of 40 mg/dL (2.2 mmol/L).
    2. Serum glucose level of 100 mg/dL (5.5 mmol/L).
    3. Serum glucose level of 140 mg/dL (7.7 mmol/L).
    4. Serum glucose level of 180 mg/dL (9.9 mmol/L).

12. The primary health care provider prescribed phenytoin 100 mg PO q.i.d. for the client. Prior to administering the second dose, the LPN/LVN observes that the client appears lethargic and has nystagmus and slurred speech. In addition to notifying the supervising RN, the LPN/LVN should do which of the following?

    1. Administer the phenytoin to prevent an impending seizure.
    2. Administer the phenytoin to prevent cardiac arrhythmia.
    3. Withhold the phenytoin due to signs of an allergic reaction.
    4. Withhold the phenytoin because client shows signs of toxicity.

13. The LPN/LVN is reviewing medication information with a female client who has been prescribed sertraline daily. Which of the following statements by the client indicates a need for further instruction?

    1. "I will continue to take my birth control pills."
    2. "If these pills don't work in 2 weeks, I will stop taking them."
    3. "I will take my pill first thing in the morning."
    4. "I will skip a missed dose if it is almost time for my next one."

Refer to the Case Study to answer the next question.

The LPN/LVN on the cardiovascular stepdown unit is caring for a client admitted for evaluation of carotid artery disease.

| Admission Notes | Radiology | Nurse's Notes |

Client describes intermittent and temporary episodes of weakness of the left side, accompanied by dizziness and loss of coordination. The client had carotid ultrasound studies last week which indicate 85% occlusion of the right carotid artery and 40% occlusion of the left carotid artery. The client is scheduled for a carotid angiogram to determine the severity of the carotid disease and occlusion. Preoperative lab work noted in medical record.

Laboratory Test	Result	Interpretation
Hematocrit	45% (0.45)	Normal
Hemoglobin	15.3 g/dL (153 g/L)	Normal
Platelets	400,000/mm^3 (400 × 10^9/L)	Normal

| Admission Notes | Radiology | Nurse's Notes |

0900: On arrival to the radiology department, the client is alert and oriented. Speech clear and follows all commands. Moves all extremities with equal strength and denies any pain in the extremities. Feet are warm and pink, with +3 pulses bilaterally. Client has an 18-gauge peripheral intravenous catheter in the left forearm infusing 0.9% normal saline at 50 mL/hour. Consent form for the angiogram is signed and witnessed. Client is given midazolam 10 mg IV prior to the insertion of the angiogram catheter in the left femoral artery.

| Admission Notes | Radiology | Nurse's Notes |

1030: Client returned to room, drowsy, but oriented × 3 when roused. Left leg positioned straight with sandbag over the insertion site in the left groin. Groin dressing dry and intact. Legs warm with +2 pedal pulses bilaterally. Capillary refill < 2 seconds on both great toes. Client denies pain at femoral insertion site.

1115: Left leg is pale and cooler than right leg. Pulses are +1 on the left and +3 on the right. Capillary refill > 3 seconds in the left great toe, and < 2 seconds in the right great toe. Client states pain at the insertion site is 3/10 on a scale of 1 to 10. Pressure dressing and sandbag intact to left groin. Stat hemoglobin and hematocrit ordered. Lab calls results: Hematocrit 31% (0.31), hemoglobin 10.1 g/dL (101 g/L).

14. Based upon the change in the client's status, which action does the LPN/LVN take **next**?

   1. Elevate the left leg.
   2. Obtain vital signs.
   3. Logroll the client to check for bleeding.
   4. Remove the sandbag from the groin.

---

15. The client comes to the urgent care clinic reporting "I've just stepped on a rusty nail at a construction site." The LPN/LVN observes a deep puncture wound on the sole of the right foot. What order would the nurse expect to receive from the primary health care provider for this client?

   1. Complete blood count.
   2. Wound culture.
   3. Tetanus vaccine.
   4. Lumbar puncture.

Chapter Quiz Answers and Explanations

1. The answer is 4

Two hours after the insertion of a Salem sump nasogastric (NG) tube, the client vomits a moderate amount of yellow-green fluid. What is the **most** appropriate action for the LPN/LVN to take?

Strategy: Read the question and answer choices to identify the topic: possible obstruction of the NG tube. As you can see, the answers are a mix of assessment and implementation actions.

Recall the best standard of care according to nursing textbooks, and consider appropriate actions that may be taken before contacting the primary health care provider. What action can be taken immediately with least risk of injury to the client?

Category: Implementation/Physiological Integrity/ Reduction of Risk Potential

(1) Injecting air into the NG tube while auscultating over the stomach is no longer an accepted standard of care for verifying NG tube placement. Eliminate.

(2) This may be a "real world" answer. Instilling a carbonated beverage to clear an NG tube obstruction is no longer an accepted standard of care. It has not been proven effective.

(3) If contacted, the primary health care provider will want to know what actions have been taken. Does another answer choice describe actions within LPN/LVN scope of practice that can taken first? Keep for consideration.

(4) CORRECT: Irrigation with normal saline is an appropriate standard of care, is a safe action, and may clear the obstruction. Select this answer.

2. The answer is 1

The LPN/LVN is caring for a client after a motor vehicle accident. The LPN/LVN observes that the client is restless, anxious, and has tremors of the hands. The family reports that the client has consumed 4 to 6 beers a day for the past 8 years. What is the **priority** action for the LPN/LVN to take?

Strategy: First, consider the symptoms described in the question: They are early signs of alcohol withdrawal. What is the priority when caring for a client during early alcohol withdrawal? Safety of the client and safety of others.

Next, determine which answer choice decreases the risk of injury to the client. When answering questions about safety, do not read into the answers or apply "real world" answers. Answer based on standards of care described in nursing textbooks.

Category: Planning/Safe and Effective Envirnoment/ Safety and Infection Control

(1) CORRECT: A client may experience hallucinations during alcohol withdrawal. Reorienting the client to the environment helps maintain client safety during hallucinations.

(2) Some light is recommended to decrease the intensity of the hallucinations. Bright lighting is not recommended, but soft lighting allows the client to observe the surroundings.

(3) Alcohol withdrawal places the client at risk for dehydration, but fluid administration does not decrease the risk of injury. Remember the topic of the question: safety.

(4) Thiamine is a vitamin (B1), and it may be administered to correct nutritional deficiencies and treat malnutrition. But it does not decrease the risk of injury.

3. The answer is 2

The LPN/LVN is preparing to administer isoniazid 300 mg PO. Which of the following is a **priority** laboratory value to monitor before administering the medication?

Strategy: The topic of the question is adverse effects of isoniazid (INH). Recall that isoniazid has the potential to cause liver injury. Which laboratory test indicates liver function?

Category: Data Collection/Physiological Integrity/ Reduction of Risk Potential

(1) B-type natriuretic peptide (BNP) is a hormone produced by the heart. Levels increase when heart failure develops or worsens. BNP is not related to liver injury.

(2) CORRECT: Aspartate aminotransferase (AST) increases in the presence of liver injury. Liver function must be monitor in clients taking isoniazid.

(3) Serum potassium levels are not affected by liver injury.

(4) Vitamin B12 levels are not affected by liver function.

4. See explanation for answers

General: Normal aging has associated common physiological changes and as an older adult, an **84-year-old client** may have increased vulnerability to common clinical diseases and conditions, including fluid and electrolyte imbalances. Additionally, completing a **bowel prep with the use of laxatives**, especially in older adults, increases the risk for a serious fluid volume deficit. INCORRECT OPTIONS: The LPN/LVN is not concerned with a mild decline in memory. This is different from cognitive impairment, such as delirium, dementia, and depression.

Neurological: The LPN/LVN is concerned with the client's **change in mental status**. The client's mental status has changed from having no prior cognitive impairments before the colonoscopy procedure to needing reorientation to time and situation after the procedure. INCORRECT OPTIONS: The LPN/LVN is not concerned that the client's pupils are equal, round, and reactive to light. The client's speech flow is not concerning, either.

Integument: The LPN/LVN is concerned with abnormal clinical findings of **hands and feet that are cool to touch**, **dry lips and oral mucous membranes**. INCORRECT OPTIONS: In older adults, uneven pigmentation is a normal assessment finding, as is skin that is intact, warm, and dry.

Cardiovascular: The LPN/LVN is concerned with the abnormal clinical finding of **1+ radial pulses**. INCORRECT OPTIONS: The client's capillary refill and heart sounds are normal, expected findings.

Vital Signs: The LPN/LVN is concerned with abnormal clinical findings of **blood pressure 90/60** and **heart rate 104**. INCORRECT OPTION: The client's pulse oximetry reading is within normal limits.

5. See explanation for answers

The LPN/LVN recognizes the client is most likely experiencing **hypovolemia**. Hypotension can result from various causes, including loss of body fluids. A bowel preparation can lead to depleted fluid and electrolytes. In hypovolemia, to sustain a normal blood pressure, the heart rate increases along with peripheral vasoconstriction. Pulse force is also affected and pulses may be weak and thready. INCORRECT OPTIONS: The client is not experiencing symptoms of orthopnea (difficulty breathing when lying flat) or orthostatic hypotension.

The LPN/LVN associates the client's blood pressure with the potential for **decreased tissue perfusion**. Hypoperfusion can occur—especially in the brain, heart, and kidneys—from hypotension. INCORRECT OPTIONS: Hypotension is not associated with the potential for potassium loss or atelectasis.

The LPN/LVN identifies the client's heart rhythm as **tachycardia**, in which the sinoatrial node increases its discharge rate to 101–180 beats/minute. Tachycardia can be clinically associated with physiologic stressors such as hypotension, hypovolemia, and exercise. INCORRECT OPTIONS: A normal sinus heart rhythm is a 60 to 100 beats/minute, and bradycardia is a heart rate below 60 beats/minute.

6. The answer is 3

CORRECT OPTION: A priority concern for the LPN/LVN is to reduce the client's risk for developing **hypovolemic shock**, a serious condition of hypoperfusion in the body. Hypovolemic shock occurs when there is insufficient fluid volume in the vascular space needed for adequate tissue perfusion and cellular metabolism.

INCORRECT OPTIONS: Hyperactive reflexes can develop in conditions that cause hypocalcemia, but they are not associated with the client's vital signs of hypotension and tachycardia. Heart failure and pulmonary edema may occur as a complication in conditions of excess intake or retention of fluids.

7. The answer is 1, 4, 5, and 6

CORRECT OPTIONS: The LPN/LVN plans goals with the RN to **restore vascular volume**, **maintain oxygenation status**, **achieve normal vital signs**, and **reduce injury from falls**. When hypotension is present due to fluid volume deficit and to maintain adequate tissue perfusion, restoring circulating volume with intravenous fluids is necessary. Maintaining oxygenation status is essential to prevent hypoxemia. Achieving normal blood pressure, heart rate, and respiratory rate are goals relating to adequate tissue perfusion and homeostasis. Reducing injury from falls is related to orthostatic hypotension, which may occur in older adults who have fluid volume deficit.

INCORRECT OPTIONS: Hypovolemia is caused by conditions of abnormal loss of body fluids, fluid shifts or inadequate intake. Antibiotics play an important role in treatment of septic shock, they are not indicated for the client at this time. Intervention for the client's hypovolemia must be immediate to avert significant complications. Caloric intake adjustments depend on changes in health status, daily activity, and other factors; hypovolemia is not one of them.

8. See explanation for answers

Indicated: **The LPN/LVN monitors an intravenous (IV) fluid bolus**, which is prescribed to correct hypovolemia. In clients with heart conditions, astute monitoring of the IV solution and flow rate is needed especially when giving large volumes. **Changes in capillary refill, peripheral pulses, and skin temperature should be reported to the RN** as these are indicators of tissue perfusion, vascular, and interstitial volume. **Changes in blood pressure, respirations, pulse rate, strength, rhythm, and pulse oximetry** are important aspects of cardiovascular assessment and should be reported to the RN. In the postanesthesia period, **continuous EKG monitoring** is recommended for clients who have a history of heart disease. Hypovolemia may cause orthostatic hypotension, so the LPN/LVN should adjust the bed to low position and **have the client dangle feet prior to standing** as a fall-prevention strategy related to dizziness. **Changes in mental status indicate cerebral hypoperfusion, and should be reported to the RN.**

Not indicated: The LPN/LVN does not provide **high-flow oxygen per the Venturi mask**. A Venturi mask is more commonly used for clients who have chronic obstructive pulmonary disease (COPD). **Epinephrine** is the first treatment for anaphylactic shock, and is not indicated for this client. **Rectal bleeding and abdominal distention** are not expected findings post-colonoscopy; these signs could indicate possible complications and should be reported to the RN.

9. See explanation for answers

Client is awake, oriented × 4. Speech is fluid and is understandable. Skin pale and cool. Chest expansion full and equal. Slight dyspnea at rest. Respiratory rate 24, regular. BP 108/70 mmHg. Heart rate 90, regular. 2⁺ radial pulses, equal. Pulse oximetry 96% on room air.

CORRECT OPTIONS: The LPN/LVN recognizes effective nursing care as indicated by normal assessments of the client being **awake and oriented × 4**, with **fluid and understandable speech**. Clear lung sounds and **full, equal chest expansion** are also normal adult assessment findings. **Full, equal radial pulses** are another improvement from the previous assessment. The **BP, HR, and pulse oximetry** are improved results.

INCORRECT OPTIONS: The client's pale, cool skin; slight dyspnea; and elevated respiratory rate are abnormal clinical findings and should be documented and reported to the physician.

10. The answer is 2

The LPN/LVN is reinforcing instructions for a client taking clopidogrel 75 mg PO daily. Which statement by the client indicates understanding of the reinforced instructions?

Strategy: The topic is client understanding of instructions about clopidogrel. You are looking for a correct statement. Eliminate incorrect answers.

Category: Evaluation/Physiological Integrity/Pharmacological Therapies

(1) Clopidogrel inhibits platelet function, however, routine blood test are not needed.

(2) CORRECT: Is there a possible interaction between garlic and clopidogrel? Yes. Both substances inhibit platelet function and increase the risk of bleeding. This statement indicates understanding.

(3) Both ibuprofen and clopidogrel inhibit platelet function and increase the risk of bleeding. This statement does not indicate understanding of the drug interaction.

(4) While there is no contraindication to a multivitamin tablet, it is not specifically recommended when a client takes an antiplatelet medication.

11. The answer is 4

The LPN/LVN is preparing a primigravid client for a primary healthcare provider examination. Laboratory test results are available. Which fasting serum glucose level result would indicate that gestational diabetes is likely?

Strategy: Recall that the normal serum blood glucose level in a pregnant client can rise to 140 mg/dL (7.7 mmol/L). Then identify the abnormal (higher) value.

Category: Evaluation/Physiological Integrity/Reduction of Risk Potential

(1) Serum glucose level of 40 mg/dL (2.2 mmol/L) indicates severe hypoglycemia; a cause should be investigated.

(2) Serum glucose level of 100 mg/dL (5.5 mmol/L) is a normal level for an adult female client.

(3) Serum glucose level of 140 mg/dL (7.7 mmol/L) is the upper limit of a normal serum glucose level for a pregnant client.

(4) CORRECT: Serum glucose level of 180 mg/dL (9.9 mmol/L); serum glucose level needs to be above 140 mg/dL (7.7 mmol/L) to suggest gestational diabetes.

12. The answer is 4

The primary health care provider prescribed phenytoin 100 mg PO q.i.d. for the client. Prior to administering the second dose, the LPN/LVN observes that the client appears lethargic and has nystagmus and slurred speech. In addition to notifying the supervising RN, the LPN/LVN should do which of the following?

Strategy: Identify the cause of the client's signs and symptoms as possible diphenylhydantoin (Dilantin) toxicity.

Category: Evaluation/Physiological Integrity/Pharmacological Therapies

(1) Lethargy, nystagmus, and slurred speech do not indicate an impending seizure.

(2) Although the phenytoin has antiarrhythmic properties, the client's findings suggest phenytoin toxicity.

(3) Lethargy, nystagmus, and slurred speech are not characteristic of an allergic reaction.

(4) CORRECT: Lethargy, nystagmus, and slurred speech suggest phenytoin toxicity. The drug should be withheld.

13. The answer is 2

The LPN/LVN is reviewing medication information with a female client who has been prescribed sertraline daily. Which of the following statements by the client indicates a need for further instruction?

Strategy: Be careful! You are looking for incorrect information.

Category: Evaluation/Physiological Integrity/Pharmacological Therapies

(1) Sertraline can cause birth defects if taken during pregnancy; the client should continue contraceptives during therapy.

(2) CORRECT: Sertraline may take 4 weeks to have a positive effect on the client's symptoms; the client should not stop taking the medication without consulting with the primary healthcare provider.

(3) It is important to take the medication at the same time each day, but it does not have to be taken in the morning.

(4) A missed dose of sertraline should be omitted if it is almost time for the next dose.

14. The answer is 3

CORRECT OPTION: After an angiogram of the left femoral artery, the client is at risk for hematoma formation at the insertion site, hemorrhage, and infection. Based upon the client's signs and symptoms and decreases in hemoglobin and hematocrit, it is a **priority to check the client for bleeding from the insertion site**. Bleeding from the insertion site may go behind the leg and back, therefore the **client needs to be rolled over** to check for bleeding.

INCORRECT OPTIONS: The client's leg should be flat, not elevated. Vital signs may be obtained, but finding the source of bleeding is the priority due to the decreases in the hemoglobin and hematocrit. The client's leg should remain flat with the sandbag on the insertion site to decrease further blood loss and hematoma formation.

15. The answer is 3

The client comes to the urgent care clinic reporting "I've just stepped on a rusty nail at a construction site." The LPN/LVN observes a deep puncture wound on the sole of the right foot. What order would the nurse expect to receive from the primary health care provider for this client?

Strategy: Consider whether testing provides any needed information about the client's status. Determine whether collecting data or implementing treatment is the priority.

Category: Planning/Physiological Integrity/ Physiological Adaptation

(1) A complete blood count is unnecessary because the client has not suffered significant blood loss.

(2) Wound culture is not necessary for a new wound.

(3) CORRECT: A deep puncture wound provides an ideal reservoir for the growth of *Clostridium tetani* (common in soils, dust, and feces and on human skin). To prevent tetanus, a potentially fatal bacterial infection, the primary health care provider would order the tetanus vaccine.

(4) A primary health care provider uses lumbar puncture to withdraw spinal fluid from the spinal column for analysis. It is used to identify conditions of the brain or spine, not to manage a puncture wound in the foot.

[CHAPTER 5]

STRATEGIES FOR PRIORITY QUESTIONS

One of the biggest challenges facing you as a candidate for practical/vocational nursing licensure is to correctly answer priority questions. You will recognize these questions because they will ask you what is the "best," "most important," "first," or "initial" response by the nurse.

Take a look at this sample question.

> An hour after admission to the nursery, the LPN/LVN observes a newborn having spontaneous, jerky limb movements. The newborn's mother had gestational diabetes mellitus (GDM) during pregnancy. Which action should the LPN/LVN take **first**?
>
> 1. Administer dextrose water.
> 2. Call the primary health care provider immediately.
> 3. Determine the blood glucose level.
> 4. Observe the newborn for associated symptoms.

As you read this question you are probably thinking, "All of these look right!" or "How can I decide what I will do first?" The panic sets in as you try to decide what the best answer is when they all seem "correct."

As a licensed practical/vocational nurse, you will be caring for clients who have multiple problems and needs. You must be able to establish priorities by deciding which needs take precedence over other needs. You probably recognized the newborn's spontaneous, jerky limb movements as a sign of hypoglycemia. Don't forget that an important part of the data collection process is *validating* what you observe. You must complete data collection before you plan and implement nursing care. The correct answer is (3).

The following situation might sound familiar: You are called to a client's room by a family member and find the client lying on the floor. The client is bleeding from a wound on the forehead, and the indwelling urinary catheter is dislodged and hanging from the side of the bed. Where do you begin? Do you call for help? Do you return the client to bed? Do you apply pressure to the cut? Do you reinsert the catheter? Do you notify the primary health care provider? What do you do *first*? This is why establishing priorities is so important.

Your nursing faculty recognized the importance of teaching you how to establish priorities. They required you to establish priorities both in clinical situations and when answering test questions. These are the type of questions that practical/vocational nursing students find most controversial.

Here is an example of a nursing school test question:

Which of the following would most concern the LPN/LVN during a client's recovery from surgery?

1. Safety.
2. Hemorrhage.
3. Infection.
4. Pain control.

A conversation in class with your instructor may then go something like this:

INSTRUCTOR: "The correct answer is (2)."

STUDENT: "Why isn't infection the correct answer? It says right here" *[pointing to textbook]* "that infection is a major complication after surgery!"

INSTRUCTOR: "Yes, infection is an important concern after surgery. But, if the client has a life-threatening hemorrhage, then the fact that the wound is infected is immaterial."

STUDENT: "But you can't count this answer wrong!"

In some situations, the faculty member will give you partial credit for your answer, or will "throw the question out" because there is more than one right answer. But you won't get the opportunity to argue about questions on the NCLEX-PN® exam. You either select the answer the test makers are looking for, or you get the question wrong. In the question given, all of the answers listed are important when caring for a postoperative client, but only one answer is the *best*.

The critical thinking required for priority questions is for you to recognize patterns in the answer choices. By recognizing these patterns, you will know which path you need to choose to correctly answer the question. This chapter will present several strategies to help you establish priorities on the NCLEX-PN® exam:

*   Maslow strategy
*   Nursing process strategy
*   Safety strategy

We will outline each strategy, describe how and when it should be used, and show you how to apply these strategies to exam-style questions. By using these strategies, you will be able to eliminate the second-best answer and correctly identify the highest priority.

Strategy One: Maslow

Maslow's hierarchy of needs (Figure 5.1) is crucial to establishing priorities on the NCLEX-PN® exam. Maslow identifies five levels of human needs: physiological, safety and security, love and belonging, self-esteem, and self-actualization.

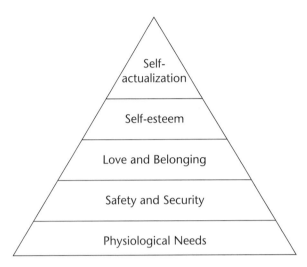

Figure 5.1 Maslow's Hierarchy of Needs

Because *physiological needs* are necessary for survival, they have the highest priority and must be met first. Physiological needs include oxygen, fluid, nutrition, temperature, elimination, shelter, rest, and sex. If you don't have oxygen to breathe or food to eat, you really don't care if you have stable psychosocial relationships!

Safety and security needs can be both physical and psychosocial. Physical safety includes decreasing what is threatening to the client. The threat may be an illness (myocardial infarction), accidents (a parent transporting a newborn in a car without using a car seat), or environmental threats (the client with COPD who insists on walking outside in 10° F [-12° C] temperatures).

To attain psychological safety, the client must have the knowledge and understanding about what to expect from others in the environment. For example, it is important to teach the client and family what to expect after a stroke. It is also important that you allow a client preparing for a mastectomy to verbalize her concerns about changes that might occur in her relationship with her partner.

To achieve *love and belonging,* the client needs to feel loved by family and accepted by others. When a client feels self-confident and useful, that client will achieve the need of *self-esteem* as described by Maslow.

The highest level of Maslow's hierarchy of needs is *self-actualization*. To achieve this level, the client must experience fulfillment and realize their potential. In order for self-actualization to occur, all of the lower-level needs must be met. Because of the stresses of life, lower-level needs are not always met, and many people never achieve this high level of functioning.

The Maslow Four-Step Process

The first strategy to use in establishing priorities is a four-step process, beginning with Maslow's hierarchy. To use the Maslow strategy, you must first recognize the pattern in the answer choices.

STEP 1. Look at your answer choices.

Determine if the answer choices are both physical and psychosocial. If they are, apply the Maslow strategy detailed in Step 2.

STEP 2. Eliminate all psychosocial answer choices. If an answer choice is physiological, don't eliminate it yet. Remember, Maslow states that physiological needs must be met first. Though pain has a physiologic component, reactions to expected pain are considered "psychosocial" on this exam and given lower priority. However, pain that is acute, severe, or not relieved as expected with treatment requires immediate assessment.

STEP 3. Look at each of the answer choices that you have not yet eliminated and ask yourself if the answer choice makes sense with regard to the disease or situation described in the question. If it makes sense as an answer choice, keep it for consideration and go on to the next choice.

STEP 4. Can you apply the ABCs?

Look at the remaining answer choices. Can you apply the ABCs? The ABCs stand for airway, breathing, and circulation. If there is an answer that involves maintaining a patent airway, it will be correct. If not, is there a choice that involves breathing problems? It will be correct. If not, go on with the ABCs. Is there an answer pertaining to the cardiovascular system? It will be correct. What if the ABCs don't apply? Compare the remaining answer choices and ask yourself, "What is the highest priority?" This is your answer.

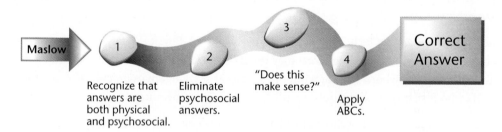

Let's apply this technique to a few sample exam-style test questions.

> A client is admitted to the hospital with a ruptured ectopic pregnancy. A laparotomy is scheduled. Preoperatively, which intervention is **most** important for the LPN/LVN to include on the client's plan of care?
>
> 1. Fluid replacement.
> 2. Therapeutic communication.
> 3. Emotional support.
> 4. Oxygen therapy.

Look at the stem of the question. The words *most important* mean:

- This is a priority question.
- There probably will be more than one answer choice that is a correct nursing action, but only one step will be the most important or highest priority action.

STEP 1. Look at the answer choices.

You see that both physical and psychosocial interventions are included. Apply the Maslow strategy.

STEP 2. Eliminate the answer choices that are psychosocial interventions.

Answer choice (2), which is therapeutic communication, should be discarded. Remember, therapeutic communication falls under psychosocial interventions on the NCLEX-PN® exam. Answer choice (3), emotional support, is also a psychosocial concern. Eliminate this answer. You have now eliminated two of the possible choices. You are halfway there!

STEP 3. Now look at the remaining answer choices and ask yourself whether they make sense.

Answer choice (1), fluid replacement, makes sense, because this client has a ruptured ectopic pregnancy. An ectopic pregnancy is implantation of the fertilized ovum in a site other than the endometrial lining, usually the fallopian tube. Initially, the pregnancy is normal, but as the embryo outgrows the fallopian tube, the tube ruptures, causing extensive bleeding into the abdominal cavity. Answer choice (4), oxygen therapy, does not make sense with a ruptured ectopic pregnancy. The obstetrical client is not likely to need respiratory care prior to surgery. Eliminate this answer choice.

You are left with the correct answer, (1). After reading this question, many students select answer choice (2) or (3) as the correct answer. They justify this by emphasizing the importance of managing this client's emotional distress or addressing her grief about losing the pregnancy. Neither answer choice takes priority over the physiological demand of fluid replacement prior to surgery.

Ready for another question? Try this one.

The LPN/LVN is implementing care for an adolescent client diagnosed with anorexia nervosa. On admission, the girl weighs 82 lb (37 kg) and is 5′4″ (162 cm) tall. Laboratory test results indicate severe hypokalemia, anemia, and dehydration. The LPN/LVN should give which nursing diagnosis the **highest** priority?

1. Body image disturbance related to weight loss.
2. Self-esteem disturbance related to feelings of inadequacy.
3. Impaired nutrition: less than body requirements related to decreased intake.
4. Deficient cardiac output related to the potential for dysrhythmias.

The first thing you should notice in this question stem is the phrase *"highest priority."* This alerts you that there may be more than one answer that could be considered correct.

STEP 1. Look at the answer choices.

You will see that both physical and psychosocial interventions are included. Apply the Maslow strategy.

STEP 2. Eliminate all psychosocial answer choices.

It is easy to see that body image disturbance, answer choice (1), is a psychosocial concern. The same is true of answer choice (2), self-esteem disturbance. Answer choices (3) and (4) are physiological. You have now eliminated all but two answer choices.

STEP 3. Ask yourself whether the remaining answer choices make sense.

Answer choice (3), "Impaired nutrition: less than body requirements related to decreased intake," does make sense. Remember, the client has anorexia nervosa, is 5'4" (162 cm) tall and weighs 82 lb (37 kg). Answer choice (4), "Deficient cardiac output related to the potential for dysrhythmias," also makes sense. Dysrhythmias are a concern for a client with severe hypokalemia, which often occurs with anorexia nervosa.

You still have work to do.

STEP 4. Can you apply the ABCs? Yes.

Deficient cardiac output is a higher priority than altered nutrition. The best answer choice is (4).

When you first read this question, you probably identified each of the answer choices as appropriate for a client with anorexia nervosa. Only one nursing diagnosis can be the highest priority. Using strategies involving Maslow and the ABCs will enable you to choose the correct answer on your NCLEX-PN® exam.

Strategy Two: Nursing Process (Data Collection Versus Implementation)

A second strategy that will assist you in establishing priorities involves the data collection and implementation steps of the nursing process. As a practical/vocational nursing student, you have been drilled so that you can recite the steps of the nursing process in your sleep—data collection, planning, implementation, and evaluation. In practical/vocational nursing school, you did have some test questions about the nursing process, but you probably did not use the nursing process to assist you in selecting a correct answer on an exam. On the NCLEX-PN® exam, you will be given a clinical situation and asked to establish priorities. The possible answer choices will include both the correct data collection action and implementation for this clinical situation. How do you choose the correct answer when both the correct mode of data collection and implementation are given? Think about these two steps of the nursing process.

Data collection is the process of establishing a data profile about the client and their health problems. The nurse obtains subjective and objective data in a number of ways: talking to clients, observing clients and/or significant others, taking a health history, evaluating laboratory results, and collaborating with other members of the health care team.

Once you collect the data, you compare it to the client's baseline or normal values. On the NCLEX-PN® exam, the client's baseline may not be given, but as a practical/vocational nursing student you have acquired a body of knowledge. On this exam, you are expected to compare the client information you are given to the "normal" values learned from your nursing textbooks.

Data collection is the first step of the nursing process and takes priority over all other steps. It is essential that you complete the data collection phase of the nursing process before you implement nursing activities. This is a common mistake made by NCLEX-PN® exam takers: don't implement before you collect data. For example, when performing cardiopulmonary resuscitation (CPR), if you don't access the airway before performing mouth-to-mouth resuscitation, your actions may be harmful!

Implementation is the care you provide to your clients. Nursing interventions may be independent, dependent, or interdependent. Independent nursing interventions are generally *not* within the scope of the LPN/LVN's nursing practice. However, the LPN/LVN can follow established care plans, standards of care, and established protocols. For example, the LPN/LVN can instruct a client to turn, cough, and deep-breathe after surgery. Dependent interventions are based on the written orders of a primary health care provider. On the NCLEX-PN® exam, you should assume that you have an order for all dependent interventions that are included in the answer choices.

This may be a different way of thinking from the way you were taught in practical/vocational nursing school. Many students select an answer on a nursing school test that is later counted wrong because the intervention requires a primary health care provider's order. Everyone walks away from the test review muttering "trick question." It is important for you to remember that there are no trick questions on the NCLEX-PN® exam. You should base your answer on an understanding that you have a primary health care provider's order for any nursing intervention described.

Interdependent interventions are shared with the RN and other members of the health care team. For instance, nutrition education would be directed and supervised by the RN and may be shared with the LPN/LVN and the dietician. Chest physiotherapy may be directed and supervised by the RN and shared with a respiratory therapist and an LPN/LVN.

The following strategy, utilizing the data collection and implementation phases of the nursing process, will assist you in selecting correct answers to questions that ask you to identify priorities.

STEP 1. Read the answer choices to establish a pattern.

If the answer choices are a mix of data collection/validation and implementation, use the Nursing Process (Data Collection vs. Implementation) strategy.

STEP 2. Refer to the question.

Determine whether you should be collecting data or implementing.

STEP 3. Eliminate answer choices, and then choose the best answer.

If after Step 2 you find that, for example, it is a data collection question, eliminate any answers that clearly focus on implementation. Then choose the best data collection answer.

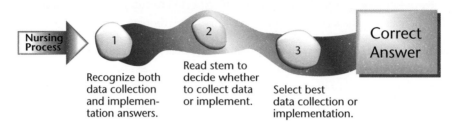

Try this strategy on the following question.

> The LPN/LVN is caring for a client who underwent abdominal surgery 6 hours ago. Which action by the LPN/LVN is **most** important?
>
> 1. Have the client use a pillow to splint the incision.
> 2. Instruct the client how to safely get out of bed.
> 3. Reinforce the dry dressing to provide more padding.
> 4. Turn the client to check for bleeding underneath the client.

THE REWORDED QUESTION: What nursing priority should the LPN/LVN identify in this scenario? What are the risks for a client after abdominal surgery?

STEP 1. Read the answer choices to establish a pattern.

There is one data collection answer, (4), and three implementation answers, (1), (2), and (3). You can use the Nursing Process (Data Collection vs. Implementation) strategy.

STEP 2. Refer to the question to determine if you should be collecting data or implementing care.

You know that bleeding is a risk for all surgical abdominal wounds. According to the nursing process, you should collect data first.

STEP 3. Eliminate answer choices, and then choose the best answer.

Eliminate answers (1), (2), and (3), which are implementation answers. You are left with only one answer choice, (4). Clients with abdominal surgical wounds often find their most comfortable position lying on their backs in bed. Fluid, namely blood, flows via gravity to dependent areas. A cursory look at the top of the dressing may reveal no drainage; however, when the client is rolled to the side, a pool of blood could be noted if the wound is hemorrhaging. Even if this had not occurred to you, you are still able to correctly answer this question using the data collection versus implementation strategy.

Let's look at another question.

> A child biking to school hit the curb and then fell, injuring the leg. The LPN/LVN was called and found the child alert and conscious, but in severe pain with a possible right femur fracture. Which is the **first** action that the LPN/LVN should take?
>
> 1. Immobilize the affected limb with a splint and ask the client not to move.
> 2. Collect data of the circumstances surrounding the accident.
> 3. Place the client in semi-Fowler position to facilitate breathing.
> 4. Check pedal pulse and blanching sign in both legs and compare the findings.

The words *"first action"* tell you that this is a priority question.

THE REWORDED QUESTION: What is the highest priority for a fractured femur?

STEP 1. Read the answer choices to establish a pattern.

The answer choices are a mix of data collection and implementation, so use the Nursing Process (Data Collection vs. Implementation) strategy.

STEP 2. Determine whether you should be collecting data or implementing.

According to the question, the LPN/LVN has determined that the child has a possible fracture. This implies that the LPN/LVN has completed the data-collection step. It is now time to implement.

STEP 3. Eliminate answer choices, and then choose the best answer.

Eliminate answers (2) and (4) because they involve data collection. This leaves you with choices (1) and (3). Which takes priority: immobilizing the affected limb, or placing the client in a semi-Fowler position to facilitate breathing? The question does not indicate any respiratory distress. The correct answer is (1), immobilize the affected limb.

Some students will choose an answer involving the ABCs without thinking it through. Students, beware. Use the ABCs to establish priorities, but make sure that the answer is appropriate to the situation. In this question, breathing was mentioned in one of the answer choices. If you had chosen the ABCs immediately without looking at the context of the question, you would have answered this question incorrectly.

Look at this question in another form.

> A child biking to school hit the curb, and then fell. The child tells the LPN/LVN, "I think my leg is broken." Which is the **first** action the LPN/LVN should take?
>
> 1. Immobilize the affected limb with a splint and ask the client not to move.
> 2. Collect data of the circumstances surrounding the accident.
> 3. Place the client in semi-Fowler position to facilitate breathing.
> 4. Check the appearance of the client's leg.

STEP 1. Determine whether you should be collecting data or implementing. In this question, the client has stated, "My leg is broken." This statement is not the LPN/LVN's data collection. This alerts the LPN/LVN that there is a problem, and the LPN/LVN should begin the steps of the nursing process. The first step is data collection.

STEP 2. Eliminate answers (1) and (3). These are implementations.

STEP 3. What takes priority? Examination of the leg takes priority over investigation into what happened to cause the accident. The correct answer is (4).

Strategy Three: Safety

LPN/LVNs have the primary responsibility of ensuring the safety of clients. This includes clients in health care facilities, in the home, at work, and in the community. Safety includes meeting basic needs (oxygen, food, fluids, etc.), reducing hazards that cause injury to clients (accidents, obstacles in the home), and decreasing the transmission of pathogens (immunizations, sanitation).

Remember that the NCLEX-PN® exam is a test of minimum competency to determine that you are able to practice safe and effective nursing care. Always think *safety* when selecting correct answers on the exam. When answering questions about procedures, this strategy will help you to establish priorities.

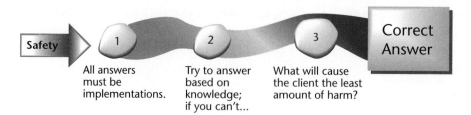

STEP 1. Are all the answer choices implementations? If so, use the Safety strategy illustrated above.

STEP 2. Can you answer the question based on your knowledge? If not, continue to Step 3.

STEP 3. Ask yourself, "What will cause my client the least amount of harm?" and choose the best answer.

Apply this strategy to the following question.

> A pediatric client undergoes a tonsillectomy for treatment of chronic tonsillitis unresponsive to antibiotic therapy. After surgery, the client is brought to the clinical unit. Which action should the LPN/LVN include in the client's plan of care?
>
> 1. Institute measures to minimize crying.
> 2. Perform postural drainage every 2 hours.
> 3. Cough and deep-breathe hourly.
> 4. Provide ice cream as tolerated.

THE REWORDED QUESTION: What should you do after a tonsillectomy?

STEP 1. Are all the answer choices implementations?

Yes.

STEP 2. Can you answer the question based on your knowledge of a tonsillectomy?

If not, continue to Step 3.

STEP 3. Ask yourself, "What will cause the client the least amount of harm?"

(1) Minimizing crying will help prevent bleeding. Keep in consideration.

(2) Postural drainage may cause bleeding. Eliminate.

(3) Coughing and deep-breathing may cause bleeding. Eliminate.

(4) Providing ice cream may cause the child to clear the throat, causing bleeding. Eliminate.

The correct answer is (1). The nurse must prevent postoperative hemorrhage, a complication seen after this type of surgery. Crying would irritate the child's throat and increase the chance of hemorrhage.

Let's try another question.

> The LPN/LVN doubts the accuracy of a medication order in the client's medication administration record (MAR). Which action should the LPN/LVN take **first**?
>
> 1. Compare order in medication administration record to order in medical record.
> 2. Contact the prescribing primary health care provider to question the order.
> 3. Consult with hospital pharmacist about the accuracy of the medication order.
> 4. Compare information about medication in nursing drug book to medication order.

THE REWORDED QUESTION: What should you do if you think the medication administration record (MAR) is incorrect?

STEP 1. Are all the answers implementations?

Yes.

STEP 2. Ask yourself the question, "What will protect my client the most?"

(1) Comparing the MAR with the original primary health care provider's order would certainly provide clarification regarding the questioned medication. Leave this choice for consideration.

(2) Calling the prescribing primary health care provider would certainly help clarify the order, but this should not be the first step. Eliminate.

(3) Consulting the hospital pharmacist can shed light on a medication, but the LPN/LVN first needs to know what the original order said. Eliminate.

(4) Looking up the medication in a nursing drug book is a good idea, but will this step help if the original order was incorrectly transcribed in the MAR? Eliminate.

Only choice (1) is left for consideration, and this is the correct answer. The NCLEX-PN® test makers want to know what decision you are going to make to protect your client, not what decision the primary health care provider will make.

Let's look at another question.

> A client admitted with a diagnosis of dementia attempts several times to remove the nasogastric tube. The LPN/LVN receives an order for wrist restraints. Which action by the LPN/LVN is **most** appropriate?
>
> 1. Attach the ties of the wrist restraints to the client's bed frame.
> 2. Perform daily range-of-motion exercises to the restrained extremities.
> 3. Remove the restraints when the client is out of bed in a wheelchair.
> 4. Explain restraint need to the family only, because the client is confused.

THE REWORDED QUESTION: "What is the safest way to apply restraints?"

STEP 1. Are all answers implementations?

Yes.

STEP 2. Can you answer this based on your knowledge?

If not, proceed to Step 3.

STEP 3. Ask yourself, "What will cause the least amount of harm to the client?"

(1) Attaching the restrain ties to the client's bed frame will not harm the client. Retain this answer.

(2) Performing daily range-of-motion exercises will not harm the client. However, they should be performed more frequently. Retain this answer.

(3) Removing the restraints when the client is out of bed in a wheelchair will be harmful to the client. Restraints should not be removed when the client is unattended. Eliminate.

(4) Explaining the need for restraints only to the family can cause harm to the client. Restraints can increase the confusion or combativeness of the client. Even though confused, the client needs to receive an explanation. Eliminate.

You are now considering answer choices (1) and (2). What will cause the least amount of harm to the client—attaching the ties of the restraint to the bed frame or performing daily range-of-motion exercises to the extremities? Range-of-motion exercises should be performed every 2 to 4 hours to prevent loss of joint mobility, not just once per day. Eliminate (2). The correct answer is (1). Attaching the ties of the restraints to the bed frame will allow the nurse to raise and lower the side rail without injury to the client.

Priority questions are an important component of the NCLEX-PN® exam. To help you select correct answers, think:

- Maslow
- The Nursing Process
- Safety

Answer the following three questions using the appropriate priority strategy. The explanations follow the questions.

Question 1

> The LPN/LVN is caring for a client with a diagnosis of stroke. The LPN/LVN is feeding the client in a chair when the client suddenly begins to choke. Which action should the LPN/LVN take **first**?
>
> 1. Check the client for breathlessness.
> 2. Leave the client in the chair and apply vigorous abdominal or chest thrusts.
> 3. Ask the client, "Are you choking?"
> 4. Return the client to the bed and apply vigorous abdominal or chest thrusts.

Question 2

> A client with a history of bipolar disorder is admitted to the psychiatric hospital. The client was found by the police attempting to climb onto the wing of a plane at the airport. A family member reports that the client has not eaten or slept in 2 days, and suspects the client has stopped taking lithium. On admission, the LPN/LVN should place the **highest** priority on which client care need?
>
> 1. Reinforcing to the client the importance of taking lithium as prescribed.
> 2. Providing the client with a safe environment with few distractions.
> 3. Arranging for food and rest for the client.
> 4. Setting limits on the client's behavior.

Question 3

> The primary health care provider orders a nasogastric (NG) tube inserted and connected to low intermittent suction for a client with an intestinal obstruction. Two hours after NG tube insertion, the client vomits 200 mL. While irrigating the NG tube, the LPN/LVN notes resistance. Which action should the LPN/LVN take **first**?
>
> 1. Replace the NG tube with a larger one.
> 2. Turn the client on the left side.
> 3. Implement continuous NG tube suction.
> 4. Continue NG tube irrigation.

Let's see if you were able to correctly determine which strategy you should use to determine priorities.

Question 1

The answer choices include both data collection and implementations. Use the Nursing Process strategy to select the correct answer.

STEP 1. Read the answer choices to establish a pattern.

Choices (1) and (3) are data collection; choices (2) and (4) are implementations.

STEP 2. Refer to the question to determine whether you should be collecting data or implementing. According to the situation, the client has begun to choke. This alerts the nurse that there is a problem. The first step of the nursing process is data collection.

STEP 3. Eliminate answer choices, and then choose the best answer.

Eliminate answer choices (2) and (4) because they are implementations. Now choose the best answer from the remaining answer choices, (1) and (3).

What takes priority—checking for breathlessness or collecting data by asking the client, "Are you choking?" Inability to speak or cough indicates airway obstruction. Breathlessness should be checked only in an unconscious client. The correct answer is (3).

Question 2

Look at the answer choices. They include both physiological and psychosocial interventions. Apply the Maslow strategy.

STEP 1. Look at the answer choices and identify which are physiological—choices (2) and (3)—and which are psychosocial—choices (1) and (4).

STEP 2. Eliminate all psychosocial answer choices—(1) and (4).

STEP 3. Ask yourself if the remaining answer choices make sense. Choice (2), providing the client with a safe environment, does make sense. Retain this answer. Choice (3), arranging for food and rest, also makes sense. Retain this answer.

STEP 4. Can you apply the ABCs to the remaining answer choices? No; neither choice refers to airway, breathing, or circulation. Since the ABCs don't apply, ask yourself "What is the highest priority—providing for a safe environment, or providing for food and rest?" According to Maslow, food and rest take highest priority. The correct answer is (3).

Question 3

This question is about a procedure: What should the nurse do when resistance is met while irrigating an NG tube? If you are unsure about a procedure, think *safety*.

STEP 1. Read the answer choices to establish a pattern. Are all the answer choices implementations? Yes.

STEP 2. Can you answer the question based on your knowledge? If not, continue to Step 3.

STEP 3. Ask yourself, "What will cause the client the least amount of harm?"

(1) Replacing the NG tube with a larger one could harm the client by damaging the mucosa. Eliminate.

(2) Turning the client to the left side would not hurt the client. Retain this answer choice.

(3) Changing the suction from intermittent to continuous is never done because it will erode the mucosa. Eliminate.

(4) Continuing the irrigation when there is resistance might be harmful. Never force an irrigation. Eliminate.

The correct answer is (2). The tip of the tube may be against the stomach wall. Repositioning the client might allow the tip to lie unobstructed in the stomach.

Strategy Recap

Here is a brief review of the strategies outlined in this chapter:

- The NCLEX-PN® exam isn't the real world, so don't rely on your real-world experience to answer NCLEX-PN® exam questions.
- To answer priority questions correctly, think Maslow, the nursing process, and safety.

Using these critical thinking strategies will help you correctly answer priority questions.

Chapter Quiz

1. The LPN/LVN is caring for a client several hours after application of a right lower extremity cast. The client reports, "My right toes feel funny." What is the **first** action the LPN/LVN should take?

    1. Elevate right leg on pillow.
    2. Administer an analgesic.
    3. Reassure the client that tingling is normal.
    4. Compare capillary refill of right and left toes.

2. The LPN/LVN is assisting a client with ambulation when the client begins to fall. What is the **most** appropriate action for the LPN/LVN to take?

    1. Grasp the client under the arms, bend at the waist, and assist the client to the floor.
    2. Place feet close together, place arms under the client's axillae, and slide the client to the floor.
    3. Place arms around the client's waist and assist the client to the closest chair or bed.
    4. Place feet wide apart, push the pelvis forward, and slide the client down one leg.

3. The LPN/LVN is observing that a client's radial pulse is now 56 beats per minute. It was 72 beats per minute 4 hours ago. What is the **most** important action for the LPN/LVN to take?

    1. Check the oxygen saturation level.
    2. Begin oxygen at 2 L/minute by nasal cannula.
    3. Obtain the client's blood pressure.
    4. Palpate bilateral pedal pulse strength.

4. A client reports to the LPN/LVN, "I just started to feel short of breath." The client has normal saline solution infusing at a rate of 75 mL/hour through a peripherally inserted central catheter (PICC). What is the **first** action the LPN/LVN should take?

    1. Obtain client's blood pressure and apical heart rate.
    2. Reassure client that shortness of breath will improve.
    3. Observe the insertion site of the PICC.
    4. Elevate the head of the bed 90 degrees.

5. The LPN/LVN at the urology clinic is obtaining a health history from an elderly male client who reports back pain during urination and difficulty starting and stopping the urine flow. Which of the following goals is **most** important for the LPN/LVN to include in the client's plan of care?

    1. Pain medication.
    2. Antibiotic administration.
    3. Physical therapy.
    4. Laboratory testing.

6. The LPN/LVN is caring for the client whose vaginal delivery resulted in a stillborn infant. Which of the following actions by the nurse is the **most** important?

    1. Be available to the client to listen to expressions of grief.
    2. Provide the client with appropriate fluid replacement.
    3. Check client's perineal pad frequently for excess bleeding.
    4. Tell client about measures to cope with severe uterine pain.

7. The primary health care provider has ordered a condom catheter for a male client. Which of the following is the **most** important question the LPN/LVN should ask the client before carrying out this order?

   1. "Do you have a latex allergy?"
   2. "Do you have a history of urinary tract infections?"
   3. "Do you have a history of frequent nocturia?"
   4. "Have you been circumcised?"

8. The client is about to be discharged home with a portable oxygen delivery system. The LPN/LVN knows that which of the following education topics is **most** important for the client's family?

   1. Correct use of prescribed nebulizers and inhalers.
   2. Prohibition of flame or heat sources in the same room.
   3. Relaxation techniques, such as visualization or meditation.
   4. Maintenance of adequate hydration and nutrition.

Refer to the Case Study to answer the next question.

The LPN/LVN is caring for a client who was diagnosed with myocardial infarction.

| Admission Notes | Nurse's Notes |

The client presented to the emergency department (ED) this morning with acute onset of chest heaviness, left shoulder and arm pain, and jaw pain that awakened the client during the night. Client awake, alert, and oriented to person, place, and time. Vital signs on admission: Temperature 100.3° F (37.9° C), pulse 86, respiratory rate 20, and blood pressure 150/100 mm Hg. In the ED, the client was placed on a cardiac monitor, and blood samples obtained for evaluation of cardiac enzymes. The results indicated elevated creatine kinase (CK-MB), lactate dehydrogenase (LDH), and troponin levels. Because of recent knee arthroplasty 6 weeks ago, the client was not eligible for thrombolytic therapy. The client was diagnosed with an acute myocardial infarction, started on a nitroglycerin infusion, and admitted to the Cardiac Care Unit (CCU).

| Admission Notes | Nurse's Notes |

CCU Day 2

Client is lethargic and difficult to arouse, then oriented to person and place only. Current vital signs: Temperature 100.5° F (38.1° C), pulse 92, respiratory rate 26, and blood pressure 90/50 mm Hg. The head of the client's bed is elevated 45°. Crackles present in the bases of both lungs. 1+ peripheral pulses with pale, cool skin. Client refusing food on tray, states, "Too hard to breathe." IV of 0.9% normal saline (NS) infusing at 50 mL/hour to right forearm. Site intact with no redness or swelling. Urine output for past 24 hours: 500 mL. Client has had a 3 lb (1.36 kg) weight gain since admission.

9. The LPN/LVN is assigned to assist the RN with the care of the client. The LPN/LVN reviews the client's medical record since admission and enters the client's room to check on the client.

   Which finding **best** indicates the client is developing left-sided heart failure? **(Select all that apply.)**

   1. Dyspnea.
   2. Peripheral edema.
   3. Jugular vein distension.
   4. Orthopnea.
   5. Frothy sputum.
   6. Crackles in the lungs.
   7. Hepatomegaly.
   8. Decreased bowel sounds.
   9. Elevated creatinine.

Refer to the Case Study to answer the next six questions.

The LPN/LVN in the internal medicine clinic assists with care of a client with a diagnosis of chronic kidney disease (CKD).

History and Physical

The client is 65 years old with a history of type 1 diabetes mellitus (DM), hypertension, peripheral vascular disease, gout, lumbar radiculopathy, gastroesophageal reflux disease (GERD), and chronic kidney disease. The client's height is 66 inches (167.64 cm) and weight is 145 pounds (63.50 kg). The client's DM is managed with twice daily doses of regular and NPH insulin, and the client is prescribed a calcium channel blocker and furosemide for hypertension management. GERD is controlled with proton pump inhibitors and dietary changes, including 6 small meals per day. On physical exam, the client is in no acute distress, but does have 2^+ pitting edema in the ankles. The client also describes decreased urine output, chronic back pain, and numbness and tingling in the feet.

10. The LPN/LVN reviews the history and physical in the client's medical record.

    The LPN/LVN recognizes which finding as a risk factor that contributed to the development of chronic kidney disease in this client? **(Select all that apply.)**

    1. Gout.
    2. Hypertension.
    3. Diabetes mellitus.
    4. Lumbar radiculopathy.
    5. Peripheral vascular disease.

History and Physical	Laboratory Results

Laboratory Test	Result (SI Information)	Interpretation
Sodium	155 mEq/L (155 mmol/L)	High
Potassium	7.2 mEq/L (7.2 mmol/L)	High
Chloride	110 mEq/L (110 mmol/L)	High
BUN	35 mg/dL (12.49 mmol/L)	High
Creatinine	2.4 mg/dL (229.84 µmol/L)	High
Glucose	300 mg/dL (16.65 mmol/L)	High

11. The physician orders stat lab work. The LPN/LVN reviews the lab results.

For each client finding, specify if the finding is consistent with hyperglycemia, hyperkalemia, or hypernatremia. Each finding may support more than one abnormality. **Each column must have at least 1 response option selected.**

Assessment Finding	Hyperglycemia	Hyperkalemia	Hypernatremia
Diarrhea	☐	☐	☐
Paresthesias	☐	☐	☐
Poor skin turgor	☐	☐	☐
Polydipsia	☐	☐	☐
Weakness	☐	☐	☐

12. Complete the following sentences by choosing from the list of options.

The client is at risk of developing [Select from list 1] due to [Select from list 2].

(1)
polyuria
cardiac dysrhythmias
seizures

(2)
elevated chloride
elevated potassium
elevated creatinine

13. Based on the client's clinical presentation and laboratory results, the physician admits the client to the hospital.

   The LPN/LVN assigned to assist with the client's care in the hospital expects an order for which medication to treat the hyperkalemia?

   1. Spironolactone.
   2. Prednisone.
   3. Naproxen.
   4. Sodium polystyrene.

14. Which nursing action is indicated for this client at this time? **(Select all that apply.)**

   1. Place the client on a cardiac monitor.
   2. Administer IV regular insulin and dextrose 5%.
   3. Maintain strict bedrest.
   4. Implement seizure precautions.
   5. Administer loop diuretics.
   6. Monitor urinary output.

15. Because of the client's history of chronic kidney disease, the LPN/LVN reviews dietary teaching related to foods high in potassium.

   Which **4** client statements indicate the client understands the information provided by the LPN/LVN?

   1. "I need to avoid grapes in my diet."
   2. "I need to restrict bananas in my diet."
   3. "I need to stop adding table salt to my food."
   4. "I should limit tomatoes and potatoes in my diet."
   5. "It is okay to eat eggs for breakfast."
   6. "Melons and oranges are high in potassium."
   7. "It is better for me to use most salt substitutes."

Chapter Quiz Answers and Explanations

1. The answer is 4

The LPN/LVN is caring for a client several hours after application of a right lower extremity cast. The client reports, "My right toes feel funny." What is the **first** action the LPN/LVN should take?

Strategy: Read the question to identify the topic: possible decrease in circulation after cast application. The client is at risk for injury from compromised circulation.

Next, read the answer choices. They are a mix of physiological and psychosocial, so apply Maslow: Rule out the psychosocial answers, and review the remaining options for sense and ABCs.

Category: Data Collection/Physiological Integrity/Basic Care and Comfort

(1) What is the outcome of leg elevation? Circulation to the right leg, foot, and toes will decrease. Is this desired? No.

(2) This is not an appropriate first action. If an analgesic is administered, it may alter some of the observations that indicate circulatory compromise.

(3) Reassuring the client is psychosocial. Physical answers are the priority; eliminate.

(4) CORRECT: By comparing capillary refill of both right and left toes, the LPN/LVN observes circulation in the casted extremity. Prolonged capillary refill may indicate decreased blood flow to the right foot and toes.

2. The answer is 4

The LPN/LVN is assisting a client with ambulation when the client begins to fall. What is the **most** appropriate action for the LPN/LVN to take?

Strategy: Read the question and answers to identify the topic. All answer choices are implementations. The topic is client safety.

Next, consider the outcome of each answer choice: Which best promotes client safety? Also consider appropriate body mechanics while assisting the client and protecting yourself from injury.

Category: Implementation/Safe and Effective Care Environment/Safety and Infection Control

(1) Bending at the waist is an example of body mechanics that increase risk of injury to the LPN/LVN. Grasping the client under the arms does not provide the greatest stability while assisting the client.

(2) This action increases the risk of injury to the LPN/LVN. The LPN/LVN should place feet wide apart to increase safety.

(3) This action increases the risk of injury to the client. It is more important to assist the client to a safe position than to place the client on a chair or bed.

(4) CORRECT: The outcome of this action is desired. The positioning of the feet (wide) and pelvis (forward) ensures stability, and sliding the client down the leg decreases the risk of injury to the client.

3. The answer is 3

The LPN/LVN observes that a client's radial pulse is now 56 beats per minute. It was 72 beats per minute 4 hours ago. What is the **most** important action for the LPN/LVN to take?

Strategy: Think about what happens when a client's heart rate decreases significantly: Cardiac output may decrease, leading to decreased perfusion of vital organs. Determine if data collection or implementation is more important.

Category: Planning/Physiological Integrity/Physiological Adaptation

(1) Oxygen saturation levels indicate the amount of oxygen attached to the red blood cells. Are oxygen saturation levels affected by cardiac output? No.

They are affected by altered respiratory function. Eliminate.

(2) Giving supplemental oxygen may be an appropriate action, but is it the priority action? More data is needed.

(3) CORRECT: If heart rate decreases, cardiac output and blood pressure decrease, decreasing blood flow to the brain and other vital organs and increasing the risk of organ damage. Select this answer.

(4) Observing bilateral pulse strength may be an appropriate action, but is it the most important? No. The priority is to gather data related to blood flow to vital organs. Eliminate.

4. The answer is 4

A client reports to the LPN/LVN, "I just started to feel short of breath." The client has normal saline infusing at a rate of 75 mL/hour through a peripherally inserted central catheter (PICC) line. What is the **first** action the LPN/LVN should take?

Strategy: The answer choices are a mix of physiological and psychosocial, so apply Maslow: Rule out the psychosocial answers, and review the remaining options for sense and ABCs.

Category: Implementation/Physiological Integrity/ Physiological Adaptation

(1) Obtaining the client's blood pressure may be an appropriate action, but is it the first action? The client reports shortness of breath, and immediate action is needed.

(2) Reassuring the client is a psychosocial answer; eliminate.

(3) What is the outcome of this answer? Observing the site of the PICC may show if infiltration or thrombophlebitis is present.

(4) CORRECT: What happens when the client is in the upright position? Chest expansion increases and respiratory status improves.

5. The answer is 4

The LPN/LVN at the urology clinic is obtaining a health history from an elderly male client who reports back pain during urination and difficulty starting and stopping the urine flow. Which of the following goals is **most** important for the LPN/LVN to include in the client's plan of care?

Strategy: Think about the consequences of each goal in light of the client's problem with his urinary system.

Category: Data Collection/Safe and Effective Care Environment/Coordinated Care

(1) The client will not benefit from pain medication, because it will not address the cause of the discomfort during urination.

(2) Without laboratory test results, it is not known if the client has an infection, so antibiotic therapy is not warranted.

(3) Physical therapy is not indicated for urological conditions.

(4) CORRECT: The client will have a urinalysis and a serum prostate-specific antigen (PSA) testing to help diagnose the condition.

6. The answer is 3

The LPN/LVN is caring for the client whose vaginal delivery resulted in a stillborn infant. Which of the following actions by the nurse is the **most** important?

Strategy: "*Most* important" indicates a priority. Maslow's hierarchy of needs prioritizes the need for physiological survival.

Category: Implementation/Safe and Effective Care Environment/Coordinated Care

(1) Although emotional support is important, it is psychosocial; physiological needs take precedence.

(2) There is no evidence of dehydration in this client.

(3) CORRECT: The nurse should check the client's perineal pad frequently for excess bleeding. Circulation is the third of the ABCs.

(4) Checking for hemorrhaging, a physiological complication, is more important than educating about pain relief.

7. The answer is 1

The primary health care provider has ordered a condom catheter for a male client. Which of the following is the **most** important question the LPN/LVN should ask the client before carrying out this order?

Strategy: Determine why you would ask each question.

Category: Data Collection/Safe and Effective Care Environment/Coordinated Care

(1) CORRECT: A latex allergy would preclude the use of some condom catheters.

(2) Research has shown that condom catheters cause fewer urinary tract infections than indwelling urinary catheters.

(3) After the primary health care provider has ordered the condom catheter, the client's voiding pattern is not an issue.

(4) Circumcision is not a contraindication to use of a condom catheter.

8. The answer is 2

The client is about to be discharged home with a portable oxygen delivery system. The LPN/LVN knows that which of the following education topics is **most** important for the client's family?

Strategy: "*Most* important" indicates a priority. Consider the outcome of each answer choice.

Category: Implementation/Safe and Effective Care Environment/Coordinated Care

(1) Treatment education is important, but basic physical safety takes priority.

(2) CORRECT: Flame or any source of heat, such as a lit cigarette, candle, or space heater, could cause a fatal fire in the presence of an oxygen delivery system.

(3) The risk of fire must be taught before addressing any concern about relaxation.

(4) Education about basic physiological needs is important, but warning about the risk of a fatal fire takes priority.

9. The answer is 1, 4, 5, 6, and 9

CORRECT OPTIONS: Clients may develop right-sided, left-sided, or "both sided" heart failure. Left-sided heart failure develops when the left ventricle is unable to pump blood to the body and backs up into the lungs. Classic signs of left-sided failure include **dyspnea**, **orthopnea**, **frothy sputum**, and **crackles** (rales). Other signs include fatigue, poor skin color, coolness, and weak pulses. Due to the decreased cardiac output, renal perfusion decreases, leading to **elevations in creatinine** and decreased urinary output.

INCORRECT OPTIONS: Right-sided failure develops when the right ventricle is unable to pump blood forward resulting in backflow into the right atrium and venous congestion. Clinical manifestations of right-sided failure include generalized edema, jugular vein distention, hepatomegaly, ascites, and decreased bowel sounds.

10. The answer is 2, and 3

CORRECT OPTIONS: Chronic kidney disease (CKD) is the progressive loss of kidney function. The most common causes of CKD are **hypertension** and **diabetes mellitus**; this is due to damage to the glomerulus caused by vascular injury (hypertension) and uncontrolled hyperglycemia.

INCORRECT OPTIONS: Gout and lumbar radiculopathy are not risk factors for the development of CKD. Clients with CKD may develop peripheral vascular disease, but it does not cause CKD.

11. See explanation for answers

Hyperglycemia: Clinical manifestations of hyperglycemia develop secondary to fluid losses associated with the effects of elevated glucose on kidney function. Fluid losses result in **poor skin turgor**. The clinical manifestations are similar to hypernatremia and include elevated temperature, **thirst (polydipsia)**, and **weakness**.

Hyperkalemia: Clinical manifestations of hyperkalemia include **diarrhea** caused by increased intestinal motility, and **paresthesias** and **weakness** that are caused by changes in nerve conduction. Bradycardia, sinus arrest, heart block, and ventricular dysrhythmias are associated with hyperkalemia.

Hypernatremia: In hypernatremia, water losses in the body lead to **poor skin turgor** as well as elevated sodium levels. Clinical manifestations of hypernatremia include elevated temperature, tachycardia, **thirst**, and **weakness**.

12. See explanation for answers

CORRECT OPTIONS: Elevated potassium levels affect the cardiac electrical conduction. Bradycardia, sinus arrest, heart block, and ventricular dysrhythmias are associated with hyperkalemia. **Cardiac dysrhythmias secondary to hyperkalemia** are potentially life threatening. These dysrhythmias are typically observed when **the potassium level exceeds 6 mEq/L (6 mmol/L)**. If hyperkalemia is not treated, it may progress to cardiac arrest.

INCORRECT OPTIONS: In this client, hyperkalemia is probably correlated with oliguria, not polyuria. Seizures are not a complication of hyperkalemia, but may be observed with hyponatremia and hyperglycemia. Clinical manifestations of elevated chloride are similar to hypernatremia and include fatigue, weakness, intense thirst, and dry mucous membranes. Elevated creatinine is observed in clients with kidney insufficiency or kidney failure as the kidneys are unable to clear creatinine.

13. The answer is 4

CORRECT OPTION: **Sodium polystyrene** lowers serum potassium levels by causing an exchange of sodium for potassium in the gastrointestinal tract that leads to excretion of potassium.

INCORRECT OPTIONS: Spironolactone is a potassium-sparing diuretic and is not indicated as it may further increase the potassium levels. Corticosteroids (e.g., prednisone) are not indicated for treatment of hyperkalemia as they lead to potassium retention. Nonsteroidal anti-inflammatory medications, like naproxen, may increase serum potassium by decreasing the kidney excretion of potassium.

14. The answer is 1, 2, 5, and 6

CORRECT OPTIONS: Placing the client on a **cardiac monitor** is indicated due to the risk of cardiac dysrhythmias secondary to hyperkalemia. The administration of **IV regular insulin with dextrose** leads the shifting of potassium into the cells, particularly in hyperkalemia secondary to metabolic acidosis. **Loop diuretics** (e.g., furosemide) are potassium-wasting diuretics and lead to increased urinary excretion of potassium. The **urinary output** is monitored for potential kidney insufficiency, which can further exacerbate hyperkalemia.

INCORRECT OPTIONS: There is no indication for limiting activity, and hyperkalemia does not increase the risk of seizures.

15. The answer is 2, 4, 5, and 6

CORRECT OPTIONS: Foods high in potassium include **bananas**, beans, **tomatoes**, **potatoes**, dried fruit, **melons**, **oranges**, and starchy vegetables. **Eggs** are not high in potassium.

INCORRECT OPTIONS: Grapes and apples are not high in potassium and are encouraged on a potassium-restricted diet. Table salt is composed of sodium chloride and is not contraindicated with hyperkalemia. However, most salt substitutes are composed of potassium and are therefore contraindicated or limited for this client.

CHAPTER 6

STRATEGIES FOR COORDINATION OF CARE QUESTIONS

The delivery of health care in the United States is an ever more integrated system, utilizing the skills of physicians; advanced practice nurses (e.g., nurse practitioners [NPs]); registered nurses (RNs); licensed practical nurses (LPNs), also called licensed vocational nurses (LVNs); and unlicensed assistive personnel (UAPs) such as certified nursing assistants (CNAs), nursing assistants, and home health aides. Each position carries its own duties and responsibilities, but coordination of all the members of the health care team is essential for the delivery of optimal care to the client. This chapter discusses the coordination of care, especially as it pertains to LPN/LVNs.

Many health care settings, including hospitals, clinics, and physician and NP private practices, are staffed by RNs and LPN/LVNs, in addition to NPs and UAPs. In most situations, it is the responsibility of the RN to coordinate the care ordered by the physician and to assign specific duties to LPN/LVNs and UAPs according to the level of knowledge and skills they possess and their legal scope of practice as set by state regulations. (In those situations in which NPs are present, the task of assigning duties to RNs and/or LPN/LVNs may fall to them.) The individual state boards of nursing set the standards that, for the most part, vary little and comply with the National Council of State Boards of Nursing (NCSBN).

In this chapter, we'll discuss the actions that the LPN/LVN is qualified to perform. We'll also review the general scope of practice of LPN/LVNs and RNs, as well as the roles of NPs and APs. You'll see questions interspersed in the discussion to illustrate the general guidelines with specific cases.

Licensed Practical Nurse/Licensed Vocational Nurse (LPN/LVN)

An LPN/LVN has specific education and skills and is licensed to work in a health care setting under the supervision of a primary health care provider, dentist, podiatrist, or, most commonly, an RN (or NP). The role of the LPN/LVN is defined by the theoretical and clinical content taught in practical/vocational nursing programs within each state and approved by the individual state board of nursing/regulatory body.

Scope of Practice/Role of the LPN/LVN

Each state has a specific scope of practice for LPN/LVNs. Under the supervision of an RN, LPN/LVNs provide care for stable clients and perform procedures with predictable outcomes.

The LPN/LVN is often the bedside nurse, providing care to stable clients. LPN/LVNs monitor vital signs, collect data, obtain lab specimens (urine, sputum, wound), monitor intake and output, check blood glucose levels, apply dressings, insert and care for indwelling urinary catheters as well as nasogastric tubes, empty Jackson-Pratt (JP) drains, maintain oxygen protocols, and administer prescribed medications. Some states restrict the administration of intravenous (IV) medications and solutions by LPN/LVNs.

Many of the duties of an LPN/LVN involve data collection. The LPN/LVN is taught to distinguish normal from abnormal findings when observing clients (for example, normal versus abnormal heart sounds) and to recognize changes from previously recorded data (for example, a sudden drop in blood pressure). The data, especially abnormal findings and changes in clinical findings, are reported to an RN (or primary health care provider) to provide the necessary information for client care.

The LPN/LVN does not perform an initial client assessment; that is the responsibility of the supervising RN (or primary health care provider). However, after the initial assessment has been made and a plan of care initiated, the LPN/LVN may collect data, reporting the findings to the supervising RN. In general, the LPN/LVN carries out the plan of care developed by or in collaboration with the RN.

LPN/LVNs may also be involved in reinforcing client teaching, such as educating pregnant women about childbirth and the care of an infant. LPN/LVNs may also practice "telephone nursing," using protocols developed by a primary health care provider. The protocols state what information to request of a caller, what to tell the caller, and how to direct the caller to proceed, depending on the condition for which the person is calling.

In some states, LPN/LVNs, with additional education and certification, may have an expanded role in IV therapy and hemodialysis under the supervision of an on-site RN. NCSBN's PN Detailed Test Plan states the LPN/LVN can monitor an IV infusion and infusion site, including a blood transfusion after the first 15 minutes; hang or change a bag of IV fluid to an existing IV line; administer IV piggyback (secondary) medications; and discontinue a peripheral IV line and perform site care. *Note: The specific situations, medications, and procedures that the LPN/LVN may perform are outlined by state and facility regulations.*

Also, in some states, LPN/LVNs assume the care of specific clients utilizing an overall plan of care developed by the RN. This situation most often arises in cases where rapid changes are not expected in the client's condition. The LPN/LVN may be assigned to monitor the client regularly while the RN is available for consultation and periodic monitoring. In long-term care facilities, the LPN/LVN may assume the "charge nurse" role with consultation of an in-house supervising RN.

Specifically, LPN/LVNs:

- Provide emotional and physical comfort for the client.
- Carry out the client plan of care initiated by the RN.
- Observe a client's signs and symptoms and report any changes to the supervising RN.
- Perform nursing procedures for which the LPN/LVN has the necessary skills and training, such as routine bedside care, data collection, dressing changes, indwelling urinary catheter insertion and care, respiratory care and suctioning, ostomy care, and medication administration.
- May assist RNs in the care of seriously ill clients in intensive care units, delivery rooms, neonatal units, etc.
- Assist with the rehabilitation of clients according to the client's plan of care.
- Provide post mortem care, but do not pronounce a client dead in most states.

LPN/LVNs may have the knowledge and training to perform additional interventions in some states, but the NCLEX® focuses on actions the LPN/LVN can perform in all states.

Let's look at a question that focuses on the scope of practice and roles of the LPN/LVN.

> Which client-care activity is appropriate for an LPN/LVN to perform?
>
> 1. Obtain detailed 24-hour diet recall from client newly admitted with a suspected eating disorder.
> 2. Obtain catheterized urine sample from client with a fever and mild lower abdominal discomfort.
> 3. Collect data for an adolescent client who is experiencing an acute asthma attack.
> 4. Care for a school-age client with a new tracheostomy for laryngotracheal bronchitis.

Strategy: Remember that LPN/LVNs perform activities concerning stable clients with predictable outcomes.

(1) A 24-hour diet history is an important part of the initial assessment of a client with suspected anorexia nervosa or other eating disorder. It helps guide the treatment plan. RNs, not LPN/LVNs, provide the initial clinical assessment. Eliminate this answer choice.

(2) LPN/LVNs routinely collect catheterized urine samples. It is a routine procedure that the LPN/LVN is qualified to perform. Keep this answer choice for consideration.

(3) An adolescent client experiencing an acute asthma attack is unstable. The care of such an unstable client with an uncertain outcome would not normally be assigned to an LPN/LVN. Eliminate this answer choice.

(4) A school-age client with a new tracheostomy for laryngotracheal bronchitis is unstable and, therefore, needs the assessment and care of an RN. Eliminate this answer choice.

The correct answer is (2).

Registered Nurse (RN)

The RN is responsible for the quality of nursing care, including the assessment of nursing needs, the planning of nursing care and its implementation, the monitoring and evaluation of the plan, and the supervision of LPN/LVNs.

Scope of Practice/Roles of the RN

The RN is responsible and accountable for making decisions based on their knowledge, competency, experience, and use of nursing processes; compliance with state laws and regulations; practice within the scope of practice for RNs in their specific state; and awareness of the scope of practice for LPN/LVNs. The decisions made must afford quality nursing care to clients and may include the assignment of specific duties to other qualified personnel (e.g., LPN/LVNs) and the appraisal of the care given by these assigned caregivers. Assignment of specific duties is essential if proper care is to be provided.

Specific responsibilities of the RN include:

- Assessing, evaluating, and making nursing judgments. These tasks cannot be delegated or assigned to LPN/LVNs or other members of the health care team.

- Assigning specific tasks to LPN/LVNs and other personnel for stable clients with predictable outcomes. If the client is unstable or the outcome of a specific procedure is unknown, the RN should personally monitor the client.

- Assigning standard activities involving unchanging procedures, such as feeding and bathing a stable client, to the appropriate member of the health care team. Feeding, bathing, and dressing a stable client are usually assigned to a UAP, while bedside monitoring following the client's individual plan of care is usually assigned to an LPN/LVN.

Coordination with LPN/LVNs

RNs and LPN/LVNs have a unique and delicate relationship within the health care setting. Although the RN assigns the LPN/LVN specific care or tasks for a specific client, the RN is ultimately responsible for the work of the LPN/LVN and how it affects the client. At the same time, the RN must recognize that LPN/LVNs are licensed by their state board of nursing or regulatory body and have completed a program of study that qualifies them to perform certain tasks and to have certain responsibilities. The LPN/LVN provides client care based on their own license.

The degree of supervision the RN exercises over the LPN/LVN is based on an evaluation of the condition of the client; of the education, skill, and training of the LPN/LVN; and of the nature of the tasks being assigned to the LPN/LVN. The supervision of the RN, physically present in the health care facility, may be a direct continuing presence or an intermittent observation and direction.

The next question may help you understand how this works in practice.

The LPN/LVN should question which assignment?

1. Obtain a stool sample for occult blood.
2. Provide nutrition information to a new mother.
3. Adjust the position of a client who has just received medication for pain relief.
4. Assess a client who has just returned to the room following abdominal surgery.

---

(1) Obtaining a stool sample is a routine procedure and thus can be performed by an LPN/LVN. Eliminate this answer choice.

(2) Providing nutrition information to a new mother is within the scope of practice of an LPN/LVN. Eliminate this answer choice.

(3) Positioning a client is within the scope of practice of an LPN/LVN. Eliminate this answer choice.

(4) An LPN/LVN cannot perform the initial assessment of a client following surgery. This is outside the scope of practice of an LPN/LVN.

The correct answer is (4).

Roles of Other Members of the Health Care Team

Let's briefly outline the roles of other possible members of the health care team. As an LPN/LVN, you may find yourself working with any or all of the following professionals:

- **Nurse practitioners (NPs)** are RNs with advanced education and training; in most states, NPs can diagnose illnesses and prescribe medications. If present in the health care setting, the NP would supervise both the RN and the LPN/LVN, or just the RN who, in turn, would assign duties to the LPN/LVN.

- **Unlicensed assistive personnel (UAPs)** include both certified nursing assistants (CNAs), who are regulated by the state boards of nursing, and nursing assistive personnel (NAPs) including nursing assistants and home health aides. UAPs aid RNs and LPN/LVNs by performing routine duties, such as feeding and bathing stable clients. Obtaining specific supplies requested by the LPN/LVN or RN for the care of a client would also be part of the duties of a UAP.

Answer the next question based on what you have learned about coordination of care and the duties of each member of the health care team.

> The nursing unit contains an RN, an LPN/LVN, and a UAP. Which client-care activity would be **most** appropriate for the LPN/LVN to perform?
>
> 1. Obtain vital signs for a client who was admitted with several fractures.
> 2. Monitor a client who had an ovarian tumor removed 2 days ago for signs of infection.
> 3. Teach a client recently diagnosed with diabetes mellitus to perform an insulin injection.
> 4. Bathe and change the clothes of a client who is recovering from an appendectomy.

(1) "Obtain vital signs for a client who was admitted with several fractures." This client is not in a stable condition and needs assessment, part of which is obtaining vital signs. An RN needs to provide the initial assessment. Eliminate this answer choice.

(2) "Monitor a client who had an ovarian tumor removed 2 days ago for signs of infection." LPN/LVNs are trained to observe a client for changes in signs and symptoms, such as an increase in temperature or other signs of infection, and to report the changes to the supervising RN. Keep this answer choice for consideration.

(3) "Teach a client with newly diagnosed diabetes mellitus to perform an insulin injection." This is not within the scope of practice of an LPN/LVN. An RN performs this type of teaching. Eliminate.

(4) "Bathe and change the clothes of a client who is recovering from an appendectomy." While an LPN/LVN could be asked to help in this situation, a UAP is more likely to be asked to perform this duty. An LPN/LVN is licensed, with specific education and training, so their services could probably be better used in another way. Eliminate.

The correct answer is (2). Although the LPN/LVN could be asked to perform the duties listed in answer choice (4), that assignment would not be the *most* appropriate.

The following is another question to help you understand coordination of care.

> Which client-care assignment is **best** for an LPN/LVN?
>
> 1. Help a client who is recovering from surgery with bathing, linen change, and ambulation to the bathroom.
> 2. Perform a head-to-toe assessment, including breath sounds, for a client admitted yesterday with pneumonia.
> 3. Assess a newly admitted client with a high fever and productive cough.
> 4. Change the dressing for a stasis ulcer in a client with diabetes mellitus.

(1) A UAP would normally be the person to help bathe and ambulate a client as well as change bed linen. Eliminate this answer choice.

(2) LPN/LVNs routinely collect head-to-toe data, including breath sounds, for stable clients. As this client is recently admitted, however, the RN should do the assessment. Eliminate this answer choice.

(3) RNs provide initial clinical assessment for newly admitted clients. Eliminate this answer choice.

(4) LPN/LVNs are qualified to change dressings in stable clients. This is the best client-care assignment.

The correct answer is (4).

Coordination of Care Questions

Here are a few more questions to test your understanding of coordination of care.

> Which client-care activity should be assigned to an LPN/LVN?
>
> 1. Auscultate breath sounds and collect sputum sample from a client with a history of respiratory problems.
> 2. Assess a client just returned from surgery to correct a spinal deformity.
> 3. Provide emergency care to a client who suffered cardiac arrhythmia during exercise.
> 4. Care for an unconscious client who is bleeding profusely from a stab wound.

(1) An LPN/LVN can auscultate breath sounds, report the findings to the RN, and collect a sputum sample for analysis. Keep this answer choice for consideration.

(2) Immediate postoperative assessment is the responsibility of the RN, especially in such a serious case as spinal surgery. The RN may subsequently ask the LPN/LVN to monitor the client, directing the LPN/LVN to be alert for specific signs/symptoms. Eliminate this answer choice.

(3) In most states, providing emergency care is outside LPN/LVN scope of practice. When LPN/LVNs are employed in emergency departments, they usually assist the RN or primary health care provider, following specific instructions. Eliminate this answer choice.

(4) An unconscious client who is bleeding profusely from a stab wound is in unstable condition and has an unpredictable outcome. An LPN/LVN does not routinely provide care for such an unstable client. Eliminate this answer choice.

The correct answer is (1).

> Which client-care activity should be assigned to an LPN/LVN?
>
> 1. Assess a new admission who is reporting severe abdominal pain.
> 2. Review the education on birthing methods provided to a pregnant client.
> 3. Provide bedside care for an infant client with a fever and obvious discomfort.
> 4. Change the dressing of a client who has undergone a partial mastectomy.

(1) Obtaining a complete assessment on a newly admitted client is the responsibility of an RN. Eliminate this answer choice.

(2) While an LPN/LVN may reinforce teaching to a pregnant client on birthing methods, only an RN can evaluate the effectiveness of the teaching. Eliminate this answer choice.

(3) Fever in an infant is a serious concern that requires careful assessment and frequent monitoring, tasks that should be performed by an RN. Eliminate this answer choice.

(4) LPN/LVNs are qualified to look for changes in the appearance of a wound and to change dressings as part of their overall monitoring of a stable client recovering from surgery. Keep this answer choice for consideration.

The correct answer is (4).

Health care in the United States involves ever more sophisticated tests, techniques, and treatments and is subject to budget constraints and frequent understaffing. It thus requires the coordination of care among licensed and unlicensed members of the health care team. Each member of the team must be called upon to contribute specific knowledge and skills so that an integrated personalized plan of care for each client is implemented. It is very important to utilize the specific education, training, and skills of an LPN/LVN, who provides bedside care for stable clients under the supervision of an RN. Doing so frees the RN to perform assessment, nursing diagnosis, development and implementation of a plan of care, and evaluation. At the same time, the assignment of time-consuming routine tasks, such as bathing and feeding stable clients, to a UAP allows the licensed members of the team to maximize the use of their skills.

An understanding of the coordination of care is essential for an LPN/LVN and for other members of the health care team. The efficient use of each member's specific knowledge and skills allows the pursuit of a common goal—the best care possible for the client.

Chapter Quiz

1. The LPN/LVN is part of the care team in a medical-surgical unit. The LPN/LVN would expect to perform which of the following client-care activities? **(Select all that apply.)**

    1. Educate the presurgical client about clean-catch urine sample procedures.

    2. Assess the client who has just returned to the room following bladder surgery.

    3. Monitor the client who had a tonsillectomy the day before.

    4. Call a code on the client found to be unresponsive.

    5. Review the effectiveness of client education about nebulizer use.

    6. Perform the initial dressing change on the client recovering from gallbladder surgery.

2. The LPN/LVN is caring for clients in the acute medical-surgical unit. The LPN/LVN should question which assignment?

    1. Monitor urine output of the client diagnosed with acute kidney injury.

    2. Perform nasotracheal suctioning for a client 4 days after a stroke.

    3. Provide tracheostomy care for the client with a cuffed tracheostomy tube.

    4. Receive hand-off report for the client being transferred from the emergency department.

Refer to the Case Study to answer the next question.

The LPN/LVN on an orthopedic unit provides care for a young adult client following surgical repair of multiple fractures of the pelvis and left lower extremity.

History	Nurse's Notes	Vital Signs

28-year-old client was involved in a motorcycle accident and sustained multiple fractures of the left leg and pelvis two days ago. The client sustained a compound fracture of the left tibia, a transverse fracture of the left upper femur, as well as a non-displaced simple fracture of the left superior pubic ramus. The client underwent open reduction and internal fixation of both fractures, and had placement of a long leg cast. The client sustained several abrasions and lacerations to the left arm and torso, and bruising to the left arm and side of the face. However, no fractures or other injuries were detected in radiological studies. Head and neck films clear.

The client has no notable medical history. No previous surgeries. The client takes no medications and has no known allergies. The client smokes 1 pack of cigarettes a day, and admits to ingestion of beer and other alcoholic beverages 1 or 2 times per week. Client is married with one child and is employed as a mechanic. Spouse is present at the bedside.

History	Nurse's Notes	Vital Signs

0730: Received change of shift report. Client has been receiving hydromorphone 2 mg IV every 4 – 6 hours for pain rated 7/10 on 10 point pain scale. Pain is located in left hip and thigh area, and left side of chest. Client has been alert, fully oriented, and cooperative with care. Vital signs have been stable. Afebrile. Skin warm and dry. Diffuse bruising present on left side of face, left wrist, and chest. Lungs clear. Using incentive spirometer to 2500 mL; non-productive cough. SpO_2 98% on room air. S1 S2 audible with no murmurs or gallops. Pedal pulses +3 bilaterally. Capillary refill less than 2 seconds on all extremities. Abdomen soft with active bowel sounds throughout. Client has been eating a regular diet. Voiding clear yellow urine to urinal. IV D5 lactated ringers (LR) at 80 mL/hour to right forearm. Left leg cast intact and left leg elevated on pillows. Client's spouse in room and unlicensed assistive personnel (UAP) present to obtain vital signs and help assist client with breakfast.

0845: UAP calls for assistance. Client is in apparent distress. Sitting up in semi-Fowler position, rapid respirations, clutching chest and reporting substernal chest pain. Client is calling for spouse and does not appear to recognize spouse who is in the room. Spouse says that client was becoming very "mean and agitated" the last few minutes, and the spouse thought the client might be in pain. Client is oriented to person and place, but not time or situation. Lungs auscultated and fine crackles noted in bases. Client has developed a light petechial rash on the central portion of the chest. Vital signs obtained.

History	Nurse's Notes	Vital Signs

Vital Signs	Results 0730	Results 0845
Temp (axillary)	99.2° F (37.3° C)	100.4° F (38° C)
BP	128/70	150/88
HR	80	112
RR	14	26
SpO_2	98% (room air)	88% (room air)

3. The LPN/LVN is reviewing the client's assessment data and vital signs.

   Complete the diagram by dragging from the choices below to specify what condition the client is most likely experiencing, 2 actions the LPN/LVN takes to address that condition, and 2 **priority** parameters the LPN/LVN monitors to assess the client's progress.

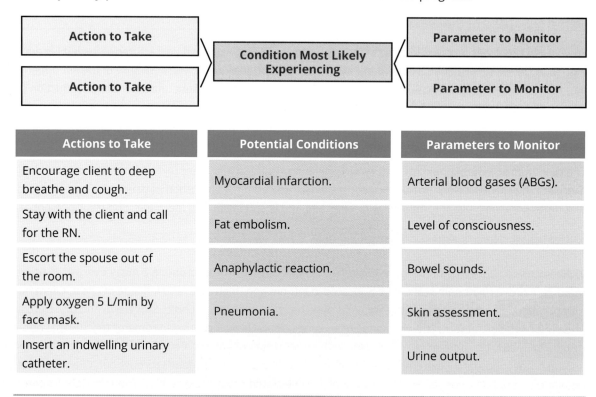

Actions to Take	Potential Conditions	Parameters to Monitor
Encourage client to deep breathe and cough.	Myocardial infarction.	Arterial blood gases (ABGs).
Stay with the client and call for the RN.	Fat embolism.	Level of consciousness.
Escort the spouse out of the room.	Anaphylactic reaction.	Bowel sounds.
Apply oxygen 5 L/min by face mask.	Pneumonia.	Skin assessment.
Insert an indwelling urinary catheter.		Urine output.

4. Which task is **most** appropriate for the unlicensed assistive personnel (UAP) to perform?

1. Reset a client's IV infusion pump when the alarm sounds.
2. Change a peripheral IV catheter insertion site dressing.
3. Observe pH of gastric secretions from enteral feeding tube.
4. Assist with the insertion of a small-bore enteral tube.

5. The LPN/LVN is caring for clients in a pediatric urgent care clinic. The supervisor indicates that the LPN/LVN will float to an adult postoperative care unit. Which is the **most** appropriate statement the LPN/LVN should make?

1. "I can't go to another unit. I don't have the proper skills to care for postoperative adult clients."
2. "I will have to work under the supervision of another LPN/LVN while on the postoperative care unit."
3. "I will need to inform the postoperative unit supervisor that my experience has been pediatric care."
4. "I am only qualified to check vital signs and document intake and output on the postoperative care unit."

6. The LPN/LVN is floating to several units in the community hospital. Which of the following client-care activities is **best** for the LPN/LVN?

1. Assisting a postsurgical client with ambulation to the bathroom.
2. Checking with family members about the effectiveness of discharge teaching.
3. Instructing newly admitted client about diagnostic test preparation.
4. Changing the purulent dressing of a client with a stage 4 pressure injury.

7. The LPN/LVN is caring for clients in the medical-surgical unit of the acute care facility. Which assignment is **most** appropriate for the LPN/LVN?

1. Observe a client who reports "tightness in the chest"; a 12-lead ECG is ordered.
2. Teach a client newly diagnosed with type 2 diabetes; the client is prescribed glyburide.
3. Change sterile dressing on the leg of a client 3 days after peripheral vascular surgery.
4. Instruct a client diagnosed with heart failure about exercise and home medications.

8. The LPN/LVN is working in the oncology unit at the pediatric hospital. Which of the following assignments, if made by the team leader, should be questioned by the LPN/LVN?

1. Providing information on chemotherapy to a parent.
2. Transporting a newly admitted client to the radiology department.
3. Finding a comfortable position for a client with post-treatment nausea.
4. Responding to a call light from a concerned parent.

9. The LPN/LVN is working in the endocrinology clinic. The LPN/LVN knows that which of the following client-care activities should be performed only by an RN?

1. Taking the medical history of the client with diabetic neuropathy.
2. Using a glucometer to test the blood glucose level of the newly diagnosed diabetic.
3. Teaching the newly diagnosed diabetic to perform an insulin injection.
4. Administering an insulin injection to the newly diagnosed diabetic.

Refer to the Case Study to answer the next six questions.

The LPN/LVN is caring for a 56-year-old client in the orthopedic unit. The staff working on the unit includes 2 RNs, 3 LPNs, and 2 unlicensed assistive personnel (UAPs).

⌐ History and Physical ⌐

History: Client is postoperative day 2 following right knee replacement. History of osteoarthritis, hypertension, hyperlipidemia, and diabetes mellitus type 2.

Body System	Findings
Neurological	Alert and oriented × 3.
Eye, Ear, Nose, and Throat (EENT)	Normocephalic, denies sore throat, nasal congestion, or vision changes. No swelling or drainage visualized.
Pulmonary	Denies shortness of breath and cough. Lung sounds clear throughout.
Cardiovascular	S1 and S2 heart sounds auscultated. Denies chest pain. Skin is warm to the touch, capillary refill < 3 seconds. No edema and peripheral pulses 2+, equal bilaterally. #18 gauge peripheral venous catheter to left forearm to saline lock. Dressing intact. Site without redness or edema.
Gastrointestinal	Reports nausea at this time and vomiting × 1 this morning. Bowel sounds active × 4 quadrants. Reports bowel movement (BM) 4 days ago.
Genitourinary	Voiding without complications.
Musculoskeletal	Full range of motion against resistance. Sitting in bedside recliner. Right knee incision clean, dry, and approximated. Incision site with redness, no swelling.

10. The LPN/LVN reviews the client's history and physical.

    Highlight below the findings that require follow-up.

Body System	Findings
Cardiovascular	<u>S1 and S2 heart sounds auscultated</u>. Denies chest pain. Skin is warm to the touch, capillary refill < 3 seconds. No edema and peripheral pulses 2+, equal bilaterally. <u>#18 gauge peripheral venous catheter to left forearm to saline lock</u>. Transparent dressing intact. Site with slight redness; no edema.
Gastrointestinal	<u>Reports nausea at this time and vomiting × 1 this morning</u>. Bowel sounds active × 4 quadrants. <u>Reports bowel movement (BM) 4 days ago</u>.
Genitourinary	Voiding without complications.
Musculoskeletal	Full range of motion against resistance. Sitting in bedside recliner. <u>Right knee incision clean, dry, and approximated.</u> <u>Redness noted to incision site, no swelling.</u>

History and Physical	Physican's Orders

- Vital signs every 4 hours.
- Encourage sips of clear liquids.
- Ambulate in halls 4 times daily and PRN.
- Instruct client on at-home therapy and care for knee replacement.
- Bisacodyl 10 mg suppository per rectum once daily PRN constipation.
- Ondansetron 4 mg IV every 4 hours PRN nausea.

11. The LPN/LVN reviews orders from the physician with the RN assigned to the client.

   For each order, specify if the order can legally be implemented by the RN, LPN/LVN, or a UAP. Each order may be implemented by more than one team member. **Each column must have at least 1 response option selected.**

Order	RN	LPN/LVN	UAP
Vital signs every 4 hours.	☐	☐	☐
Ambulate in halls 4 times daily and PRN.	☐	☐	☐
Instruct client on at-home therapy and care for knee replacement.	☐	☐	☐
Ondansetron 4 mg IV every 4 hours PRN nausea.	☐	☐	☐
Bisacodyl 10 mg suppository once daily PRN constipation.	☐	☐	☐

12. The LPN/LVN talks with the UAP about the client's care.

   Complete the following sentences by choosing from the list of options.

   The LPN/LVN can delegate [Select from list 1] to the UAP. The LPN/LVN can also instruct the UAP to [Select from list 2]. The LPN/LVN will need to [Select from list 3].

(1)	(2)	(3)
vital signs	administer the bisacodyl suppository	restart the client's IV
home care instruction	assist the client to ambulate in the hall	perform surgical incision care
care of the IV site	assess the client's abdomen	teach the client about signs and symptoms of an infection

13. The client falls while ambulating with the UAP. The LPN/LVN and RN are notified and the client is assessed.

For each client finding below, specify the potential nursing interventions that are appropriate for the care of the client. **Each client finding may support more than 1 potential nursing intervention.**

Client Finding	Potential Nursing Interventions
2 cm laceration with scant bleeding to right forearm.	☐ The LPN/LVN will apply pressure with sterile gauze. ☐ The UAP will notify the physician. ☐ The RN will cleanse skin around laceration.
Ecchymosis and swelling to right shoulder.	☐ The LPN/LVN will immobilize the joint to prevent movement. ☐ The RN will request an order for an X-ray of the shoulder. ☐ The UAP will complete an incident report.
Small amount of emesis to client's chest and gown.	☐ The LPN/LVN will administer ondansetron IV push. ☐ The UAP will bathe the client and change the client's gown. ☐ The UAP will provide mouth care.

14. The client's x-ray is negative for fracture or dislocation.

The LPN/LVN is performing a dressing change to the client's forearm laceration. Which action does the LPN/LVN delegate to the UAP?

1. Apply sterile gauze to the laceration site.
2. Teach the client about care of the laceration.
3. Hand over supplies during the dressing change.
4. Assess client's peripheral pulse after dressing application.

15. The LPN/LVN reinforces teaching to the client regarding laceration care. Which client statement indicates the need for **further** education? **(Select all that apply.)**

1. "If I notice a change in color or increased amount of drainage, I should let the doctor know."
2. "I should keep the wound clean and dry to promote healing."
3. "If I experience pain, I can apply a heat pack to the wound."
4. "If the wound is itchy in a couple days, I need to come to the emergency department."
5. "Once a scab has formed over the wound, I can keep it open to air."
6. "It is important for me to clean the wound with hydrogen peroxide every day."

Chapter Quiz Answers and Explanations

1. The answer is 1, 3, 4, and 6

The LPN/LVN is part of the care team in a medical-surgical unit. The LPN/LVN could expect to perform which of the following client-care activities? (**Select all that apply.**)

Strategy: Think about the skill level involved in each client-care activity.

Category: Implementation/Safe and Effective Care Environment/Coordinated Care

(1) CORRECT: The LPN/LVN can educate pre- and postsurgical clients about laboratory test sample collection procedures.

(2) Performing the initial assessment of a client following surgery is outside the scope of LPN/LVN practice. An RN would perform this task.

(3) CORRECT: LPN/LVNs are trained to observe stable clients for changes indicating complications. One day after a tonsillectomy, the client would be considered in stable condition.

(4) CORRECT: LPN/LVNs can call a code on an unresponsive client.

(5) The LPN/LVN can provide medication instruction, but only an RN can evaluate the effectiveness of the teaching.

(6) CORRECT: LPN/LVNs are qualified to examine a surgical incision for problems as part of their overall monitoring of stable postsurgical clients. The LPN/LVN is caring for clients in the acute medical-surgical unit.

2. The answer is 4

The LPN/LVN is caring for clients in the acute medical-surgical unit. The LPN/LVN should question which assignment?

Strategy: Remember that LPN/LVNs perform activities concerning stable clients with predictable outcomes. LPN/LVNs can reinforce teaching after RN has done initial teaching. Be careful! You are looking for an incorrect action.

Category: Evaluation/Safe and Effective Care Environment/Coordinated Care

(1) Monitoring urine output is within LPN/LVN scope of practice. LPN/LVNs can monitor urine output and report observations to the RN. Eliminate.

(2) Providing nasotracheal suctioning for this client is within LPN/LVN scope of practice. LPN/LVNs can do nasotracheal suctioning in stable clients with predictable outcomes. Eliminate.

(3) Providing tracheostomy care for this client is within LPN/LVN scope of practice. LPN/LVNs can do tracheostomy care in stable clients with predictable outcomes. Eliminate.

(4) CORRECT: Receiving hand-off report is not within LPN/LVN scope of practice. Also, a client that is being admitted to the client care area from the emergency department is unstable and requires assessment and evaluation by an RN. LPN/LVNs care for stable clients with predictable outcomes.

3. See explanation for answers

Potential Condition	
Fat embolism.	☑

CORRECT OPTION: The client's history and symptoms are highly suggestive of **fat embolism.** The client is young and sustained long bone and pelvic fractures. The rapid change in the client's personality and level of orientation, coupled with chest pain, tachypnea, hypoxia, tachycardia, and low-grade fever, are suggestive of fat embolism syndrome (FES).

INCORRECT OPTIONS: The symptoms of myocardial infarction are not usually as sudden and severe as FES. The client may report intense chest pain, but there is usually not an immediate change in the level of consciousness or development of a petechial rash. A client experiencing an anaphylactic reaction might have sudden symptoms of respiratory distress, but there is no indication the client was receiving medications at the time of the incident. Anaphylactic rashes may be on the trunk but are not usually petechial. A client who is experiencing anaphylaxis is more likely to have wheezes and stridor, not fine crackles. This client may develop pneumonia, but the sudden development of respiratory symptoms is indicative of embolism.

Actions to Take	
Stay with the client and call for the RN.	☑
Apply oxygen 5 L/min by face mask.	☑

CORRECT OPTIONS: The client's symptoms and vital signs indicate the client is in respiratory distress, so the LPN/LVN must think ABCs (airway, breathing, circulation). The client's SpO$_2$ has fallen dramatically, so the **LPN/LVN should quickly apply oxygen**. The LPN/LVN should also **stay with the client and either call the RN to the room** or have the UAP get the RN to come to the room. If a Rapid Response Team is available, they should be notified, along with the client's physician. However, the LPN/LVN's priority is to support the airway and obtain the RN's assistance.

INCORRECT OPTIONS: Having the client deep breathe and cough will not help the situation. The client needs more aggressive assistance. If the client's spouse needs support or needs to leave the room, the UAP can be assigned to that task. The client will likely need strict monitoring of intake and output and may need an indwelling urinary catheter, but not at this time.

Parameters to Monitor	
Arterial blood gases (ABGs)	✓
Level of consciousness	✓

CORRECT OPTIONS: It is crucial that respiratory status and neurologic status are carefully monitored when a client develops a fat embolism. Treatment for FES is supportive. The client may become extremely hypoxemic and develop acute respiratory distress syndrome. Monitoring the client's **ABGs** can help determine what kind of support the client needs to prevent respiratory failure. The client's neurologic status can quickly deteriorate to coma and the client can develop seizures, so it is very important to monitor the **client's level of consciousness.**

INCORRECT OPTIONS: The client with FES can develop dysfunction of the microcirculation and thrombocytopenia. This can cause such issues as bowel infarction and acute kidney failure. While it is important to monitor bowel sounds and urine output, neither takes precedence over respiratory and neurologic monitoring. The petechial skin rash is due to issues with microcirculation; it is asymptomatic and there is no treatment, so monitoring the skin is not a priority.

4. The answer is 4

Which task is **most** appropriate for the unlicensed assistive personnel (UAP) to perform?

Strategy: Remember that UAPs can assist clients with activities of daily living and perform standard, unchanging procedures.

Category: Evaluation/Safe and Effective Care Environment/Coordinated Care

(1) Resetting a client's IV infusion pump alarm requires assessment and evaluation; it is not within UAP scope of practice. Eliminate.

(2) Changing a peripheral IV catheter insertion site dressing is not within UAP scope of practice. Eliminate.

(3) Observing the pH of gastric secretions requires assessment and evaluation; it is not within UAP scope of practice. Eliminate.

(4) CORRECT: Assisting with the insertion of a small-bore enteral tube is within UAP scope of practice. UAPs may assist with procedures.

5. The answer is 3

The LPN/LVN is caring for clients in a pediatric urgent care clinic. The supervisor indicates that the LPN/LVN will float to an adult postoperative care unit. Which is the **most** appropriate statement the LPN/LVN should make?

Strategy: Remember that skills are transferable during the care of clients. Float nurses should know and be able to perform core competencies in the new unit to meet legal obligations as an LPN/LVN.

Category: Implementation/Safe and Effective Care Environment/Coordinated Care

(1) Skills are transferable. The LPN/LVN should be familiar with and prepared to perform core competencies. Eliminate.

(2) Rules of delegation should be followed. The LPN/LVN should inform the supervisor of previous experience and request an orientation. Eliminate.

(3) CORRECT: The LPN/LVN should inform the supervisor of previous experience and request an orientation.

(4) Float nurses should know and be able to perform core competencies on the new unit to meet legal obligations as an LPN/LVN. Eliminate.

6. The answer is 3

The LPN/LVN is floating to several units in the community hospital. Which of the following client-care activities is **best** for the LPN/LVN?

Strategy: *"Best"* indicates that discrimination is required to answer the question.

Category: Implementation/Safe and Effective Care Environment/Coordinated Care

(1) An unlicensed assistive personnel (UAP) would be an appropriate member of staff to assist a postsurgical client to the bathroom.

(2) Evaluating the effectiveness of discharge teaching is within the scope of RN practice, not LPN/LVN duties.

(3) CORRECT: LPN/LVNs are trained to provide client education and physical preparation for diagnostic tests.

(4) LPN/LVNs are qualified to change dressings in stable clients. A client with a stage 4 pressure injury is not considered stable.

7. The answer is 3

The LPN/LVN is caring for clients in the medical-surgical unit of the acute care facility. Which assignment is **most** appropriate for the LPN/LVN?

Strategy: Remember that LPN/LVNs perform activities concerning stable clients with predictable outcomes. LPN/LVNs can reinforce teaching after an RN has done the initial teaching.

Category: Planning/Safe and Effective Care Environment/Coordinated Care

(1) This client is not stable and requires assessment and evaluation by an RN.

(2) The LPN/LVN can reinforce initial teaching done by an RN.

(3) CORRECT: The LPN/LVN can administer prescribed therapies such as dressings.

(4) The LPN/LVN can reinforce initial teaching done by an RN.

8. The answer is 1

The LPN/LVN is working in the oncology unit at the pediatric hospital. Which of the following assignments, if made by the team leader, should be questioned by the LPN/LVN?

Strategy: "Should be questioned" signals you to look for an outlier. Identify the assignment that is beyond the scope of practice of the LPN/LVN.

Category: Planning/Safe and Effective Care Environment/Coordinated Care

(1) CORRECT: The RN is the team member who would communicate information about chemotherapy.

(2) Although transportation is often assigned to unlicensed assistive personnel (UAPs), an LPN/LVN would not need to question this task.

(3) LPN/LVNs are knowledgeable about positioning options.

(4) LPN/LVNs routinely answer call lights.

9. The answer is 3

The LPN/LVN is working in the endocrinology clinic. The LPN/LVN knows that which of the following client-care activities should be performed only by an RN?

Strategy: Look at each answer choice in terms of the appropriate scope of practice. You are looking for an answer that is outside that scope.

Category: Implementation/Safe and Effective Care Environment/Coordinated Care

(1) LPN/LVNs are trained to take medical histories.

(2) LPN/LVNs are trained to use glucometers to obtain accurate blood glucose readings.

(3) CORRECT: Teaching a newly diagnosed diabetic to perform insulin injections is not within the scope of LPN/LVN practice. An RN performs this type of teaching.

(4) LPN/LVNs are trained in insulin injection techniques.

10. See explanation for answers

Body System	Findings
Cardiovascular	S1 and S2 heart sounds auscultated. Denies chest pain. Skin is warm to the touch, capillary refill < 3 seconds. No edema and peripheral pulses 2⁺, equal bilaterally. #18 gauge peripheral venous catheter to left forearm to saline lock. Transparent dressing intact. Site with slight redness; no edema.
Gastrointestinal	Reports nausea at this time and vomiting × 1 this morning. Bowel sounds active × 4 quadrants. Reports bowel movement (BM) 4 days ago.
Genitourinary	Voiding without complications.
Musculoskeletal	Full range of motion against resistance. Sitting in the bedside recliner, at this time. Right knee incision clean, dry, and approximated. Redness noted to incision site, no swelling.

CORRECT OPTIONS: **Nausea with vomiting** and **constipation** are common in the postoperative period; however, they should be managed adequately to identify and prevent a postoperative ileus. The client has not had a BM since prior to surgery. The fact that bowel sounds are active is a positive sign, but further investigation is necessary to determine if the client is experiencing flatus or if the client is constipated.

INCORRECT OPTIONS: S1 and S2 heart sounds are normal findings. If IV fluids are discontinued, the client would have the IV converted to a saline lock to retain IV access as needed. Right knee incision clean, dry, and approximated is a desired outcome. Redness to the incision site in the first few days is normal. Local inflammation to promote wound healing causes vasodilation and red appearance.

11. See explanation for answers

RN: The RN is responsible for any actions that require clinical judgment, assessment, and teaching. The RN is able to perform all of the interventions listed.

LPN/LVN: The LPN/LVN can provide care to a stable client with predictable outcomes. The LPN/LVN is able to obtain vital signs, ambulate the client, and administer medications. However, the LPN/LVN cannot administer an IV push medication or provide initial teaching or instruction.

UAP: The UAP can perform interventions that have a standard procedure. The UAP can take vital signs and ambulate the client in the hall. The UAP cannot administer medications and cannot provide teaching or instruction.

12. See explanation for answers

The LPN/LVN can delegate standard procedures to the UAP; in this case, taking **vital signs** and **assisting with ambulation** can be performed by the UAP. INCORRECT OPTIONS: Home care instruction requires the judgment of the RN and is not appropriate delegation. Additionally, care of the IV site and medication administration do not fall within the scope of practice of the UAP.

The LPN/LVN is able to administer rectal medications, **perform incision site care or dressing changes**, and monitor the client's IV site. INCORRECT OPTIONS: The RN would restart the client's IV, if needed, and teach the client about signs and symptoms of a surgical site infection. The LPN/LVN can reinforce teaching and instruction presented by the RN. Only the RN can assess the client's abdomen; the LPN/LVN can neither take this action nor delegate it to the UAP.

13. See explanation for answers

2 cm laceration with scant bleeding to right forearm: Hemostasis is the first step in wound healing and **applying pressure** will promote this in a new laceration. Additionally, **ensuring the skin is clean will prevent infection**. The RN or LPN/LVN could provide this care. INCORRECT OPTION: If the physician needs to be notified, the RN would perform that action, not the UAP.

Ecchymosis and swelling to right shoulder: Ecchymosis and swelling are visible signs of potential tissue damage. **Immobilizing the shoulder will prevent further injury** until an x-ray is performed to determine the full extent of the damage. The LPN/LVN may immobilize the shoulder, and **the RN should call the physician to obtain an order for an x-ray**. An **incident report will need to be completed** due to the client's witnessed fall and subsequent injuries. The UAP witnessed the fall and may complete the incident report.

Small amount of emesis to client's chest and gown: In order to maintain skin integrity, it is important to **keep the skin clean and dry and change the client's gown**. The UAP can assist the client with this. It is important to provide **mouth care** to the client who has vomited. The UAP can provide this care. INCORRECT OPTION: It would be beneficial to administer an antiemetic to prevent further nausea and vomiting. Because it is an IV push medication, the RN, not the LPN/LVN, needs to perform this action.

14. The answer is 3

CORRECT OPTION: It is within the UAP's scope of practice to **assist the LPN/LVN with a dressing change by handing over supplies.**

INCORRECT OPTIONS: Applying sterile gauze requires in-depth knowledge of maintaining sterility. Teaching and assessment are not appropriate to delegate to the UAP as these require nursing judgment and should be performed by the RN.

15. The answer is 3, 4, and 6

CORRECT OPTIONS: The client's statements indicate further education is needed. Pain with a healing wound is not uncommon; **applying heat will bring more blood flow to the area and could increase pain**. It is also **common for clients to experience itching with healing skin**, so coming to the emergency department is unnecessary. **Hydrogen peroxide can cause tissue destruction** and should not be used to clean a laceration. The client should use mild soap and water.

INCORRECT OPTIONS: The client understands the instructions and does NOT need further education. During wound healing, a change in color or increased amount of drainage could indicate infection and would be important to report to the physician. Correct wound care includes keeping the skin clean and dry by allowing it to remain open to air, if the skin is approximated.

[CHAPTER 7]

STRATEGIES FOR POSITIONING QUESTIONS

Because many illnesses affect body alignment and mobility, you must be able to safely care for these clients in order to be an effective LPN/LVN. These topics are also important on the NCLEX-PN® exam. The successful test taker must correctly answer questions about impaired mobility and positioning.

Immobility occurs when a client is unable to move about freely and independently. To answer questions on positioning, you need to know the hazards of immobility, normal anatomy and physiology, and the terminology for positioning.

Many graduate LPN/LVNs are not comfortable answering these questions because:

- They don't understand the "whys" of positioning.
- They don't know the terminology.
- They have difficulty imagining the various positions.

If you have difficulty answering positioning questions, the following strategy will assist you in selecting the correct answer.

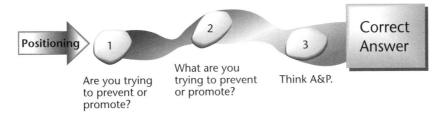

STEP 1. Decide if the position for the client is designed to prevent something or promote something.

STEP 2. Identify what it is you are trying to prevent or promote.

STEP 3. Think about anatomy, physiology, and pathophysiology ("A&P").

STEP 4. Which position best accomplishes what you are trying to prevent or promote?

Does this sound a little confusing? Hang in there.

Let's walk through a question using this strategy.

> Immediately after a percutaneous liver biopsy, the LPN/LVN should place the client in which position?
>
> 1. Supine.
> 2. Right side-lying.
> 3. Left side-lying.
> 4. Semi-Fowler.

Before you read the answers, let's go through the four steps.

STEP 1. By positioning the client after a liver biopsy, are you trying to prevent something or promote something? Think about what you know about a liver biopsy. You position a client after this procedure to prevent something.

STEP 2. What are you trying to prevent? The most serious and important complication after a percutaneous liver biopsy is hemorrhage.

STEP 3. Think about the principles of A&P. What do you do to prevent hemorrhage? You apply pressure. Where would you apply pressure? On the liver. Where is the liver? On the right side of the abdomen under the ribs.

STEP 4. How should the client be positioned to prevent hemorrhage from the liver, which is on the right side of the body? Look at your answer choices.

(1) Supine. If you lay the client flat on the back, no pressure will be applied to the right side. Eliminate.

(2) Right side-lying. If you lay the client in a right side-lying position, will pressure be applied to the right side? Yes. Keep it in for consideration.

(3) Left side-lying. No pressure is applied to the right side. Eliminate.

(4) Semi-Fowler. If you lay the client on the back with head partially elevated, no pressure is applied to the right side. Eliminate.

The correct answer is (2). Some students select (3) because they don't know normal anatomy and physiology. Some students select (4) because semi-Fowler position is used for so many different reasons.

Things to Remember

- Even if you didn't memorize what position to use before, during, and after a procedure, think about the question for a moment. You can figure out what position is needed.

- You cannot figure out the correct position if you do not know what the terms (such as *supine* or *Fowler*) mean.

- You cannot figure out a correct position if you do not know anatomy and physiology. If you think the liver is on the left side of the body, you are in trouble!

- You cannot figure out a correct position if you do not know what you are trying to accomplish. If you couldn't remember that a complication after a liver biopsy is hemorrhage, you will simply be taking a random guess at the correct answer.
- If you think in images, you should form a mental image of each position. Picture yourself placing the client in each position, and then see if the position makes sense.

Let's try another question using the strategies for positioning.

> An angiogram is scheduled for a client with decreased circulation in the right leg. After the angiogram, the LPN/LVN should place the client in which position?
>
> 1. Semi-Fowler with right leg bent at the knee.
> 2. Side-lying with a pillow between the knees.
> 3. Supine with right leg extended.
> 4. High Fowler with right leg elevated.

Let's go through the steps.

STEP 1. By positioning the client after an angiogram, are you trying to prevent something or promote something? You are trying to promote something.

STEP 2. What are you trying to promote? Adequate circulation of the right leg.

STEP 3. Think about the principles of A&P. What promotes adequate circulation in the right leg? Keeping the leg at or below the level of the heart so blood flow is not constricted.

STEP 4. How will the client be positioned after an angiography to prevent constriction of vessels and keep the right leg at or below the level of the heart? Look at the answer choices.

(1) "Semi-Fowler with the right leg bent at the knee." The head of the bed is elevated 30–45 degrees in this position. The leg is lower than the heart. If the right leg is bent at the knee, this could constrict arterial blood flow. Eliminate.

(2) "Side-lying with a pillow between the knees." Use of a pillow in this position could create pressure points in the right leg. You don't want the knees bent. Eliminate.

(3) "Supine with leg extended." In this position, the leg is at the level of the heart. Circulation will not be constricted because the leg is straight. Keep this answer in for consideration.

(4) "High-Fowler with right leg elevated." The head of the bed is elevated 60–90 degrees in this position. Elevating the leg promotes venous return. Eliminate.

The correct answer is (3). The client is on bed rest for 8–12 hours in a supine position after an angiogram.

If you didn't know the specific positioning needed after an angiogram, you could apply your knowledge to select the correct answer by just thinking about it.

Let's look at another question.

> The LPN/LVN is caring for a client after a lumbar laminectomy. Which statement **best** describes the method of turning a client following a lumbar laminectomy?
>
> 1. The head of the bed is elevated 30 degrees; the client locks the knees when turning.
> 2. A pillow is placed between the client's legs; the body is turned as a unit.
> 3. The client straightens the back and grasps the side rail on the opposite side of the bed.
> 4. The head of the bed is flat; the client bends the knees and rolls to the side.

This question isn't about positioning after a procedure. It asks how to turn the client after surgery.

STEP 1. When turning the client after a laminectomy, are you trying to prevent or promote something? Promote.

STEP 2. What are you trying to promote? A straight back. The client can't bend or twist the torso.

STEP 3. Think about the principles of anatomy, physiology, and pathophysiology (A&P). A laminectomy is removal of one or more vertebral laminae. After a laminectomy, the back should be kept straight.

STEP 4. How should the client be turned in order to keep the back straight?

(1) If the head of the bed is elevated 30 degrees, the back will not be straight. Eliminate.

(2) If a pillow is placed between the legs and the body is rolled as a unit, the client's back will be kept straight. Keep in for consideration.

(3) If the client grabs the opposite side rail, the client's torso will twist. The back will not be straight even though the client straightened the back before turning and twisting. Eliminate.

(4) If the head of the bed is flat, the client's back will be straight. If the client bends the knees and rolls to the side, the back will not be kept straight. Eliminate.

The correct answer is (2). That is a textbook description of log-rolling. But if you didn't recall log-rolling, you were able to select the correct answer by thoughtfully considering each answer choice.

Sometimes a positioning question will be difficult to identify, such as in the following example.

> The LPN/LVN is caring for a client after an appendectomy. The client continues to report discomfort to the nurse shortly after receiving an analgesic. Which measure by the LPN/LVN would be **most** appropriate?
>
> 1. Notify the primary health care provider
> 2. Place the client in Fowler position.
> 3. Massage the client's abdomen.
> 4. Provide the client with reading material.

As you can see, not all of the answer choices involve positioning. How should you approach this question?

First, reword the question so that you know what to focus on in the answer choices. The question really being asked is, "What should the LPN/LVN do to help this client with pain relief?" Let's look at the answer choices.

(1) Notifying the primary health care provider, as you know, is almost never the right answer. See if another answer choice is more appropriate.

(2) Fowler position. Why change this client's position? To promote pain relief. Will Fowler position decrease the client's pain? Yes, by relieving pressure on the client's abdomen. This answer is a possibility.

(3) Massaging the client's abdomen will increase the client's pain. Eliminate.

(4) Providing the client with reading materials might distract the client from discomfort, but this is not an appropriate intervention for a client in pain. Eliminate.

The correct answer is (2).

Positioning is an important part of the NCLEX-PN® exam. You must be able to answer these questions correctly in order to prove your competence. If you use the strategies just discussed, you will be thinking about nursing principles and you will select correct answers!

Essential Positions to Know for the NCLEX-PN® Exam

POSITION	THERAPEUTIC FUNCTION
Flat (supine)	Avoids hip flexion, which can compress arterial flow
Dorsal recumbent	Supine with knees flexed; more comfortable
Side lateral	Allows drainage of oral secretions
Side with leg bent (Sims)	Allows drainage of oral secretions; used for rectal exam
Head elevated (Fowler) • High Fowler: 60–90 degrees • Fowler: 45–60 degrees • Semi-Fowler: 30–45 degrees • Low Fowler: 15–30 degrees	Increases venous return; allows maximal lung expansion
Feet and legs elevated	Increases blood return to heart
Feet elevated and head lowered (Trendelenburg)	Used to insert central venous pressure (CVP) line, or for treatment of umbilical cord compression
Feet elevated 20 degrees, knees straight, trunk flat, and head slightly elevated (modified Trendelenburg)	Increases venous return; may be used to prevent shock
Elevation of extremity	Increases venous return; decreases blood volume to extremity
Flat on back, thighs flexed, legs abducted (lithotomy)	Increases vaginal opening for examination
Prone	Promotes extension of hip joint; not well tolerated by persons with respiratory or cardiovascular difficulties
Knee-chest	Provides maximal visualization of rectal area

Chapter Quiz

1. The LPN/LVN is caring for a client diagnosed 6 months ago with a 6th thoracic (T6) spinal cord injury. The client reports a "throbbing headache," and the client's face, neck, and upper chest are flushed and diaphoretic. Which action should the LPN/LVN take **first**?

    1. Loosen the client's upper body clothing.
    2. Check the client for fecal impaction.
    3. Remove the indwelling urinary catheter.
    4. Sit the client in an upright position.

2. The LPN/LVN is assisting with the care of a client diagnosed 2 weeks ago with a right-sided stroke. When assisting the client with meals, it is **most** important for the LPN/LVN to take which action?

    1. Encourage the client to swallow each bite of food 4 times.
    2. Assist the client to use a straw to drink fluids with the meal.
    3. Instruct the client to sit in a chair for 30 minutes after the meal.
    4. Provide 8 oz (240 mL) of milk with every meal and at bedtime.

3. The LPN/LVN is assisting with the care of a client 48 hours after a right total hip arthroplasty. Which observation requires an intervention by the LPN/LVN?

    1. The client is positioned in a high Fowler position during meal times.
    2. The right and left legs are slightly abducted when client is supine.
    3. The head of the bed is elevated 50 degrees during morning oral care.
    4. The unlicensed assistive personnel (UAP) places a pillow between client's legs before turning client.

Refer to the Case Study to answer the next question.

| History | Nurse's Notes |

Older adult client with history of osteoarthritis, chronic obstructive pulmonary disease (COPD), and anxiety. Underwent right total knee replacement yesterday afternoon. Client tolerated surgery well, pain well controlled with oral hydrocodone/acetaminophen, 7.5/325 mg and ice packs to knee. Pulmonologist managing oxygenation and home medications. Client currently awake, alert, and fully oriented on oxygen at 2L/min per nasal cannula with SpO_2 93–95%. Has been very pleasant and cooperative with post-operative instructions. Using incentive spirometer hourly while awake. Lung sounds diminished but clear with non-productive cough. Right knee dressing intact and dry. Bulb suction drain removed this morning. Client eating a regular breakfast with no nausea, voiding clear yellow urine to bedside commode. Active bowel sounds; passing flatus. Plan to discharge to skilled nursing facility later this afternoon. Physical therapy to ambulate client and instruct in walker use.

| History | Nurse's Notes |

1000: Physical therapy ambulating in hall with client and instructing client on walker use. Client states, "It feels good to be out of bed, but I may need some pain medication when I get back to my room!" Client using portable oxygen while ambulating. Slight dyspnea with exertion.

1045: Client back to bed. Requested pain medication for "throbbing" right knee pain, rated 6/10. Hydrocodone/acetaminophen, 7.5 mg/325 mg PO given for pain.

1130: Entered room to bring client's lunch tray. Client attempting to ambulate to bathroom with walker. Client wearing socks with no shoes and holding cell phone in one hand. Client watching feet carefully. Client has removed oxygen in order to ambulate and is diaphoretic, with RR 22 and shallow. Client instructed to ask for assistance before getting out of bed. Portable oxygen placed on client and client assisted to bathroom.

1145: Client rings bathroom alarm for assistance. Discovered client pulling up on walker to stand from being seated on toilet. Client states, "I needed to get up, and I couldn't wait any longer." Peri care provided and client assisted back to bed.

4. The LPN/LVN reviews the client's history and the nurse's notes and prepares to provide care to the client.

Complete the diagram by dragging from the choices below to specify what condition the client is **most** likely experiencing, 2 areas of education the LPN/LVN will reinforce, and 2 client statements that indicate the client needs **further** education.

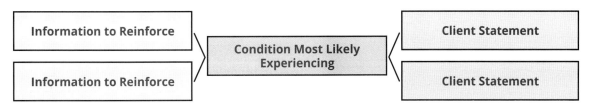

Information to Reinforce	Potential Conditions	Client Statements
Use the walker very carefully to pull up to standing from sitting on a toilet or chair.	Hearing deficit.	"I will take a step forward only when all four legs of the walker are level on the ground."
Avoid using the walker when you are short of breath.	Knowledge deficit.	"I should lock my arms when putting my weight on the walker."
When using the walker on stairs, grip the handles firmly.	Noncompliance.	"When walking, I will lean forward over the walker and look down to make sure my feet don't slip on anything."
Wear sturdy, non-skid shoes while walking.	Dementia.	"When I step forward, I should move my right leg first, followed by my left."
Use a bag or pouch on the walker to hold items.		"I will lift the walker up and place it 2–3 inches (5.1–7.6 cm) in front of me, then walk toward it."

5. The LPN/LVN in the long-term care facility is assisting the client with chronic obstructive pulmonary disease and varicose veins. Before breakfast is served, the LPN/LVN places the client in Fowler position. Which of the following **best** describes why Fowler position would be used in this client?

    1. It straightens the neck, which allows client to swallow more effectively.
    2. It pulls the diaphragm downward, which permits greater chest expansion.
    3. It puts the back in a natural position, which relieves muscle tension.
    4. It increases venous return, which improves the circulation to the legs.

6. The LPN/LVN is preparing the client with hemorrhoids for a rectal examination. Depending on the physical limitations of the client, the nurse should put the client in which of the following positions? **(Select all that apply.)**

    1. Prone.
    2. Supine.
    3. Knee-chest.
    4. Trendelenburg.
    5. Sims.
    6. Fowler.

Refer to the Case Study to answer the next six questions.

The LPN/LVN is providing care to an older adult client on a medical-surgical unit.

| Admission Notes | Nurse's Notes |

The client is admitted from home for evaluation of findings related to the right lower leg. The client is accompanied by an adult child. For the past 24 hours the client has been experiencing unilateral right lower leg swelling, with 3+ pitting edema. Additionally, there is tenderness, erythema, and warmth of the right posterior calf. The client lives with the adult child, who reports, "My parent had a viral respiratory illness three weeks ago and was confined to bed for about four days." The client and adult child also recently returned from a long car trip in which the client was immobile and sitting for prolonged periods without exercise.

Past history includes type 2 diabetes, hypertension, coronary artery disease (CAD), osteoarthritis, and varicose veins. Home medications:

- Hydrochlorothiazide 25 mg PO every day.
- Losartan 25 mg PO every day.
- Metformin 500 mg PO every day.
- Atorvastatin 20 mg PO every day.

| Admission Notes | Nurse's Notes |

Assessment	Client Finding
General	Appears chronically ill. Slightly agitated.
Neurological	Awake, alert, oriented × 4. PERRL.
Integument	Skin intact, pale, warm, and dry.
Cardiovascular	S_1 and S_2, regular rhythm, no murmurs. Capillary refill less than 2 seconds. 2+ radial pulses, equal. Right lower leg with erythema and 3+ pitting edema. Tender, warm posterior right calf upon palpation. Left leg no edema, 2+ pedal pulses.
Respiratory	Bronchovesicular breath sounds bilaterally. Non-labored breathing.
Abdomen	Soft, rounded, non-tender. Normoactive bowel sounds.
Musculoskeletal	Moves all extremities. Right hip and knee joint pain and stiffness. Muscle strength, 4/5 bilaterally.

Vital Signs/Pain/BMI	Results
BP	118/80 mmHg
Heart rate	112, regular
Respiratory rate	20, regular
Temperature (oral)	98.9° F (37.16° C)
Pulse oximetry	96% on room air
Pain score (0/10)	5/10 right lower leg
Body Mass Index (BMI)	32 kg/m^2 (obese)

7. The LPN/LVN reviews the admission notes and the nurse's notes.

    Which **4** client findings concern the LPN/LVN?

    1. Pain 5/10 right lower leg.
    2. Heart rate 112, regular.
    3. Temperature 98.9° F (37.16° C).
    4. Tender, warm posterior right calf upon palpation with 3+ pitting edema.
    5. Recent period of prolonged immobility.
    6. Right hip and knee joint pain and stiffness.
    7. Bronchovesicular breath sounds.

8. Complete the following sentence by choosing from the list of options.

    The client is at risk for developing [Select from list 1] due to [Select from list 2] and [Select from list 3].

(1)	(2)	(3)
peripheral arterial disease	osteoarthritis	immobility
deep vein thrombosis	thrombocytopenia	intermittent claudication
diabetes-related neuropathy	obesity	hyperlipidemia

9. The LPN/LVN recognizes that deep vein thrombosis (DVT) increases the client's risk to develop which complication?

    1. Pneumothorax.
    2. Polycythemia vera.
    3. Severe anemia.
    4. Pulmonary embolism.

10. The client's diagnostic venous duplex ultrasound is positive for right leg deep vein thrombosis below the knee. The client is prescribed the anticoagulant, rivaroxaban, 15 mg PO twice a day with food.

Drag the choices below to fill in each blank in the following sentence. Each choice will only be used once.

The LPN/LVN and the RN develop the plan of care with goals to _____ [Select from the list], _____ [Select from the list], and _____ [Select from the list].

provide pain relief
restore fluid balance
teach medication safety
supplement dietary protein
reduce the risk for bleeding

11. Which action does the LPN/LVN implement while caring for the client? **(Select all that apply.)**

1. Encourage use of soft bristle toothbrushes and electric razors.
2. Report changes in blood pressure, heart rate, respiratory rate, and pulse oximetry to the RN.
3. Reinforce that reddish color urine and darker stools are expected effects of rivaroxaban.
4. Reinforce teaching about the dosage, action, and effects of rivaroxaban therapy.
5. Instruct to use the call light before getting out of bed.
6. Encourage frequent ambulation and repositioning as prescribed.
7. Administer pain relief medications by subcutaneous or intramuscular injections.
8. Elevate legs and remind the client to perform frequent flexion and extension of feet and legs while awake.

12. On the day of discharge, the LPN/LVN reviews the client findings documented by the RN.

Which findings indicate that nursing care has been effective? Highlight correct sections.

Documentation	Client Findings
Client Statements	"I understand I need to make big changes to eating leafy greens and salad due to my new medication." "Setting a timer when I'm home will help me remember to get up and move around."
Vital signs	Pain score 2/10 Heart rate 88, regular
Cardiovascular	Right lower leg 1+ edema No erythema or warmth of right lower leg
Respiratory	Bronchovesicular breath sounds bilaterally No adventitious lung sounds
Client activity	Uses call light for assistance to ambulate in hall × 3 Keeps legs dependent when sitting in chair

13. The home-care LPN/LVN is visiting the frail client with type 2 diabetes, osteoporosis, and nighttime drooling. The client sleeps in the prone position. The nurse recognizes which of the following as an advantage of this position for the client? **(Select all that apply.)**

    1. It allows full extension of the hip and knee joints.
    2. It produces lordosis in most people.
    3. It causes plantar flexion.
    4. It keeps saliva drainage flowing from the mouth.
    5. It promotes better breathing.
    6. It prevents hypoglycemia.

14. The LPN/LVN in the postsurgical unit cares for the client immediately after an L4-L5 spinal fusion. The primary health care provider's order calls for the client to be turned every hour. Arrange the following steps in the order that the nurse should perform them. **All options must be used**.

    1. Place the pillow between the client's legs.
    2. Remove the pillow from under the client's head.
    3. Perform hand hygiene.
    4. Document the client's repositioning.
    5. Firmly grasp the client's draw sheet with both hands.
    6. Move the client's body as a unit.

15. The LPN/LVN is caring for the obstetrical client who is in active labor. Suddenly the fetus's umbilical cord can be seen protruding from the vagina. The LPN/LVN will immediately place the client in which of the following positions?

    1. Trendelenburg.
    2. Sims.
    3. Prone.
    4. Semi-Fowler.

Chapter Quiz Answers and Explanations

1. The answer is 4

The LPN/LVN is caring for a client diagnosed 6 months ago with a 6th thoracic (T6) spinal cord injury. The client reports a "throbbing headache," and the client's face, neck, and upper chest are flushed and diaphoretic. Which action should the LPN/LVN take **first**?

Strategy: As you can see, not all the answers involve positioning. Read the question and answers to identify the topic, and note the level of the spinal cord injury. What complication of spinal cord injury do these symptoms describe? Autonomic dysreflexia is a potential complication when a client has a spinal cord injury of T6 or above. The topic is the *first* action to take when autonomic dysreflexia is suspected.

Autonomic dysreflexia is an emergency. Immediate action must be taken to prevent severe hypertension and a stroke. Think about which action will decrease blood pressure most quickly.

Category: Implementation/Physiological Integrity/ Reduction of Risk Potential

(1) Loosening the upper body clothing is an appropriate action when autonomic dysreflexia occurs, but is it the first action? Keep for consideration.

(2) Checking for fecal impaction is an appropriate action, as fecal impaction may be a cause of autonomic dysreflexia. The impaction should be removed, but is it the first action? Keep for consideration.

(3) Removing the indwelling urinary catheter is an appropriate action. Bladder distension may be a cause of autonomic dysreflexia. If the catheter is obstructed, it should be removed. Is this the first action? Keep for consideration.

(4) CORRECT: What happens if you sit the client upright? The client's blood pressure will immediately decrease. Remember that autonomic dysreflexia is an emergency and immediate action must be taken to decrease blood pressure. This action will prevent a further increase in blood pressure. Select this answer.

2. The answer is 3

The LPN/LVN is assisting with the care of a client diagnosed 2 weeks ago with a right-sided stroke. When assisting the client with meals, it is **most** important for the LPN/LVN to take which action?

Strategy: Identify the topic of the question: All answers relate to swallowing and eating. Recall that clients diagnosed with stroke often have difficulty swallowing and are at risk for aspiration. The question asks you to select the priority, or "*Most* important" action—preventing aspiration. Consider each answer choice and determine if the action will decrease the risk of aspiration.

Category: Implementation/Physiological Integrity/ Physiological Adaptation

(1) Swallowing each bite of food more than once will help clear the oropharynx and decreases the risk of aspiration. Is it necessary for the client to swallow each bite of food 4 times? No. Eliminate.

(2) Use of a straw and drinking thin liquids both increase the risk of choking and aspiration. Thin liquids are more difficult to swallow. The risk of choking and aspiration is increased. Eliminate.

(3) CORRECT: What happens when a client sits in an upright position after a meal? Gravity increases the passage of food into the stomach. Will this help prevent aspiration? Yes. Keep for consideration.

(4) Milk and milk products increase production of saliva and make swallowing more difficult. The client is at greater risk for aspiration. Eliminate.

3.   The answer is 1

The LPN/LVN is assisting with the care of a client 48 hours after a right total hip arthroplasty. Which observation requires an intervention by the LPN/LVN?

Strategy: Identify the topic: appropriate positioning after a total hip arthroplasty. Recall the goals for clients after a total hip arthroplasty. One goal is to prevent subluxation (partial dislocation) or total dislocation of the prosthesis.

The question asks which answer *requires an intervention*. Review the answers and determine if each action is correct or incorrect. Be careful! You are looking for an incorrect action.

Category: Evaluation/Physiological Integrity/Physiological Adaptation

(1)   CORRECT: When a client is in high Fowler position, the degree of elevation is 60–90 degrees. What is the effect of this position? It increases the risk of prosthesis dislocation. This action is incorrect.

(2)   What is the effect of slight abduction of the involved hip and leg? It decreases the risk of prosthesis dislocation. This is a desired outcome.

(3)   Elevating the head 60 degrees or less does not increase the risk of prosthesis dislocation. (By contrast, if the head is elevated more than 60 degrees, the risk of subluxation and dislocation is increased.) This action is correct.

(4)   Placing a pillow between the legs while turning maintains slight abduction of the involved hip and leg. This action is correct.

4. See explanation for answers

Potential Condition	
Knowledge deficit.	☑

CORRECT OPTION: The client is most likely exhibiting a **knowledge deficit**. The client was just instructed on the use of the walker, and will need reinforcement of teaching and demonstration of learning before education can be considered effective. The client may have misunderstood. The client has a history of anxiety, and may not have fully comprehended all of the new information received. The older adult client was also medicated with an opioid analgesic, which can contribute to the client not fully understanding what was taught.

INCORRECT OPTIONS: There is no indication or information to suggest the client has a hearing deficit. The client has been alert and cooperative. Non-compliance indicates the client has the opportunity and knowledge to do what has been instructed but chooses not to do so. There may be factors, such as socioeconomic issues, that preclude a client from following a plan of care, or being non-compliant. This client was just given new information and has had very little opportunity to process it. There is no indication the client has dementia; the client is described as being alert, oriented, and cooperative.

Information to Reinforce	
Wear sturdy, non-skid shoes while walking.	☑
Use a bag or pouch on the walker to hold items	☑

CORRECT OPTIONS: The client should always wear **sturdy, non-skid shoes** with a flexible sole. A walker can provide the client with some stability to stand and walk but it will not prevent the client from slipping. In addition, the client should not try to carry anything in the hands while using the walker. The client needs both hands free. The client can **use a bag or pouch** that attaches to the walker to carry needed items like glasses, tissues, or a cell phone.

INCORRECT OPTIONS: The client should NEVER pull up on the walker to move from sitting to standing. The walker can easily tip over, causing the client to fall. The client can use the arms of a chair, grab bars, or a counter to pull up to standing from being seated, then firmly grab the hand grips of the walker. This client has a diagnosis of COPD. It is not practical to tell the client not to use the walker when short of breath. The client may need to rest and will need extension tubing for oxygen, or portable oxygen when using the walker to ambulate. The client should never use the walker on stairs. The client should have someone take the walker up or down stairs, and allow the client to use the handrails on the stairs or the assist of another person to navigate stairs.

Client Statements	
"I should lock my arms when putting my weight on the walker."	☑
"When walking, I will lean forward over the walker and look down to make sure my feet don't slip on anything."	☑

CORRECT OPTIONS: The **elbows should bend at a comfortable angle of about 15 degrees** when the client is ambulating with the walker. While ambulating, the client should **maintain an upright posture and look forward**, rather than leaning forward over the walker and looking down at the feet.

INCORRECT OPTIONS: These options indicate the client understands and does not need further teaching. The client should not advance using the walker until all four legs are firmly on the ground. The device is well balanced in this position and the client is less likely to fall. The client should step in or move the injured or surgical leg into the walker before the unaffected leg. The client can support part of the weight through the hands as the unaffected leg is brought into the walker box. The walker should be moved forward a short distance of about 2–3 inches (5.1–7.6 cm) at a time. If the client moves the walker too far forward, the client is more likely to lose balance and fall.

5. The answer is 2

The LPN/LVN in the long-term care facility is assisting the client with chronic obstructive pulmonary disease and varicose veins. Before breakfast is served, the LPN/LVN places the client in Fowler position. Which of the following **best** describes why Fowler position would be used in this client?

Strategy: *"Best"* indicates that discrimination is required to answer the question. Remember the ABCs.

Category: Implementation/Physiological Integrity/Basic Care and Comfort

(1) A client in Fowler position can use a pillow to moderately flex the neck. This would not impede, and might help, the client's swallowing ability.

(2) CORRECT: Gravity pulls the diaphragm downward, increasing space for lung expansion. The client can breathe easier.

(3) There is no "natural" back position.

(4) Fowler position promotes venous return; however, the reason this client is placed in Fowler position is to increase chest expansion to help the client breathe.

6. The answer is 3 and 5

The LPN/LVN is preparing the client with hemorrhoids for a rectal examination. Depending on the physical limitations of the client, the nurse should put the client in which of the following positions? (**Select all that apply.**)

Strategy: Visualize the client ready for the examination. Then consider each answer choice.

Category: Planning/Reduction of Risk Potential

(1) In the prone position, where the client lies on the abdomen, the rectal area cannot be readily accessed.

(2) In the supine position, where the client lies on the back, there is no access to the rectal area.

(3) CORRECT: The knee-chest position allows for visualization of the rectal area.

(4) The Trendelenburg position has the client lying on the back, which gives no access to the rectal area.

(5) CORRECT: In Sims position, the client is lying on one side with the upper leg bent. This position allows access to the rectal area.

(6) Fowler position has the client lying on the back, which gives no access to the rectal area.

7. The answer is 1, 2, 4, and 5

CORRECT OPTIONS: The LPN/LVN is concerned with abnormal clinical findings of **pain in the right lower leg, tachycardia, warmth and tenderness of the posterior right calf upon palpation, and 3+ pitting edema of that extremity**. Because of physiological changes which may occur with immobility, the LPN/LVN is also concerned with the client's **recent period of prolonged immobility.**

INCORRECT OPTIONS: The client's temperature is normal for an adult. Right hip and knee joint pain and stiffness are findings consistent with the client's history of osteoarthritis. Bronchovesicular breath sounds bilaterally and absence of adventitious (abnormal) lung sounds are normal adult respiratory assessment findings.

8. See explanation for answers

CORRECT OPTIONS: The LPN/LVN identifies the client's right lower leg findings as most likely related to **deep vein thrombosis (DVT)**. Clinical findings which may occur in DVT range from no obvious physical changes in the affected extremity to unilateral leg edema, pain, tenderness with palpation, warm skin, and erythema. Venous stasis, hypercoagulability of blood and endothelial damage (Virchow's triad) are the primary risk factors associated with DVT and venous thromboembolism (VTE). Venous stasis can occur in clients who are **obese** or are **immobile** for long periods, such as traveling on long trips without exercise.

INCORRECT OPTIONS: Peripheral arterial disease is a condition that results from narrowing of arteries in the upper and lower extremities caused by atherosclerosis. Clinical findings include intermittent claudication or ischemic muscle pain that occurs with exercise. Diabetes-related neuropathy is the loss of protective sensation in the lower extremities due to diabetes associated metabolic imbalances. Osteoarthritis, thrombocytopenia, intermittent claudication, and hyperlipidemia are not risk factors associated with DVT. Osteoarthritis is a condition that involves the loss of cartilage in the synovial joints. Impaired production, increased destruction, or abnormal distribution of platelets can lead to thrombocytopenia, a reduction of circulating platelets. Intermittent claudication is ischemic muscle pain that occurs in peripheral arterial disease. Hyperlipidemia refers to high levels of serum lipids including fats, triglycerides, and cholesterol that is a major risk factor for coronary artery disease.

9. The answer is 4

CORRECT OPTION: The LPN/LVN recognizes that DVT, a thrombus that forms in the deep veins, increases the client's risk to develop **pulmonary embolism.** A thrombus may detach from the vein wall as an embolus and move through the venous circulation to the heart and obstruct pulmonary circulation. This results in impaired or absent gas exchange in the affected area.

INCORRECT OPTIONS: Pneumothorax, polycythemia vera, and severe anemia are not complications of DVT. A pneumothorax occurs when air enters the pleural space causing the lung to collapse. Polycythemia vera is a blood disorder characterized by the presence of increased numbers of red blood and white blood cells. Polycythemia vera can lead to hyperviscosity and hypervolemia, impairing blood circulation and increasing a client's risk for DVT. Severe anemia is also a risk factor for VTE.

10. See explanation for answers

CORRECT OPTIONS: The LPN/LVN and the RN develop the of plan of care with goals to **provide pain relief, teach medication safety, and reduce risk for bleeding**. Decreasing discomfort associated with DVT is a key nursing concern and a necessary adjunct to therapy. Client and caregiver teaching regarding medication dosage, actions, and adverse effects is essential safety information to provide when a client is taking an anticoagulant. Nursing management of DVT includes actions to monitor the effectiveness and reduce the risk for bleeding associated with anticoagulant therapy.

INCORRECT OPTIONS: The plan of care does not include goals to restore fluid balance and supplement dietary protein. Examples of conditions associated with fluid imbalances include heart failure, kidney disease, gastrointestinal losses and other abnormal gains or losses of body fluids. The addition of supplemental protein would be important for wound healing but is not indicated at this time for the acute treatment of DVT.

11. The answer is 1, 2, 4, 5, 6, and 8

CORRECT OPTIONS: The LPN/LVN encourages use of **soft bristle toothbrushes and electric razors** as these minimize bleeding risk to gums and skin. **Changes in blood pressure, heart rate, respiratory rate, and pulse oximetry should be reported to the RN** because these are clinical signs that can indicate bleeding. **Reinforcing teaching about the dosage, actions, and effects of rivaroxaban therapy** is information that should be included in the teaching plan for a client receiving anticoagulant therapy. **Instructing to use the call light before getting out of bed** is a safety precaution to decrease the risk of falls and bleeding when taking an anticoagulant. **Encouraging frequent ambulation and repositioning** can result in decreased edema and limb discomfort and is effective in increasing venous flow. The LPN/LVN will **elevate the client's legs and remind the client to perform frequent flexion and extension of the feet and legs while awake**. These actions reduce the client's discomfort and increases venous flow.

INCORRECT OPTIONS: Reddish color urine and darker stools are not expected effects of treatment and may indicate bleeding. The client should be instructed to report these findings immediately. Subcutaneous and intramuscular injections should be avoided when taking anticoagulants due to the bleeding risk.

12. See explanation for answers

Documentation	Client Findings
Client Statements	"I understand I need to make big changes to eating leafy greens and salad due to my new medication." "Setting a timer when I'm home will help me remember to get up and move around."
Vital signs	Pain score 2/10 Heart rate 88, regular
Cardiovascular	Right lower leg 1+ edema No erythema or warmth of right lower leg
Respiratory	Bronchovesicular breath sounds bilaterally No adventitious lung sounds
Client activity	Uses call light for assistance to ambulate in hall × 3 Keeps legs dependent when sitting in chair

CORRECT OPTIONS: The client's statement about **setting a timer** to remind the client to get up and move around indicates client understanding about mobility and preventing venous stasis. The **pain score is improved** and the **heart rate is an accepted value** for an adult. The description of the client's **right lower leg indicates improvement** from the client's admission findings. **Bronchovesicular breath sounds bilaterally** and **absence of adventitious lung sounds** are normal adult respiratory assessment findings. The **use of the call light** to ambulate indicates client understanding of bleeding and fall precautions while taking an anticoagulant.

INCORRECT OPTIONS: The client receiving rivaroxaban should not modify the dietary intake of vitamin K or leafy green vegetables. The client's dependent leg position while in a sitting position does not promote venous flow and can contribute to venous stasis.

13. The answer is 1 and 4

The home-care LPN/LVN is visiting the frail client with type 2 diabetes, osteoporosis, and nighttime drooling. The client sleeps in the prone position. The nurse recognizes which of the following as an advantage of this position for the client? **(Select all that apply.)**

Strategy: Remember this client's characteristics and the benefits of a prone position. Consider each answer choice keeping both facts in mind.

Category: Evaluation/Physiological Integrity/Basic Care and Comfort

(1) CORRECT: Allowing full extension of the hip and knee joints is an advantage of the prone position.

(2) Producing lordosis (inward curvature of the spine) is a disadvantage, because it puts strain on the client's back.

(3) Causing plantar flexion is a disadvantage, because it overstretches the foot muscles.

(4) CORRECT: Allowing saliva drainage to flow from the mouth is an advantage of the prone position.

(5) The prone position does not promote better breathing. It inhibits chest expansion, which is a disadvantage.

(6) The prone position has no effect on the client's blood glucose level; this is neither an advantage nor a disadvantage.

14. The answer is 3, 2, 1, 5, 6, 4

The LPN/LVN in the postsurgical unit is caring for the client immediately after an L4-L5 spinal fusion. The primary health care provider's order calls for the client to be turned every hour. Arrange the following steps in the order that the nurse should perform them. **All options must be used.**

Strategy: Picture the client with a surgical wound in the lumbar region. It must not be distorted when moving the client.

Category: Implementation/Physiological Integrity/Basic Care and Comfort

(3) Perform hand hygiene.

(2) Remove the pillow from under the client's head.

(1) Place the pillow between the client's legs.

(5) Firmly grasp the client's draw sheet with both hands.

(6) Move the client's body as a unit.

(4) Document the client's repositioning.

15. The answer is 1

The LPN/LVN is caring for the obstetrical client who is in active labor. Suddenly the fetus's umbilical cord can be seen protruding from the vagina. The LPN/LVN will immediately place the client in which of the following positions?

Strategy: Consider the outcome of placing the client in each position.

Category: Planning/Reduction of Risk Potential

(1) CORRECT: The Trendelenburg position, with the client's head down, will shift the weight of the body upward, relieving pressure on the prolapsed cord.

(2) Sims position does not alter pressure on the prolapsed cord.

(3) The prone position puts pressure on the client's abdominal area.

(4) The Semi-Fowler position puts pressure on the client's vaginal area.

CHAPTER 8

STRATEGIES FOR COMMUNICATION QUESTIONS

Communication is emphasized on the NCLEX-PN® exam because it is critical to your success as a beginning practitioner. Therapeutic communication means listening to and understanding the client while promoting clarification and insight. It enables the practical/vocational nurse to form a working relationship with both the client and the health care team, using both verbal and nonverbal communication. Remember that nonverbal communication is the most accurate reflection of attitude.

Therapeutic responses include the following.

RESPONSE	GOAL/PURPOSE
Using silence	Allows the client time to think and reflect; conveys acceptance. Allows the client to take the lead in conversation.
Using general leads or broad opening	Encourages the client to talk. Indicates your interest in the client. Allows the client to choose the subject.
Clarification	Encourages recall and details of a particular experience. Encourages description of feelings. Seeks explanation; pinpoints specifics.
Reflecting	Paraphrases what client says. Reflects on what client says, especially the feelings conveyed.

Eliminate Answer Choices

There are many questions on the NCLEX-PN® exam that require you to select the correct therapeutic communication response. As with other NCLEX-PN® exam questions, one of the biggest errors that students commit when trying to answer this type of question is to look for the correct answer. Remember, you are selecting the *best* answer from the four possible answers that you are given. To select the best answer, you must eliminate answer choices. Let's look at some of the different answer choices you can eliminate:

- *"Don't worry" answers:* Eliminate answer choices that offer false reassurance. This type of responses discourages communication between the LPN/LVN and the client by not allowing the client to explore their own ideas and feelings. False reassurance also discounts what the client is feeling. Examples include:
  - "It is going to be OK."
  - "Don't worry. Your doctors will do everything necessary for your care."

- **"Let's explore" answers:** Another incorrect answer choice that many graduate practical/vocational nurses select is the choice that includes the word "explore." On the NCLEX-PN® exam, avoid being a junior psychiatrist. It isn't the practical/vocational nurse's role to delve into the reasons why the client is feeling a particular way. The client must be allowed to verbalize the fact that they are sad, angry, fearful, or overwhelmed. Examples include:
  - "Let's talk about why you didn't take your medication."
  - "Tell me why you really injured yourself."

- **"Why" questions:** Eliminate answer choices that include "why" questions: ones that seek reasons or justification. "Why" questions imply disapproval of the client, who may become defensive. A "why" question can come in many forms and need not always begin with "why." Any response that puts the client on the defensive is nontherapeutic and therefore incorrect. Examples include:
  - "What makes you think that?"
  - "Why do you feel this way?"

- **Authoritarian answers:** Eliminate answer choices in which the LPN/LVN is telling the client what to do without regard to the client's desires or feelings. Examples include:
  - Insisting that the client follow unit rules
  - Insisting that the client do what you command, immediately

- **Nurse-focused answers:** Eliminate answer choices in which the focus of the comment is on the LPN/LVN. Be careful, because these answer choices may sound very empathetic. The focus of your communication should always be on the client. Examples include:
  - "That happened to me once."
  - "I know from experience this is hard for you."

- **Closed-ended questions:** Eliminate answer choices that include closed-ended questions that can be answered with yes, no, or another monosyllabic response. Closed-ended questions discourage the client from sharing thoughts and feelings. Examples include:
  - "Are you feeling guilty about what happened?"
  - "How many children do you have?"

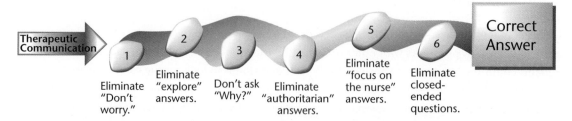

Eliminating these types of nontherapeutic responses that appear as answer choices is a very effective strategy when answering therapeutic communication questions. Don't simply look for the specific words that you see here; you may need to "translate" the answer choices into the above errors of therapeutic communication.

Select the Correct Response

So, how do you select the correct response? By choosing from the answer choices that are left! The correct response will usually contain one or both of the following elements:

- *Gives correct information.* Offering information encourages further communication from the client. Examples of giving correct information include:
  - "You are experiencing acute alcohol withdrawal; you may see and feel things that aren't real."
  - "There are many reasons for memory loss; tell me more about what you have noticed."
- *Is empathetic and reflects the client's feelings. Empathy* is the ability to perceive what another person experiences using that person's frame of reference. *Reflection* communicates to the client that the LPN/LVN has heard and understands what the client is trying to communicate. When reflecting feelings, the LPN/LVN focuses on the feelings and not the content of what is said. Examples of empathetic, reflective statements include:
  - "I can see that you are frightened about being here."
  - "You seem very upset. Tell me how you're feeling."

Let's practice with a few exam-style questions.

> A client is admitted to the telemetry unit with a diagnosis of acute myocardial infarction. The client tells the LPN/LVN, "I'm scared, I think I'm going to die." Which response by the LPN/LVN would be **most** appropriate?
>
> 1. "Everything is going to be fine. We'll take good care of you."
> 2. "I know what you mean. I thought I was having a heart attack once."
> 3. "I'll call your primary health care provider so you can discuss it."
> 4. "It's normal to feel frightened. We're doing everything we can for you."

STEP 1. Eliminate incorrect answer choices.

(1) "Everything is going to be fine. We'll take good care of you." This is a "don't worry" response. There is no acknowledgment of the client's fears. Eliminate it.

(2) "I know what you mean. I thought I was having a heart attack once." The focus of this response is on the LPN/LVN, not the client. Eliminate it.

(3) "I'll call your primary health care provider so you can discuss it." It is within the scope of nursing practice for the LPN/LVN to respond to the client's feelings. Don't pass the responsibility to the primary health care provider. Eliminate it.

(4) "It's normal to feel frightened. We're doing everything we can for you." This answer choice responds to feelings and provides information. Keep it in consideration.

STEP 2. Select an answer from the remaining choices.

One answer was not eliminated: (4). This is the correct answer. The LPN/LVN both acknowledges that the client feels frightened and provides information.

Let's try another question.

> A client is to undergo a breast biopsy. The client tells the LPN/LVN, "If I lose my breast, I know my husband will no longer find me attractive." Which response by the LPN/LVN would be **most** appropriate?
>
> 1. "You don't know if you are going to lose your breast. They are just doing the biopsy now."
> 2. "You should focus on your children right now. They are young and they need you."
> 3. "You seem to be concerned that your relationship with your husband might change."
> 4. "Why don't you wait and see what your husband's reaction is before you get upset."

STEP 1. Eliminate answer choices.

(1) "You don't know if you are going to lose your breast. They are just doing the biopsy now." This response gives false reassurance and discounts the client's feelings. Eliminate it.

(2) "You should focus on your children right now. They are young and they need you." This response is authoritarian: the LPN/LVN tells the client what to do. Eliminate it.

(3) "You seem to be concerned that your relationship with your husband might change." This response reflects the fears of the client. The response is open-ended and allows the client to express personal feelings. Keep it in for consideration.

(4) "Why don't you wait and see what your husband's reaction is before you get upset." This response dismisses the feelings that the client is experiencing and gives advice. Eliminate it.

STEP 2. Select an answer from the remaining choices.

You have eliminated three of the four answer choices. The correct answer is the only answer choice remaining, (3).

Let's look at one more question.

> A client in the psychiatric unit asks the LPN/LVN, "Am I in a special radioactive shelter? When was it last checked for radioactivity?" Which response by the LPN/LVN would be **most** appropriate?
>
> 1. "This is a hospital, and we do not have a nuclear medicine department here."
> 2. "Don't worry, you're safe. There's no radioactivity here."
> 3. "I'm sure your safety is of concern to you, but this is a hospital."
> 4. "Please share with me what makes you think there is radioactivity here."

STEP 1. Eliminate answer choices.

(1) "This is a hospital, and we do not have a nuclear medicine department here." This response provides information. Leave it in for consideration.

(2) "Don't worry, you're safe. There's no radioactivity here." This response offers false reassurances. Eliminate it.

(3) "I'm sure your safety is of concern to you, but this is a hospital." This response reflects the client's concern about safety and provides information. Keep it in for consideration.

(4) "Please share with me what makes you think there is radioactivity here." This response allows the client to verbalize, but you don't want to encourage a client with psychological problems to talk about hallucinations or delusions. Rather, you want your discussion to focus on the feelings that accompany them. Eliminate this choice.

STEP 2. Select an answer from the remaining choices.

You have more than one possible answer choice: (1) and (3). Look for the answer choice that reflects feelings and gives information. The correct answer is (3).

Strategy Recap

Here are some points to remember about selecting correct answers to therapeutic communication questions:

- No matter how confident you are about an answer choice, read all of the choices before selecting an answer.
- Even if you would never say any of the responses given in the answer choices, choose the "textbook" answer.
- When you first read the answer choices, don't look for the correct answer. Always eliminate answer choices first.

If you follow the Kaplan strategies for therapeutic communication, you will be able to select the correct answers to this question type on the NCLEX-PN® exam.

Chapter Quiz

1. The LPN/LVN is having a long discussion with a client diagnosed with diabetes who requires an amputation. At times during the conversation, the LPN/LVN continues looking at the client but becomes silent. Which of the following is the **best** advantage of this approach?

   1. It gives the client time to think and reflect on what was said.
   2. It gives the client the opportunity to end the conversation.
   3. It allows the client to recall other tasks needing attention.
   4. It prompts the client to fill in the silence with information.

2. The client says to the LPN/LVN, "I really like you and I think you really like me. Would you like to go on a date with me after I am discharged?" What is the **most** appropriate response by the LPN/LVN?

   1. "This is a hospital, and I am here to take care of you during your illness."
   2. "Why do you think I am available? I have been married for 10 years."
   3. "Our policy requires that I report this comment to the hospital administrator."
   4. "I have been asked out by clients before. I am not sure what I do to cause it."

3. The LPN/LVN is caring for a client recently diagnosed with type 1 diabetes mellitus. The client says, "I just can't believe that I am going to have to give myself shots every day." What is the **priority** statement for the LPN/LVN to make?

   1. "I have cared for people who had to learn how to inject insulin. They adapted well after time."
   2. "Do you have any family members who can help you with the daily insulin injections?"
   3. "I have to go see another client, but I want to talk with you about this. I will be right back."
   4. "Tell me more about how you plan to take care of yourself when you return home."

4. The LPN/LVN is working in the hospice unit. The client's partner approaches the nurse and says, "I won't be able to face life without my partner of over 50 years." Which of the following would be an appropriate response by the LPN/LVN? **(Select all that apply.)**

   1. "Fifty years! That's a wonderful accomplishment!"
   2. "Make every moment you have together really count."
   3. "You seem to be upset, anticipating your partner's death."
   4. "We'll make sure quality time is allotted for your goodbyes."
   5. "You should focus on the good years you have had."
   6. "I sense that you are looking ahead, to being alone."

5. The unlicensed assistive personnel (UAP) tells the LPN/LVN, "I want to change my assignment for today. I will not take care of a client diagnosed with AIDS." What is the **most** appropriate statement for the LPN/LVN to make?

   1. "Haven't you taken care of clients diagnosed with AIDS before?"
   2. "Don't worry. I have taken care of clients diagnosed with AIDS with no problem."
   3. "This is your assignment for today and you have to go through with it."
   4. "What is your understanding about care of clients diagnosed with AIDS?"

6. The client in the adolescent psychiatric unit asks the LPN/LVN, "Do you hear those voices? They sound so frightening." Which of the following responses by the LNP/LVN would be the **most** appropriate?

   1. "The voices around here sound friendly to me."
   2. "Are they men's voices or women's voices?"
   3. "I don't hear voices, but I can understand why that would scare you."
   4. "Let's turn up the volume of the music, and that will distract you."

7. Family members of the client with dementia are visiting the memory care unit for the first time. They express concern to the LPN/LVN caring for their relative about the client's unobserved wandering. Which of the following responses by the LPN/LVN would be **most** appropriate?

   1. "It's all right. We will take care of your relative's safety."
   2. "We use wrist bands that signal if clients exit our doors."
   3. "I worried about the same thing with my parent for years."
   4. "We have a superb staff-to-client ratio, so that can't happen."

8. The LPN/LVN is caring for a client 5 days after a colostomy procedure. During colostomy care, the LPN/LVN observes the client vigorously rubbing the skin around the stoma before applying the colostomy pouch. What is the **most** appropriate statement for the LPN/LVN to make?

   1. "Do you think you are ready to care for the colostomy after you go home?"
   2. "Is there a family member who can help you care for the colostomy at home?"
   3. "There is a step of colostomy care we need to review. Start at the beginning and show me how you do the care."
   4. "Do you think that you should read the written instructions about colostomy care before you try again?"

Refer to the Case Study to answer the next six questions.

The LPN/LVN in a long term care facility is providing care for an adult client with a diagnosis of end-stage liver disease (ESLD).

History and Physical

The client was diagnosed with alcoholic cirrhosis of the liver 2 years ago. The client developed severe ascites and has undergone numerous paracentesis procedures to relieve abdominal discomfort and dyspnea. Despite severe debilitation, the client has continued to drink alcohol. Two weeks ago, the client began to experience increasing abdominal girth, abdominal pain, nausea, vomiting, and shortness of breath (SOB). The client came to the emergency department (ED). The client underwent paracentesis with removal of 4 liters of ascitic fluid. Computed tomography (CT) scan of the abdomen detected numerous neoplasms in the liver, and the client was diagnosed with cancer of the liver. The client was discharged after an overnight observation.

Yesterday, the client was readmitted to the ED with gastrointestinal bleeding, acute confusion, and declining neurologic status. Ammonia level was elevated at 104.5 μg/dL (74.61 μmol/L), and the client was diagnosed with hepatic encephalopathy. Client is periodically awake and confused, calling out, but unable to converse.

The client is divorced and has no children. The client has one younger sibling who is active in the client's care. The medical team has explained that the client's condition is extremely serious and is rapidly deteriorating. The medical team discusses hospice care with the client's sibling. The sibling agrees to a hospice referral, and states that the client "has been living with me, but I cannot provide care in my home. I have to work." The client has no advance directive on file. Social services has been contacted to facilitate placement in a long term care facility as soon as the client's medical condition has stabilized.

9. The LPN/LVN reviews the client's history before providing the client's care.

    Complete the following sentences by choosing from the list of options.

    The LPN/LVN knows that in order for the client to receive hospice care, [Select from list 1]. The focus of hospice care is [Select from list 2]. It is routine for the hospice team to provide [Select from list 3].

(1)	(2)	(3)
the client must have an advance directive completed	to manage the client's symptoms	additional nursing staff for the long term care facility
the client must have insurance to pay for care	to hasten the client's death	family and spiritual support
the client's family must agree to a "Do Not Resuscitate" order	to make all decisions at end of life	legal and financial advice
two physicians must certify the client has 6 months or less to live	to keep the client sedated	24-hour care

| History and Physical | Hospice Admission |

Client admitted to hospice in long term care facility. Client's sibling is present. Client lying on hospital bed with head elevated 60 degrees. Skin color and sclerae yellow; skin hot and dry. Oral mucous membranes dry. Client opens eyes to name and will groan loudly and grimace, but does not speak clearly. Respirations labored and lung sounds diminished throughout. Heart sounds audible. Abdomen large, very protuberant. Hypoactive bowel sounds. 3+ edema in hands, forearms, lower legs, and feet. Client taking small amount of ice chips. Client is diapered and voiding moderate amount dark yellow urine. Vital signs: BP 90/62, HR 108, axillary temp 102.6° F (39.22° C), RR 22, SpO$_2$ 94% on room air.

At the request of the client's sibling, physician completes an order for "Do Not Resuscitate" for the client. The client's sibling states that the client wants to be cremated at death and has no religious affiliation. Chaplain made aware of client's preferences.

10. The LPN/LVN enters the client's room as the hospice nurse completes the initial assessment.

    Drag the choices below to fill in each blank in the following sentence. Each choice will only be used once.

    The LPN/LVN is **most** concerned about the nurse's assessment findings of _____ [Select from the list], _____ [Select from the list], and _____ [Select from the list].

| yellow skin color |
| dry oral mucous membranes |
| groaning and grimacing |
| labored respirations |
| large abdomen |
| 3+ edema |
| dark yellow urine |
| HR 108 |
| axillary temp 102.6° F (39.22° C) |

11. The LPN/LVN reviews the client's plan of care.

    Which treatment from the client's care plan will the LPN/LVN provide **first**?

    1. Administer acetaminophen 650 mg rectal suppository.
    2. Administer 0.5 mL oral liquid morphine 20 mg/mL.
    3. Provide mouth care with oral sponges and water.
    4. Change the client's diaper and provide perineal care.

History and Physical	Hospice Admission	Nurse's Notes

LPN/LVN Notes Day 4:

Client minimally responsive. Occasionally opening eyes. Does not obey commands. Skin cool and deeply jaundiced. Hands and feet mottled. Bilateral legs mottled to upper thighs. Oral mucous membranes dry. Eyes appear sunken. Respirations deep and rapid, then slow with 10–15 second periods of apnea. Client making a gurgling sound when exhaling. Client had 1 large dark bloody stool last night, and is voiding scant amounts of dark urine.

12. The LPN/LVN provides care for the client a few days later and documents findings.

    Which findings indicate the client is in the last stages of dying? Highlight correct sections.

    Client minimally responsive to any stimuli. Occasionally opening eyes. Does not obey commands. Skin cool and deeply jaundiced. Hands and feet mottled. Bilateral legs mottled to upper thighs. Oral membranes dry. Eyes appear sunken. Respirations deep and rapid, then slow with 10–15 second periods of apnea. Client making a gurgling sound when exhaling. Client had 1 large dark bloody stool last night, and is voiding very scant amounts of dark urine in diaper.

13. The client's sibling enters the room and remarks that the client "sounds terrible." The sibling is very concerned about the client's breathing and states, "My sibling needs oxygen. You nurses need to suction all of that drainage out of there!"

    Which response is therapeutic for the LPN/LVN to make? **(Select all that apply.)**

    1. "Those gurgling sounds are very difficult for family members to hear."
    2. "It may help if we elevate your sibling's head. Let's try that first."
    3. "Clients frequently make those sounds right before death."
    4. "It would be pointless to place oxygen on your sibling now."
    5. "Noisy respirations occur when the jaw and mouth relax and do not mean your sibling is struggling to breathe."
    6. "I will get a suction catheter to suction your sibling's mouth."
    7. "Using oxygen right now will just prolong your sibling's suffering."
    8. "You may need to leave the room if the noises bother you too much."

14. A few hours later, the LPN/LVN enters the client's room to turn the client.

    Which **2** findings indicate the client has expired?

    1. No movement or breathing.
    2. Unresponsiveness.
    3. Cool mottled skin.
    4. Absence of an apical pulse.
    5. Absence of audible blood pressure.
    6. Dilated pupils.

Refer to the Case Study to answer the next question.

The LPN/LVN is caring for a client transferred to the behavioral health unit from the intensive care unit (ICU) after a drug overdose.

History	Nurse's Notes	Vital Signs

Client reports increasing despondency over the last month after being fired from a janitorial job due to multiple unexcused absences. Client reports a 10 pound (4.54 kg) weight loss over the past 2 weeks, difficulty sleeping, and a lack of interest in previously enjoyed activities. Client reports the third divorce 6 months ago and denies having close friends. The client also reports a lack of family support due to longstanding issues with alcohol abuse. The client has maintained sobriety from alcohol for 7.5 months.

When asked about the suicide attempt, the client responded, "Death would be a relief. I'm disappointed that the thirty 5 mg tablets of diazepam I took didn't help me get to a better place."

History	Nurse's Notes	Vital Signs

1300: Client is alert and oriented to person, place, and time; is calm and cooperative; and presents with a logical thought process. Client is noted to be sitting at the edge of the bed, dressed in a hospital gown, slumped over, and making minimal eye contact. Client's speech is slowed with limited verbalizations.

History	Nurse's Notes	Vital Signs

Vital Sign	Result 1315
BP	152/94
HR	96
RR	18
Temp (oral)	98.9°F (37.1°C)

15. The LPN/LVN is reviewing the client's history and assessment data with the nurse to prepare the client's plan of care.

Complete the diagram by dragging from the choices below to specify what condition the client is **most** likely experiencing, 2 **priority** actions the LPN/LVN should take to address that condition, and 2 parameters the LPN/LVN should monitor to assess the client's progress.

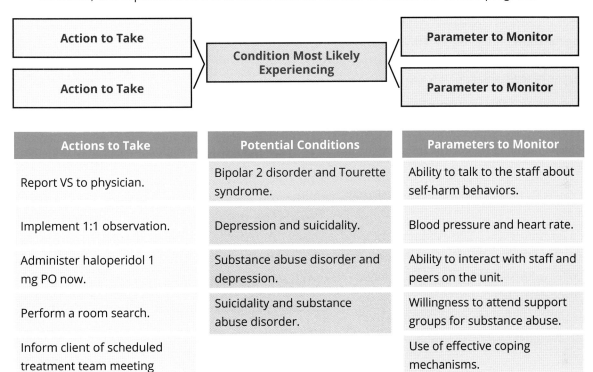

Actions to Take	Potential Conditions	Parameters to Monitor
Report VS to physician.	Bipolar 2 disorder and Tourette syndrome.	Ability to talk to the staff about self-harm behaviors.
Implement 1:1 observation.	Depression and suicidality.	Blood pressure and heart rate.
Administer haloperidol 1 mg PO now.	Substance abuse disorder and depression.	Ability to interact with staff and peers on the unit.
Perform a room search.	Suicidality and substance abuse disorder.	Willingness to attend support groups for substance abuse.
Inform client of scheduled treatment team meeting at 1300.		Use of effective coping mechanisms.

Chapter Quiz Answers and Explanations

1. The answer is 1

The LPN/LVN is having a long discussion with a client diagnosed with diabetes who requires an amputation. At times during the conversation, the LPN/LVN continues looking at the client but becomes silent. Which of the following is the **best** advantage of this approach?

Strategy: "Best" indicates that there may be more than one response that appears correct.

Category: Implementation/Psychosocial Integrity

(1) CORRECT: Rather than feel pressured to respond, the client can relax for a moment and reflect on the conversation.

(2) The reason for using silence is to make the conversation more productive, not to end the dialogue.

(3) The reason for using silence is to allow quiet focus, not to provide distraction.

(4) Silence should not be used to make the client feel pressured to respond.

2. The answer is 1

The client says to the LPN/LVN, "I really like you and I think you really like me. Would you like to go on a date with me after I am discharged?" What is the **most** appropriate response by the LPN/LVN?

Strategy: Eliminate incorrect answer choices.

Category: Implementation/Psychosocial Integrity

(1) CORRECT: This response provides realistic information and is not confrontational.

(2) "Why" questions can be confrontational. Even though realistic information is offered in this response, the opening statement implies disapproval and might put the client on the defensive.

(3) This response is confrontational. The LPN/LVN should be able to take care of the situation right now. If the comment needs to be reported, the LPN/LVN should report it to the direct supervisor and follow the chain of command.

(4) This response puts the focus on the nurse and is not therapeutic communication. Focus should remain on the client.

3. The answer is 4

The LPN/LVN is caring for a client recently diagnosed with type 1 diabetes mellitus. The client says, "I just can't believe that I am going to have to give myself shots every day." What is the **priority** statement for the LPN/LVN to make?

Strategy: Eliminate incorrect answer choices.

Category: Implementation/Psychosocial Integrity

(1) This statement takes the focus away from the client and dismisses the client's feelings.

(2) This is a "yes/no" question, which does not allow the client to give information or express feelings. It also assumes that the client cannot care for self.

(3) In this response, the focus is on the nurse. Remember that on the NCLEX, you have the time to provide emotional support *right now*.

(4) CORRECT: Even though it is a statement, this response is open-ended and encourages the client to discuss feelings. The client has expressed concern about the insulin injection but may need to discuss feelings about the diagnosis of diabetes.

4. The answer is 3 and 6

The LPN/LVN is working in the hospice unit. The client's partner approaches the nurse and says, "I won't be able to face life without my partner of over 50 years." Which of the following would be an appropriate response by the LPN/LVN? **(Select all that apply.)**

Strategy: For each response, remember the principles of therapeutic communication. Eliminate nontherapeutic responses to identify the best answer. You may need to "translate" responses to identify errors in therapeutic communication.

Category: Implementation/Psychosocial Integrity

(1) The client's partner is not in the mood to celebrate; this response ignores the partner's grief.

(2) This is an authoritarian response that instructs the client's partner to behave in a certain way, your way.

(3) CORRECT: This response is empathetic and reflects the partner's feelings.

(4) This response is a version of "Don't worry."

(5) This is an authoritarian response that instructs the partner to think in a certain way, your way.

(6) CORRECT: This response is empathetic and reflects the partner's feelings.

5. The answer is 4

The unlicensed assistive personnel (UAP) tells the LPN/LVN, "I want to change my assignment for today. I will not take care of a client diagnosed with AIDS." What is the **most** appropriate statement for the LPN/LVN to make?

Strategy: Eliminate incorrect answer choices.

Category: Implementation/Psychosocial Integrity

(1) This is a "yes/no" question and can be interpreted as confrontational.

(2) This response gives false reassurance and does not address the concerns of the AP.

(3) This response is authoritarian and argumentative, and it does not address the concerns of the AP.

(4) CORRECT: This response is open-ended and allows the UAP to express feelings about care of a client diagnosed with AIDS. It seeks more information about the UAP's knowledge of the care needed.

6. The answer is 3

The teenage client in the adolescent psychiatric unit asks the LPN/LVN, "Do you hear those voices? They sound so frightening." Which of the following responses by the nurse would be the **most** appropriate?

Strategy: "*Most* appropriate" indicates that discrimination is required to answer the question. Remember therapeutic communication as well as scope of practice.

Category: Implementation/Psychosocial Integrity

(1) This response contradicts the client's experience and also moves the focus from the client to the nurse.

(2) This response affirms the client's delusions and is exploratory; outside the scope of LPN/LVN practice.

(3) CORRECT: This response gives correct information and is empathetic, reflecting the client's feelings.

(4) This response is unnecessarily authoritative and removes focus from the client's needs.

7. The answer is 2

Family members of the client with dementia are visiting the memory care unit for the first time. They express concern to the LPN/LVN caring for their relative about the client's unobserved wandering. Which of the following responses by the LPN/LVN would be **most** appropriate?

Strategy: Remember therapeutic communication: Focus on assuring good client care.

Category: Implementation/Psychosocial Integrity

(1) This "Don't worry" response discounts what the family members feel.

(2) CORRECT: This response provides factual information and encourages further communication.

(3) This response moves the focus from the client to the LPN/LVN.

(4) The response negates the family members' concern and discourages further communication.

8. The answer is 3

The LPN/LVN is caring for a client 5 days after a colostomy procedure. During colostomy care, the LPN/LVN observes the client vigorously rubbing the skin around the stoma before applying the colostomy pouch. What is the **most** appropriate statement for the LPN/LVN to make?

Strategy: Eliminate incorrect answer choices.

Category: Data Collection/Psychosocial Integrity

(1) Asking the client for an explanation may be deemed confrontational. Also, this is a "yes/no" question, which does not encourage the client to give information or express feelings.

(2) This question is closed-ended and judgmental. It assumes that the client does not have the ability to care for the colostomy.

(3) CORRECT: This statement gives factual information. There is an increased risk of damage to the skin if the area around the stoma is rubbed vigorously. With this approach, the LPN/LVN can provide positive reinforcement for the steps of the procedure done correctly and give suggestions for improvement.

(4) This question assumes that the client has not read the written instructions. The priority is to have the client demonstrate all steps of colostomy care.

9. See explanation for answers

CORRECT OPTIONS: In order to elect hospice care, a client must be certified as terminally ill with a prognosis of 6 months or less to live. This certification comes from **two physicians**, one of whom is the medical director of the hospice. The client may continue to receive hospice care beyond 6 months as long as the client continues to meet hospice criteria for the terminal illness. The focus of hospice care is to **manage the client's symptoms, provide family and spiritual support,** and provide a dignified death.

INCORRECT OPTIONS: A client does not have to have an advance directive or insurance to receive hospice care. The client also does not have to have a "Do Not Resuscitate" order to receive hospice care. Most hospice clients do, however, decide to allow a natural death and forgo aggressive resuscitation efforts. The focus of hospice care is not to hasten or postpone the client's death, or to keep the client sedated. The hospice facilitates the client's preferences for end of life care and end of life decisions, but does not decide for the patient. When a client receives hospice care in a long term nursing facility, the hospice is not allowed to provide additional staff for the care of other clients in the facility. Hospice staff are utilized to provide needed care for the hospice client in addition to the usual care provided by the nursing staff at the facility. Hospice does not provide financial or legal advice, but can provide resources to clients and families. Hospice does not routinely provide 24-hour care. This type of hospice care may be provided if the client's symptoms warrant continuous care, and it is carefully documented when provided.

10. See explanation for answers

CORRECT OPTIONS: The client's non-verbal behavior of **groaning and grimacing** indicates the client is in pain. **Labored respirations** indicate the client is having increased work of breathing. The client's temperature indicates a **high fever**, which may contribute to the client's discomfort. A client's temperature may be very erratic as the client approaches death. These are the most concerning client findings at this time.

INCORRECT OPTIONS: Findings which are expected for the client in ESLD include jaundice, a large abdomen due to ascites, 3+ peripheral edema, and dark yellow urine. Dry mucous membranes and a HR of 108 are consistent with an elevated temperature.

11. The answer is 2

CORRECT OPTION: **Liquid oral morphine** is widely used in hospice care as a pain reliever and to relax pulmonary smooth muscle and facilitate breathing. The LPN/LVN can administer this oral narcotic medication.

INCORRECT OPTIONS: Administering acetaminophen is necessary to reduce temperature, but is not the most important intervention at this time; addressing pain and dyspnea is the priority. Providing mouth care and perineal care is also necessary and will provide comfort to the client, but these actions are not the priority actions to take. They may also be delegated to an unlicensed assistive personnel (UAP).

12. See explanation for answers

Client minimally responsive to any stimuli. Occasionally opening eyes. Does not obey commands. Skin cool and deeply jaundiced. Hands and feet mottled. Bilateral legs mottled to upper thighs. Oral membranes dry. Eyes appear sunken. Respirations deep and rapid, then slow with 10–15 second periods of apnea. Client making a gurgling sound when exhaling. Client had 1 large dark bloody stool last night, and is voiding very scant amounts of dark urine in diaper.

CORRECT OPTIONS: Clients approaching death within a few hours are typically **minimally responsive** to unresponsive, exhibit **mottling** of the extremities, have **erratic breathing** patterns and **periods of apnea**, and may make **gurgling sounds** when breathing. This breathing is sometimes called the "death rattle" and can be very disconcerting to family members.

INCORRECT OPTIONS: The client's skin may be cool or may be extremely hot at the time of death, due to issues of poor temperature regulation. Jaundice is due to the client's terminal liver disease. While some clients will defecate immediately preceding or at the time of death, having a large bloody stool does not signify active dying.

13. The answer is 1, 2, 5, and 6

CORRECT OPTIONS: The LPN/LVN should **acknowledge** that the situation may be very difficult and distressing for the client's family. Offering interventions to address the distressing symptoms help the family see that concerns are not being ignored or disregarded. **Changing the client's position** may help. Raising the head or turning the client on the side may allow air to move more freely in the airway. It may sound like the client is choking and struggling to breathe, but the issue is the **loss of muscle tone in the back of the jaw and throat**, and the collection of oral secretions in the oropharynx which the client can no longer swallow. Providing **oral suction at the bedside** may alleviate some of the gurgling, and may help the family feel they are doing something positive for the client. Deep tracheal suctioning will not be of use in this situation.

INCORRECT OPTIONS: While the LPN/LVN is correct in saying that clients frequently experience noisy respirations immediately before death, this statement is not worded in a therapeutic manner. Oxygen is not beneficial in this situation, as the client is not really exchanging oxygen and CO_2, and the issue is not hypoxia. However, in some situations, oxygen may be used as a comfort for the family if they are insistent. The nurse should not tell the family what can NOT be done, but should focus on doing something positive and acknowledging their concerns. The nurse should also not tell a family member to leave.

14. The answer is 1 and 4

CORRECT OPTIONS: Definitive signs of death are an **absence of breathing** and **absence of apical pulse**. However, an LPN/LVN cannot pronounce death. A registered nurse with hospice may pronounce the client's time of death in most states.

INCORRECT OPTIONS: Unresponsiveness alone is not an indication of death. While cool mottled or grey skin may be present when the client has expired, it may be present while the client is still alive in the last few hours of life. A client may not have an audible blood pressure for many hours before death. The client's peripheral circulation becomes very erratic, and peripheral pulses and blood pressure may be difficult or impossible to detect. The client's pupils may dilate prior to actual death.

15. See explanation for answers

Potential Condition	
Depression and suicidality.	☑

CORRECT OPTION: Based on presenting factors, client history, and client statement, this client is exhibiting symptoms of **depression and suicidality**.

INCORRECT OPTIONS: Bipolar 2 disorder is characterized by mood swings from depression to hypomania. Unlike mania, hypomania never contains psychosis. Tourette syndrome is a disorder characterized by motor and verbal tics. This client does not meet the criteria for these diagnoses. While this client has a history of alcohol abuse, there is no evidence of a current problem.

Actions to Take	
Implement 1:1 observation.	☑
Perform a room search.	☑

CORRECT OPTIONS: This client is at risk for self-harm based on recent overdose attempt and has expressed disappointment of failed attempt. Client safety is the number one priority on the behavioral health unit. A **1:1 observation** provides this client with constant observation, ensuring the client does not harm self. A **room search** creates a safe environment by removing potentially harmful objects from client access, such as belts, ties, and sharp objects.

INCORRECT OPTIONS: The only VS that is abnormal is the BP. While this should be reported to the physician, client safety is a higher priority. Haloperidol is an antipsychotic. This client shows no signs of psychosis. While attending a treatment team meeting is part of the nursing care plan, client safety is a higher priority.

Parameters to Monitor	
Ability to talk to the staff about self-harm behaviors.	☑
Ability to interact with staff and peers on the unit.	☑

CORRECT OPTIONS: Clients who participate in a safety plan demonstrate the desire for help by **talking to a staff member when the client feels a desire to harm self**, rather than carrying out the plan to harm self. This client has a history of isolative social behaviors, which contribute to depression and suicidality. The client's **ability to appropriately interact with staff and peers** indicates an improvement in the condition.

INCORRECT OPTIONS: Monitoring the client's BP, willingness to attend support groups, and use of effective coping mechanisms are important to include in the plan of care. However, safety is a higher priority.

PART THREE

PREPARING FOR THE NCLEX-PN® EXAM

[CHAPTER 9]

HOW TO STUDY FOR THE NCLEX-PN® EXAM

Now that you've read about the various Kaplan test taking strategies, you are probably thinking, "Wow! This is great!" Most of you have started identifying why you are having difficulty answering application/analysis-level test questions. Some of you have already formulated a plan to master your NCLEX-PN® exam questions using the strategies outlined in this book, and are confident that you will pass the exam. Others are thinking, "This sounds great, but can I really answer questions using these strategies?"

The authors of this book work for Kaplan, the oldest test prep company in the nation. We have been preparing graduate nurses and international nurses for licensure exams for more than 40 years. We know what works to prepare for the exam and what doesn't work.

Ineffective Ways to Prepare

Here are a few of the biggest mistakes some NCLEX-PN® exam test takers make before Test Day.

Relying on False Hopes

Some students use what is knows as the "hope" method of study. "I hope that I don't have questions about chest tubes on the test." "I hope that I don't have questions about medication on my test." "I hope that I have questions about electrolytes because I did great on that test in school." The "hope" method usually doesn't work very well. The test pool contains thousands of questions. How many topics do you "hope" won't be on your test?

Lacking Respect for the Exam

Many candidates for the NCLEX-PN® exam are good students in school. Because of their school success, they expect to pass the exam with minimal preparation. After all, it's just a test of minimum competency. These students do some studying, but they really believe there is no chance they might fail this exam. You might think that you can't possibly fail, but if you do not respect this exam and prepare for it correctly, you run the risk of failure!

All students know why they take the NCLEX-PN® exam. However, after interviewing hundreds of students, we have discovered that many have no idea what the exam content is. How can you effectively study for a test if you don't know what content the exam tests? Learn what is on the NCLEX-PN® exam and then you will realize that preparation with a planned method of study is essential.

Cramming

Some students completed nursing school with a minimal understanding of nursing content. These students studied long and hard on the night before a nursing school test, cramming as many facts into their heads as they could remember. Because the test questions primarily involved recognition and recall, cramming worked for tests in nursing school. But as we said earlier, the NCLEX-PN® exam is not an exam about facts. It tests your ability to apply the knowledge that you have learned and to think critically. Recognition and recall will not work!

Planning Poorly

As with all standardized exams, you must work on your areas of weakness. This is hard to do because there's usually a reason you're weak in an area. Some graduate practical/vocational nurses, for example, profess a weakness in or dislike for obstetrical nursing. Some students didn't understand the theory, while other students had a poor clinical experience or didn't get to see many deliveries; still other students simply didn't like this rotation. Whatever the reason, it causes you to have a weakness in a particular area. In order to pass a standardized test, you must work on your areas of weakness.

Some students don't establish a plan of study. Other students establish a plan of study but don't follow it. You can buy review books, but if you don't apply yourself, they will do you no good.

Effective Methods of Preparation

To pass the NCLEX-PN® exam, you not only need to know nursing content, you also need to be able to apply the critical thinking skills we've just reviewed. Next, you need to be an expert on the content of the exam. What topics are usually included on the NCLEX-PN® exam? How is the content organized? And finally, you need to create a study plan, and make sure that you are able to cope with the testing experience.

So let's start by talking about some of the issues that you may be asking yourself.

QUESTION: "I'm terrible at standardized tests. Is this really going to help me?"

ANSWER: Yes, these strategies will help you choose more correct responses when you take the NCLEX-PN® exam. Read this book—more than once if necessary—to learn the strategies. Then practice, practice, practice. Use the strategies to answer many, many test questions, and you will find yourself answering more and more questions correctly. Tear out the Chart of Critical Thinking Paths in Appendix A and consult it while you are answering practice test questions. This will help you become more comfortable with putting the strategies into practice. As you answer more and more questions, put the diagram aside and rely on your memory to identify and implement a critical thinking strategy.

QUESTION: "Am I going to have enough time when I take the NCLEX-PN® exam to figure out which strategy to use?"

ANSWER: Timing is a concern on the NCLEX-PN® exam. You need to maximize your efforts on each test question. Practice answering test questions using the various strategies we've outlined. As you get more proficient, you will discover that it takes you less time to identify the strategy or path that will lead you to the correct answer.

QUESTION:	"I don't have to use these strategies on every question, do I? I think I'll use them only when I can't figure out the correct answer on my own."
ANSWER:	Wrong! You should use critical thinking to answer every question on the NCLEX-PN® exam to make sure that you pass. Follow the steps that we have outlined for every practice question that you answer as you prepare for the exam. If you practice these steps, you will not need to randomly guess the correct answer on the NCLEX-PN® exam.
QUESTION:	"So all I have to do is memorize the strategies, right?"
ANSWER:	Just memorizing the various strategies will not ensure your success on the NCLEX-PN® exam. Remember, the exam does not test your ability to memorize either critical thinking strategies or the nursing content. The NCLEX-PN® exam tests your ability to think critically and use the nursing knowledge that you have. It's relatively easy to just memorize nursing content. The hard part is figuring out how to use this knowledge to make nursing decisions. It's relatively easy to memorize the critical thinking strategies. The hard part is to figure out which strategy to use on each and every question. That takes practice.
QUESTION:	"What if I use the strategies but still can't figure out the correct answer?"
ANSWER:	It's not unusual that students will read a question, read the answers, and think "Huh? Something is missing." If you feel like something is missing, reread the question to determine if you have correctly identified what the question is asking. If you have identified the question correctly, then read the answer choices to make sure that you haven't missed the nursing concept contained in the answer choices.
QUESTION:	"Will these strategies work on every practice question that I answer?"
ANSWER:	The critical thinking strategies discussed in this book will enable you to answer all kinds of multiple choice test questions. The critical thinking strategies apply to test questions written at the application/analysis level and do not work with knowledge-based test questions. If you feel that the strategies don't work with the practice questions you are answering, determine the level of difficulty of the questions you are working with. Are the practice questions knowledge-based, or are they at the application/analysis level of difficulty? Remember, the majority of questions that are of a passing level of difficulty on the NCLEX-PN® exam are at the application/analysis level of difficulty.

It's time for you to start your successful preparation for the NCLEX-PN® exam. Begin by identifying your strengths and weaknesses, as follows:

- Take as many diagnostic exams as you can.
- Identify your weaknesses in nursing content.
- Identify your weaknesses in test taking skills.

Next, decide if you need to take a review course. If you decide that this is the best way for you to prepare, ask yourself these questions:

- Is the course mainly a review of nursing content or memory techniques? This type of review won't help you put it all together on Test Day. You can know everything about heart failure, but if you don't know how to use this information to answer a question about heart failure correctly on the NCLEX-PN® exam, you will have difficulty on the exam. Are the strategies specific for the NCLEX-PN® exam?

- Are there plenty of opportunities for practice testing? You need to prove your competence by answering NCLEX-PN® exam-style test questions, so you should practice answering these questions. If the exam were about opening a sterile pack, what would you spend your time doing to prepare for the exam? Reading about opening a sterile pack or practicing opening a sterile pack? Are there exam-style questions included in the course? Do the questions require recall and recognition of facts or application of nursing care principles? Remember, your NCLEX-PN® exam will consist mainly of analysis/application-level questions.

- What do students who have taken the course have to say about how it helped them prepare for the exam? If a review course boasts of a particularly high pass rate, ask to see their statistics. Be an informed consumer.

- Is there a guarantee? There are guarantees and there are empty promises. Make sure the course you are considering puts the guarantee in writing. Study the small print. Is your total tuition refunded? Do you have to fail the exam more than once?

- How much does it cost? This sounds easy, but "extras" can add up. Are there additional charges for books? Software? Registration fees?

- Is this course right for me?

And finally, create a realistic study schedule that works for you. Then make a vow to stick to that plan and reward yourself when you do. Spend at least 3 weeks before your exam date preparing. Don't cram! Your content focus should be in understanding the principles of nursing care, not memorizing facts.

Stay away from people who are "prophets of doom." You know the type. With the proper preparation you can and will pass the NCLEX-PN® exam. Keep a positive attitude.

You may need to consider some techniques for battling stress and managing the Test Day experience. Do any of these statements apply to you?

> *"I always freeze up on tests."*

> *"I need to pass to get my new job/promotion/commission."*

> *"My best friend/girlfriend/sister/brother did really well, but I won't."*

> *"My hospital/family/parents won't like it if I fail."*

> *"I'm afraid of losing concentration."*

> *"I'm afraid I'm not spending enough time preparing."*

If these sound familiar, you may want to mentally prepare yourself by understanding ways to manage test stress. Forcing yourself to identify and face fears may make you edgy at first but will significantly alleviate test stress in the long run by adding another dimension to your preparation.

Mental Preparation*

1. Visualize

You have probably learned how to do this with clients; now it's your turn. Sit back and let your shoulders and arms relax. Close your eyes and imagine yourself in a relaxing situation—it can be fictional, but a real-life memory is best. Make it as detailed as possible. Think about the sights, the sounds, the smells, even the tastes that you associate with the relaxing situation. Keep your eyes shut; keep sinking back into your chair. Now that you're in that situation, start bringing your test in—think about the experience of taking the test while *in* that relaxing situation. Imagine how much easier it would be if you could take your test in that situation. Notice how much easier your test seems in that situation.

Here's another variation. Close your eyes and think about a situation in which you did well on a test. If you can't come up with one, pick a situation in which you did some good academic work that you were really proud of, or some other kind of genuine accomplishment. Not a fiction, mind you: it has to be from real life. Make it as detailed as possible. Think about the sights, the sounds, the smells, even the tastes that you associate with this experience of academic success. Now think about your test in line with that experience. Don't make comparisons between them. Just imagine taking your test with that same feeling of relaxed control.

2. Exercise

Whether it be jogging, walking, yoga, push-ups, or a pickup basketball game, physical exercise is a great way to stimulate the mind and body and improve one's ability to think and concentrate. A surprising number of those who prepare for standardized tests don't exercise regularly because they spend so much time preparing. Sedentary people—this is a medical fact—get less oxygen in the blood, and therefore to the brain, than active people.

3. Do the Following on Exam Day:

- *Keep moving forward.* You don't need to get everything right to pass, so don't linger on a question that is going nowhere. The best test takers don't get bothered by difficult questions because they accept that everyone encounters them on the NCLEX-PN® exam. You can achieve the the ability to keep moving forward by doing enough preparation with practice questions by Test Day that it becomes an instinct to move on instead of getting bogged down by one difficult question.

- *Disregard negative words and behavior.* Don't be distracted by the ignorant babble or the behavior of other, less-prepared, less-skilled candidates around you. Negative thoughts lead to negative feelings and may interfere with performing your best on Test Day.

- *Ignore the pace of other test takers.* Don't be anxious if others seem to be working harder or answering questions more quickly. Continue to spend your time patiently but persistently thinking through your answers; it's going to lead to higher-quality test taking and better results. Set your own pace and stick to it.

---

*Some of these methods were originally conceptualized by Dr. Emile Coué, who in the 1920s told everyone that the key to a happy life was to constantly repeat the phrase, "Every day in every way I am getting better and better." As advice to test takers, that isn't bad at all!

- *Keep breathing!* Weak standardized test takers tend to share one major trait: forgetting to breathe steadily as the test proceeds. They do not know the value of proper breathing. They start holding their breath without realizing it, or begin breathing erratically or arrhythmically. This can hurt confidence and accuracy. Do what you can to instill an awareness of proper breathing before and during each study or testing section.

- *Do some quick isometrics during the test.* This is especially helpful if your concentration is wandering or energy is waning. For example, put your palms together and press intensely for a few seconds.

To effectively prepare for the NCLEX-PN® exam, first identify your strengths and weaknesses, and then choose an effective method of study that works for you. Practice using mental preparation techniques to alleviate stress and manage your Test Day experience.

[CHAPTER 10]

THE LICENSURE PROCESS

The process of obtaining an American nursing license requires a definite sequence of actions by the candidate. Because this may be your first experience with the LPN/LVN licensure process, and because there are no established test dates, you may have difficulty knowing exactly how to complete the paperwork and go through the process. This chapter will give you a checklist to follow when planning to take the NCLEX-PN® exam. This is a general list, so you must individualize it according to the requirements for the state or province in which you wish to become licensed. We will outline the questions that you need to ask, and the steps you need to take to complete the licensure process.

How to Apply for the NCLEX-PN® Exam

During your last semester of nursing school, you will be given the following applications:

(1) Application for licensure that goes to your state board of nursing/regulatory body.

(2) Application for the NCLEX-PN® exam that goes to Pearson VUE.

On a predetermined date, you will submit the completed forms and the required licensure fees to your nursing school.

Application Fees

- The NCLEX-PN® examination fee is $200 ($360 CAD). Additional licensure fees are determined by each state nursing board. Refer to your state board of nursing's website to determine your state's fee.

- You are responsible for submitting the completed test application and the $200 fee to Pearson VUE. All applications will be processed by phone or online.

The Registration Process

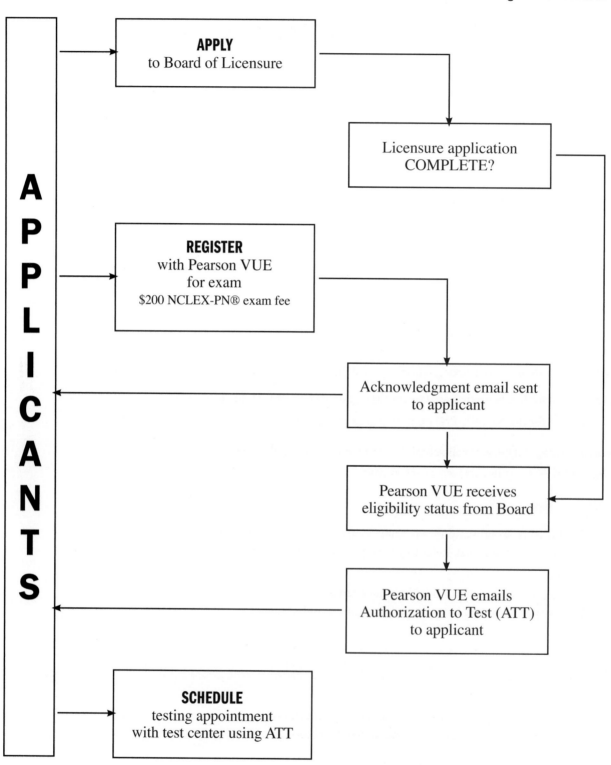

Applicant must APPLY, REGISTER, and SCHEDULE

Registration

You can register for the NCLEX-PN® with Pearson VUE using either of the following two methods:

(1) *Internet registration:* To register online, go to **nclex.com** (the NCLEX candidate website). Payment is by credit, debit, or prepaid card (using Visa, MasterCard, or American Express only).

(2) *Telephone registration:* Call VUE NCLEX Candidate Services at 1-866-496-2539 (1-866-49-NCLEX). To register by phone, you must pay using a Visa, MasterCard, or American Express credit or debit card. Even if you register by phone, you must provide an email address to recieve communications from Pearson VUE about your registration.

Pearson VUE does not accept exam registrations submitted by mail.

Some states require that the testing application form and fee be sent along with the licensure application and fee.

For more information, visit **nclex.com/prepare.page** and download the most recent *NCLEX Candidate Bulletin*. For questions regarding registering to take the NCLEX-PN® exam, your Authorization to Test (ATT), acceptable forms of identification, or comments about the test center, visit the NCLEX candidate website (**nclex.com**) or contact:

> NCLEX Candidate Services
> 1-866-49-NCLEX
> **https://www.ncsbn.org/exam-contacts.htm**
>
> NCLEX-PN® Examination Program
> Pearson Professional Testing
> 5601 Green Valley Drive
> Bloomington, MN 55437-1099
> **pvamericascustomerservice@pearson.com**

How Do You Know Your Application Has Been Received?

You will receive a card from your state board confirming that all of your information has been received.

Potential Problems with Licensure Application

Some states require that your permanent transcript be mailed with your application.

Here is a checklist to follow to avoid problems with your application:

- Have you met all requirements for graduation? Do you have any electives still outstanding?
- Has your nursing school received a permanent transcript for any credits that you transferred from another institution?
- Do you owe any fines or have any unpaid parking tickets? (This can delay the release of your permanent transcript. Check at your nursing school office, just to be sure.)

- Some states require that a statement be sent from your nursing school stating that you have met all requirements for graduation.
- Did you change your mind about the state to which you want to apply for licensure? If so, you must apply to the new state—and forfeit the original application fee.

What If You Want to Apply for Licensure in a Different State?

If you plan to apply for licensure in a different state from the one in which you are attending practical/vocational nursing school, contact the state board of nursing in the state in which you wish to become licensed.

Here's a checklist for obtaining a license in another state:

- Contact the state board of nursing of that state and find out what their requirements are for licensure.
- Find out what their fees are.
- Request a new candidate application for licensure.

After you pass the NCLEX-PN® exam, you will receive your nursing license from the state in which you applied for licensure regardless of where you took your exam. For example, if you applied for licensure in Michigan, you can take the test in Florida if you wish. You would then receive a license to practice as an LPN in Michigan because that is where you applied for licensure.

When Can You Schedule Your NCLEX-PN® Exam?

Pearson VUE will send you a document entitled "Authorization to Test" (ATT). The ATT will be sent to you via email at the email address you provided when you registered. You will be unable to schedule your test date until you receive this form.

On the ATT is your assigned candidate number; you will need to refer to this when scheduling your exam. Your ATT is valid for a time determined by the individual state board of nursing/regulatory body, and you must test before your ATT expires. If you don't, you will need to reapply to take the exam and pay the testing fees again. With your ATT, you will receive a list of test centers. You can schedule your NCLEX-PN® exam using the following procedures:

- Log on to the NCLEX Candidate Website at **nclex.com**
- Call NCLEX Candidate Services

    United States and Canada: 1-866-496-2539 (1-866-49-NCLEX) (toll-free)
    Asia Pacific Region: +852-3077-4923 (pay number)
    Europe, Middle East, Africa: +44-161-855-7445 (pay number)
    India: 91-120-439-7837 (pay number)
    All other countries not listed above: 1-952-905-7403 (pay number)

Candidates with hearing impairments who use a Telecommunications Device for the Deaf (TDD) can call the U.S.A. Relay Service at 1-800-627-3529 (toll-free) or the Canada & International Inbound relay service at 1-605-224-1837 (pay number).

Those with special testing requests, such as persons with disabilities, must call the NCLEX-PN® Program Coordinator at NCLEX Candidate Services at one of the numbers listed above. If you require special accommodations, you cannot schedule your exam through the NCLEX Candidate Website.

There is a space on the ATT for you to record the date and time of your scheduled exam. You will also receive confirmation of your scheduled date and time.

Potential Rescheduling Problems

- You must test prior to the expiration date of your ATT. If you miss your appointment, you forfeit your testing fees and must reapply to both the state board of nursing/regulatory body and Pearson VUE.
- If you wish to change your appointment, you must notify Pearson VUE during business hours, at least 24 hours prior to your scheduled appointment. Call one of the numbers listed above or go the NCLEX candidate website (**nclex.com**). If your test date is on a Saturday, Sunday, or Monday, make sure to call on or before Friday.

Do not call the test site directly or leave a message if you are unable to take your test on the scheduled date. You must follow the procedure outlined here.

When Will You Take the Exam?

The earliest date on which you can take the NCLEX-PN® exam varies depending on your state, but the majority of students test approximately 45 days after the date of their graduation. Variables include when you submit the applications and fees, the length of time the ATT is valid, personal factors (weddings, births, vacations), and job requirements. Each state determines the requirements for graduate practical/vocational nurses, licensure pending. If you are working as a graduate practical/vocational nurse, you must be knowledgeable about the rules in your state.

Taking the Exam

What Happens on the Day of My NCLEX-PN® Exam?

Arrive at the test center at least 30 minutes before your scheduled test time. Wear layered clothing—the rooms may be cool in the morning but can warm up as the day progresses.

Here's a checklist of things to bring on the day of the exam:

- Your Authorization to Test (ATT). (Although your ATT is no longer required for admission to your exam, you may wish to refer to it.)
- One form of unexpired, government-issued, signed identification (ID) that includes a picture. It must exactly match the first and last names you provided when registering. If you have changed your hair color, lost weight, or grown a beard, have a new picture ID made before Test Day. Acceptable forms of ID include driver's license, state/territorial/provincial identity card, passport, and U.S. military ID.
- A snack and something to drink.
- *Do not* bring any study materials to the test center.

Check-in procedure:

- Present a valid, acceptable form of ID.
- Provide your digital signature, take a palm vein scan, and have your photograph taken.
- Agree to the Candidate Statement via digital signature.
- Seal all electronic devices in a plastic bag provided by the test center.
- Place all other personal belongings in secure storage outside the testing room. This includes watches, large jewelry, scarfs and hats, lip balm, food and drink, and medical devices.

Earplugs are available on request. Request them, in case you find yourself distracted by background noise.

You will be provided an erasable note board for scratch work.

Where Will I Take My Test?

You will be in a room separate from the rest of the test center. Many testing sites consist of a room with 10 to 15 computers placed around the outside walls. Each computer sits on a full-size desk, with an adjustable chair for you to sit on. There are dividers between desks, but you will be able to see the person sitting next to you. There is a picture window from which the proctor will observe each person testing. There are also video cameras and sound sensors mounted on the walls to monitor each candidate.

What Will the Computer Screen Look Like?

The number of the question you are answering is located in the lower-right side of your computer screen. In the upper-right corner is a digital clock that counts down from 5:00:00—representing the 5 hours you have to complete the short tutorial that begins the exam, the exam itself, and all breaks.

If the question is a traditional four-option, text-based, multiple choice question, the question stem is located in the top half of the screen and the four answer choices are located in the lower half of the screen (Figure 10.1). Radio buttons are in front of each answer choice.

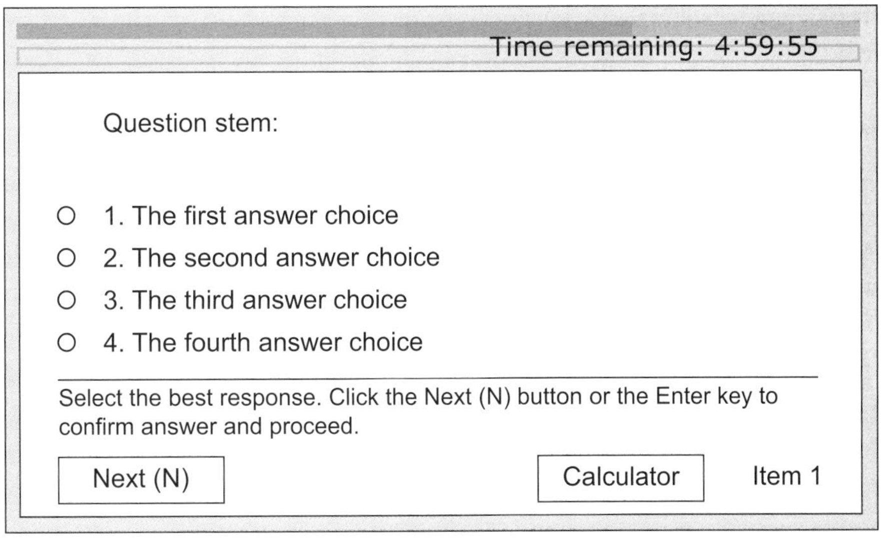

Figure 10.1

You will notice that there are two buttons at the bottom of the computer screen. You use the Next (N) button to confirm your answer selection and move to the next question. Click the Calculator button to display a drop-down calculator that can be used to perform computations.

If the question is an alternate format question that may have more than one correct answer, you will see the phrase "Select all that apply" between the stem of the question and five to nine answer choices. A small box is in front of each answer choice. The Next (N) button and Calculator button are at the bottom of the computer screen.

If the question is a hot spot alternate format question, the screen will contain a graphic or a picture. The Next (N) button and Calculator button are at the bottom of the computer screen.

If the question is a fill-in-the-blank alternate format question, a text box will be under the question. The Next (N) button and Calculator button are at the bottom of the computer screen.

If the question is a drag-and-drop/ordered response alternate format question, the unordered options will be under the question and to the left. The space for the ordered response will be to the right of the unordered options. The Next (N) button and Calculator button are at the bottom of the computer screen.

If the question is a chart/exhibit alternate format question, it will include the following prompt after the question stem: "Click on the Exhibit button below for additional client information." The Exhibit button is located at the bottom of the computer screen between the Next (N) button and the Calculator button. Click on the Exhibit button to display a pop-up box containing three tabs. Click on each of the tabs to display information needed to answer the question.

If the question is an audio alternate format question, the question will contain an audio clip that you must listen to in order to answer the question. Click on the Play button (a right-pointing arrow) to listen to the clip. A slider bar allows you to adjust the volume at which you hear the clip. If you want to listen to the audio clip more than once, you can click on the Play button again.

If the question is a graphics alternate format question, each of the four answer choices will be a graphic instead of text.

How Do I Use the Calculator?

Using the mouse, click on the Calculator button, and a drop-down calculator will appear on the computer screen. Use the mouse to click on the calculator keys. Remember, the diagonal or slash (/) key is used for division. When you are through with your calculations, click on the Calculator button again, and the calculator will disappear.

How Do I Select an Answer Choice for Traditional Four-Option, Multiple Choice Questions?

You will use a two-step process to answer each question. Read the question and select an answer by using the mouse to click on the radio button preceding your answer choice. Your answer is now highlighted. When you are certain of your answer, click on the Next (N) button or press the Enter key to confirm your answer. Your answer is now locked in and a new question will appear on the screen. *You are not able to change your answer after clicking on the Next (N) button or pressing the Enter key, so be certain of your answer before you do so.*

After your answer is entered into the computer, the computer selects a new question for you based on the accuracy of your previous answer and the components of the NCLEX-PN® exam test plan. If you answer a question correctly, the next question selected by the computer is more difficult. If you answer a question incorrectly, the next question selected by the computer is easier.

What If I Want to Change the Answer That I Have Highlighted?

If you want to change the highlighted answer, click on a different answer choice. Your answer is not locked in until you click on the Next (N) button or press the Enter key.

Even if you've never used a computer before, don't panic. You will be given instructions at the beginning of the test, and you will have to answer three tutorial questions before your test begins. These questions allow you to practice using the mouse to select an answer.

How Do I Select an Answer Choice for Select All That Apply Questions?

Read the question and click on the small box in front of the answer choice you want. A small check will appear in the box. Click on each answer choice that answers the question.

What If I Want to Change an Answer That I Have Checked?

If you change your mind and don't want an answer choice that you have selected, just click again on the small box in front of that answer choice and the check will disappear. When you are certain of your answer, click on the Next (N) button or press the Enter key to confirm your answer. Your answer is now locked in and a new question appears on the screen.

How Do I Select an Answer Choice for Hot Spot Questions?

To answer a hot spot alternate format question, just click on the area of the graphic or picture that answers the question.

What If I Want to Change the Area That I Have Selected?

If you change your mind and want to select another area of the graphic or picture, just use your mouse to click on the area that you want and the original selection disappears. When you are certain of your answer, click on the Next (N) button or press the Enter key to confirm your answer. Your answer is now locked in and a new question appears on the screen.

How Do I Enter an Answer Choice for Fill-in-the-Blank Questions?

To enter an answer for a fill-in-the-blank question, just use the keyboard to select the numbers or letters you want. If a unit of measurement already appears next to the answer box on the screen, be sure you enter *numbers* only into the answer box; adding a unit of measurement may cause your answer to be wrong.

What If I Want to Change What I Have Entered in the Text Box?

If you change your mind and want to enter another answer in the text box, just backspace over the answer you entered and then use the keyboard to enter another answer. When you are certain of your answer, click on the Next (N) button or press the Enter key to confirm your answer. Your answer is now locked in and a new question appears on the screen.

How Do I Select Options for Drag-and-Drop/Ordered Response Questions?

To put the responses in the correct order, click on the option you think should come first, hold down the button on the mouse, and drag the option over to the box on the right side of the screen. You may also highlight the option in the box on the left side and then click the arrow key that points to the box on the right side to move the option. Do the same with each response in the proper order.

What If I Want to Change the Order of My Responses?

If you change your mind about the order of a response, click on it with the mouse and drag it back to the left side of the screen or use the arrow key as described above. To complete the question, you must move all options from the box on the left side of the screen to the box on the right side. When you are certain of your answer, click on the Next (N) button or press the Enter key to confirm your answer. Your answer is now locked in and a new question appears on the screen.

How Do I Enter or Change an Answer Choice for Chart/Exhibit, Audio, and Graphics Alternate Format Questions?

Chart/exhibit, audio, and graphics alternate format questions all use a four-option, multiple choice format, so you can enter or change your answer choices just as you would for a traditional text-based, four-option, multiple choice question.

Do I Get Any Breaks?

You will receive an optional break at the end of 2 hours of testing. There will be a pre-programmed prompt offering you a break. Leave the testing room, stretch your legs, and eat your snack. Take some deep, cleansing breaths and get yourself ready to go back into the testing room. The computer will offer you another optional break after 3½ hours of testing. We recommend that you take it unless you feel you're on a roll.

You may take a break at any time during your test, but the time that you spend away from your computer is counted as a part of your five hours of total testing time. Kaplan recommends that you take a short (2–5 minute) break if you are having trouble concentrating. Take time to go to the restroom, eat your snack, or get a drink. This will enable you to maintain or regain your concentration for the test. Remember, every question counts! If you need to take a break, raise your hand to notify the test administrator. You must leave the testing room, and you will be required to take a palm vein scan before you are allowed to resume your test.

How Will I Know When My Test Ends?

A screen will appear on your computer that states, "Your test is concluded." You will then be required to answer several exit questions. These are a few multiple choice questions about your response to the examination experience. They do not count toward your results.

How Long Will It Take to Receive My Results?

Your results are sent to you by your state board of nursing. Each state board determines when the NCLEX-PN® exam results are released. In the following jurisdictions, you may access your "unofficial" results two business days after taking your examination via the NCLEX® candidate website (for a $7.95 fee):

> Alaska, Arizona, Arkansas, Colorado, Connecticut, District of Columbia, Florida, Georgia, Hawaii, Idaho, Illinois, Indiana, Iowa, Kansas, Kentucky, Maine, Maryland, Massachusetts, Michigan, Minnesota, Mississippi, Missouri, Montana, Nebraska, Nevada, New Jersey, New Mexico, New York, North Carolina, North Dakota, Northern Mariana Islands, Ohio, Oklahoma, Oregon, Pennsylvania, Rhode Island, South Carolina, South Dakota, Tennessee, Texas, U.S. Virgin Islands, Utah, Vermont, Virginia, Washington, West Virginia, Wisconsin, Wyoming

For most states, you will receive your official results approximately 6 weeks after your test date.

CHAPTER 11

TAKING THE TEST MORE THAN ONCE

Some people may never have to read this chapter, but it's a certainty that others will. The most important advice we can give to repeat test takers is: Don't despair. There is hope. We can get you through the NCLEX-PN® exam.

You Are Not Alone

Think about that awful day when the big brown envelope arrived. You just couldn't believe it. You had to tell family, friends, your supervisor, and coworkers that you didn't pass the NCLEX-PN® exam. When this happens, each unsuccessful candidate feels like the only person who has failed the exam.

How to Interpret Unsuccessful Test Results

Unsuccessful candidates on the NCLEX-PN® exam will usually say, "I almost passed." Some of you *did* almost pass, and some of you weren't very close. If you fail the exam, you will receive a Candidate Performance Report from NCSBN. In this profile, you will be told how many questions you answered on the exam. The more questions you answered, the closer you came to passing. The only way you will continue to get questions after you answer the first 85 is if you are answering questions close to the level of difficulty needed to pass the exam. If you are answering questions far above the level needed to pass or far below the level needed to pass, your exam will end at 85 questions.

Figure 11.1 on the next page shows a representation of what happens when a candidate fails in 85 questions. This student does not come close to passing. In 85 questions, this student demonstrates an inability to consistently answer questions correctly at or above the level of difficulty needed to pass the exam. This usually indicates a lack of nursing knowledge, considerable difficulties with taking a standardized test, or a deficiency in critical thinking skills.

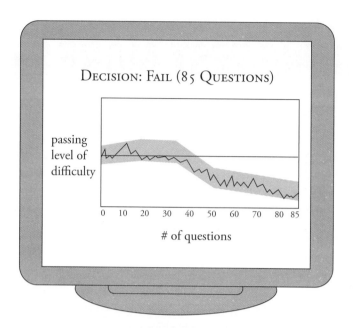

Figure 11.1

Figure 11.2 shows what happens when a candidate takes all 150 questions and fails. This candidate "almost passed." The candidate answers question 149 and the computer does not make a determination when it selects the last question. If the candidate's final ability estimate is at or above the passing standard after answering question 150, the candidate passes. If the final ability estimate is below the passing standard, the candidate fails.

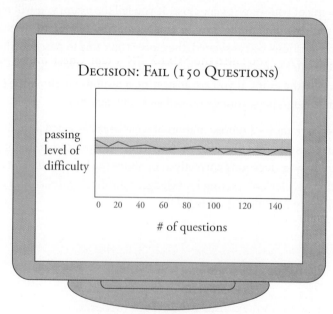

Figure 11.2

If you took a test longer than 85 questions and failed, you were probably familiar with most of the content you saw but you may have difficulty using critical thinking skills or taking standardized tests.

The information contained on the Candidate Performance Report helps you identify your strengths and weaknesses on this particular NCLEX-PN® exam. This knowledge will help you identify where to concentrate your study when you prepare to retake the NCLEX-PN® exam.

Should You Test Again?

Absolutely! You completed your nursing education to become an LPN/LVN. The initial response of many unsuccessful candidates is to declare, "I'm never going back! That was the worst experience of my life! What do I do now?"

When you first received your results, you went through a period of grieving—the same stages that you learned about in nursing school. Three to four weeks later, you find that you want to begin preparing to retake the NCLEX-PN® exam.

How Should You Begin?

You should prepare in a different way this time. Whatever you did to prepare last time didn't work well enough. The most common mistake made by candidates who failed is to assume that they did not study hard enough or learn enough content. For some of you, that's true. But for the majority of you, memorizing more content does not mean more right answers. It could simply mean more frustration for you.

The first step in preparing for your next exam is to make a commitment that you will test again. Decide when you want to schedule your test and allow yourself enough time to prepare. Mark this test date on your calendar. You can do all of this before you send in your fees and receive your authorization to test. Remember, you cannot retake the NCLEX-PN® exam for 45 to 90 days, depending on your state board of nursing/regulatory body, so you may as well use this time wisely.

The next step is to figure out why you failed the NCLEX-PN® exam. Check off any reasons that pertain to you:

- ☐ I didn't know the nursing content.
- ☐ I memorized facts without understanding the principles of client care.
- ☐ I had unrealistic expectations about the NCLEX-PN® exam test questions.
- ☐ I had difficulty correctly identifying THE REWORDED QUESTION.
- ☐ I had difficulty staying focused on THE REWORDED QUESTION.
- ☐ I found myself predicting answer choices.
- ☐ I did not carefully consider each answer choice.
- ☐ I am not good at choosing answers that require me to establish priorities of care.
- ☐ I answered questions based on my real-world experiences.
- ☐ I did not cope well with the computer-adaptive experience.
- ☐ I thought I would complete the exam in 85 questions.
- ☐ When I got to question 120, I totally lost my concentration and just answered questions to get through the rest of the exam.

After determining why you failed, the next step is to establish a plan of action for your next test. Remember, you should prepare differently this time. Consider the following when setting up your new plan of study.

You've seen the test.

You may wish that you didn't have to walk back into the testing center again, but if you want to be a licensed practical/vocational nurse, you must go back. This time you will have an advantage over the first-time test taker: you've seen the test! You know exactly what you are preparing for, and there are no unknowns. The computer will remember what questions you took before, and you will not be given any of the same questions. However, the content of the questions, the style of the questions, and the kinds of answer choices will not change. You will not be surprised this time!

Study both content and test questions.

By the time you retest, you will be out of nursing school for 6 months or longer. Remember that old saying, "What you are not learning, you are forgetting." Because this is a content-based test about safe and effective nursing care, you must remember all you can about nursing theory in order to select correct answers. You must study content that is integrated and organized like the NCLEX-PN® exam.

You must also master exam-style test questions. It is essential that you be able to correctly identify what each question is asking. You will *not* predict answers. You will *think* about each and every answer choice to decide if it answers the reworded question. In order to master test questions, you must practice answering them. We recommend that you answer hundreds of exam-style test questions, especially at the application level of difficulty.

Know all of the words and their meanings.

Some students who have to learn a great deal of material in a short period of time have trouble learning the extensive vocabulary of the discipline. For example, difficulty with terminology is a problem for many good students who study history. They enjoy the concepts but find it hard to memorize all of the names and dates that allow them to do well on history tests. If you are one of those students who have trouble memorizing terms, you may find it useful to review a list of the terminology that you must know to pass the NCLEX-PN® exam. There is a list of those words at the end of this book.

Practice test taking strategies.

There is no substitute for mastering the nursing content. This knowledge, combined with test taking strategies, will help you to select a greater number of correct answers. For many students, the strategies mean the difference between a passing test and a failing test. Using strategies effectively can also determine whether you take a short test (85 questions) or a longer test (up to 150 questions).

Evaluate your testing experience.

Some students attribute their failure to the testing experience. Comments we have heard include:

"I didn't like answering questions on the computer."

"I found the background noise distracting. I should have taken the earplugs!"

"I looked up every time the door opened."

"I should have taken a snack. I got so hungry!"

"After 2½ hours I didn't care what I answered. I just wanted the computer to shut off!"

"I didn't expect to be there for 4 hours!"

"I should have rescheduled my test, but I just wanted to get it over with!"

"I wish I had taken aspirin with me. I had such a headache before it was over!"

Do any of these comments sound familiar? It is important for you to take charge of your testing experience. Here's how:

- Choose a familiar testing site.
- Select the time of day that you test your best. (Are you a morning person or an afternoon person?)
- Accept the earplugs when offered.
- Take a snack and a drink for your break.
- Take a break if you become distracted or fatigued during the test.
- Contact the proctors at the test site if something bothers you during the test.
- Plan on testing for 5 hours. Then, if you get out early, it's a pleasant surprise.
- Say to yourself every day, "I will pass the NCLEX-PN® exam."

CHAPTER 12

ESSENTIALS FOR INTERNATIONAL NURSES

Many of you have years of nursing experience in your home country. Now you are preparing for the NCLEX-PN® exam so you can be licensed to practice your profession in the United States. Because of Kaplan's extensive experience preparing nurses who were educated in other countries, we are very aware of the special issues that you face when trying to pass the NCLEX-PN® exam. Your special concerns will be discussed in this chapter.

Many nurses educated outside of the United States have not had the experience of taking a test that combines objective multiple choice questions with alternate format questions. Your testing experience may have been limited to oral exams or writing answers to essay and short answer questions. Multiple choice tests are used in the United States because they measure knowledge more objectively and are easier to administer to large groups of people. In order to pass the NCLEX-PN® exam, you must demonstrate that you are a safe and effective nurse by correctly answering predominantly multiple choice questions along with alternate format question types.

NCLEX-PN® Exam Administration Abroad

NCSBN administers the NCLEX-PN® exam in selected international locations including Australia, Canada, England, Hong Kong, India, Japan, Mexico, the Philippines, and Taiwan. (Testing is temporarily unavailable in Germany.) Please see **nclex.com** to locate a test center near you.

International sites provide greater convenience for international nurses to take the NCLEX-PN® exam. The international administration does not circumvent any regulations posed by the state boards of nursing, and the test sites are subject to the same security and procedures followed in U.S. test sites. If you choose to take the test at one of these sites, you must pay an additional $150 international scheduling fee plus a Value Added Tax (VAT) where applicable.

The CGFNS® Certificate

In order to apply for licensure as an LPN/LVN in the United States, many U.S. state boards of nursing require internationally educated LPN/LVNs to obtain a certificate from the Commission on Graduates of Foreign Nursing Schools (CGFNS®). Some states require that this process be completed prior to taking the NCLEX-PN® exam. The process of obtaining a CGFNS® certificate includes (1) a review of your secondary and nursing education credentials and original nursing program, (2) passing the CGFNS® exam that tests nursing knowledge, and (3) obtaining a minimum score on a designated English language proficiency exam.

The CGFNS® exam is a two-part test of nursing knowledge. Nurses who pass this exam have been shown to be more likely to pass the NCLEX-PN® exam on the first try than nurses who have not passed the CGFNS®. This exam can be taken overseas at a number of international testing sites run by CGFNS® or at selected sites in the United States.

Applications for the CGFNS® exam are free, and you may apply online at **cgfns.org**. Go to **cgfns.org** for further information. Only online applications for the CGFNS® Certification Program are accepted. On the CGFNS® website, you will also find application deadlines and test dates. With an online application, you can submit your educational and professional documentation, choose a location and date for your exam, and pay fees by credit card. The online CGFNS Qualifying Exam® is administered in March, July, September, and November during a 5-day testing window in each of these months.

To find out about a particular state's requirements for international nurses, call that state's board of nursing and request an application packet for initial licensure as an internationally educated LPN/LVN. You can also visit your chosen state's website using the key words "Board of Nursing" and the state name.

Regarding the CGFNS® English proficiency requirements, the following information will help you register for the appropriate exams. Remember that these exam results are usually only valid for 2 years, so plan accordingly to avoid retakes. For more information about preparing for these exams, see the Kaplan English Programs section at the end of this chapter.

> TOEFL®, TWE®, and TSE®
> Educational Testing Service
> P.O. Box 6151
> Princeton, NJ 08541-6151
> Phone: 1-800-468-6335 (United States, U.S. Territories, Canada)
> Phone: 1-609-771-7100 (all other locations)
> Fax: 1-610-290-8972
> Website: **www.ets.org/toefl**
>
> TOEIC® Testing Program
> Educational Testing Service
> Rosedale Road
> Princeton, NJ 08541
> Phone: 1-609-771-7170
> Fax: 1-610-628-3722
> Email: **toeic@ets.org**
> Website: **www.ets.org/toeic**
>
> IELTS® International
> Website: **www.ielts.org**

Work Visas

For the most current information on visa requirements, contact the nearest U.S. embassy or consulate in your home country or the nearest regional office of the U.S. Citizenship and Immigration Services if you already live in the United States. You can also contact CGFNS® by telephone at 1-215-222-8454 or through its website at **cgfns.org**.

Nursing Practice in the United States

Some international LPN/LVNs find nursing in the United States similar to nursing as they learned it in their country. For others, nursing in the United States is very different from what they learned or experienced in their home country. The NCLEX-PN® exam may ask you questions about procedures that are unfamiliar to you. You may be asked questions about diets and foods that are new to you. In order to be successful on the NCLEX-PN® exam, you must be able to correctly answer questions about nursing as it is practiced in the United States.

Here is an overview of services and skills that LPN/LVNs are expected to perform:

- LPN/LVNs are involved with prevention, early detection, and treatment of illness for people of all ages.
- LPN/LVNs care for the whole person, not just an illness. Their focus is on client needs; that is, how a client will respond to an illness.
- LPN/LVNs are professionals who are responsible for their actions.
- LPN/LVNs must communicate with clients and all the members of the health care team: RNs, unlicensed assistive personnel (UAPs), physicians, dietitians, pharmacists, therapists, technicians, and social workers.
- LPN/LVNs serve as clients' advocates; that is, they counsel clients and make sure their rights are protected.
- LPN/LVNs help clients understand the health care system and assist them to make decisions about their health care.
- LPN/LVNs are assertive and ask questions of other health care professionals when necessary, including physicians. Their style of communication is polite and professional but very direct.
- LPN/LVNs are responsible for meeting the needs of clients whose care involves high-tech equipment.
- LPN/LVNs are responsible for basing their actions on knowledge and acceptable nursing practice.
- LPN/LVNs, not families, are responsible for all the hands-on nursing care for clients in the hospital setting.
- LPN/LVNs are responsible for teaching clients and their families how to manage their health care needs.

U.S.-Style Nursing Communication

An issue of special concern for international nurses is therapeutic communication. Correctly answering the questions about communication can be difficult for some nurses educated in the United States. These questions become a special challenge to test takers for whom English is a second language, or for test takers who do not yet fully understand American-style communication.

Key features of U.S.-style communication in nursing:

- *Validate the client's experience and feelings by responding to the client verbally.* Ask questions that relate directly to what the client says.

- *Direct the client's behavior to promote comfort and well-being.* Do not patronize or reject the client by imposing a value judgment.

- *Maintain eye contact with the client, especially during conversation.* Lean forward to face the client. Nod, smile, or frown to demonstrate agreement or disagreement while listening.

Responses used in U.S. nursing are based on an assessment of the client's needs and are designed to foster growth and establish mutually formulated goals.

NCLEX-PN® exam questions concerning communication are best answered by:

- Conveying *respect* and *warmth*, making the client feel accepted and respected as an individual regardless of their words, actions, or behavior. This means that the LPN/LVN:
  - Assumes that all client behavior is purposeful and has meaning even though it may not make sense to others
  - Defines the social, physical, and emotional boundaries of the nurse-client relationship
  - Develops a contract with the client
  - Structures time to develop a nurse-client relationship
  - Creates a safe and secure environment
  - Accepts the dependency needs of the client while encouraging, assisting, and supporting movement toward health and independence
  - Intervenes when a client behaves inappropriately to directly reject the behavior but not the client
  - Intervenes directly to respond to the client, not to reinforce an inappropriate behavior
- Demonstrating *active listening* and *genuineness*. This means that the LPN/LVN:
  - Asks questions that relate directly to what the client says
  - Maintains good eye contact
  - Leans forward in the chair to face the client
  - Nods, smiles, or frowns to show agreement or disagreement
  - Understands that the personal feelings and past experiences of the nurse can negatively or positively affect relationships with clients

- Communicating *interest* and *empathy* by allowing the client to comfortably communicate concerns and behave in new ways. This means that the LPN/LVN:
  - Focuses conversation on the client's feelings
  - Understands that clients respond to the behavioral expectations of the nursing staff
  - Validates the client's feelings
  - Analyzes both verbal and nonverbal behavioral clues
  - Anticipates that there might be some difficulty as the client learns new behaviors

LPN/LVNs create barriers in the communication process when they demonstrate a poor understanding of the basics in therapeutic communication. They must convey respect, warmth, and genuineness through active listening and communicating interest and empathy about the concerns of clients, families, or staff.

Examples of barriers to communication:

- Minimizing concerns
- Giving false reassurance
- Giving approval
- Rejecting the person, not the behavior
- Choosing sides with the client, family member, or staff member in a conflict
- Blaming the external environment for the situation
- Disagreeing or arguing with the client or family member
- Offering advice about a situation
- Pressuring the client or family member for an explanation
- Defending one's own actions or behavior
- Belittling concerns of the client, family member, or staff
- Giving one-word responses to questions
- Using denial
- Interpreting or analyzing both verbal and nonverbal behavioral clues to the client in the situation
- Shifting the focus of the conversation away from the concerns of the client, family member, or staff
- Using jargon or medical terminology without explanation in conversation with the client and/or family
- Invalidating the client's, family member's, or staff's feelings
- Offering unrealistic hope for the future
- Ignoring client clues to help the client set appropriate limits on their behavior

The following are some questions that will allow you to practice the right approach.

Sample Questions

> ***Directions:*** Carefully read the question and all answer choices. Determine whether each option is an appropriate response. In the space at the right, record your decision ("Correct" or "Incorrect") along with the reason you believe that the nurse's response is correct or incorrect.

Questions	Reason the Option is Correct/Incorrect

1. A client has been hospitalized for two days for treatment of hepatitis A. When the LPN/LVN enters the client's room, the client says, "Leave me alone and stop bothering me." Which response by the LPN/LVN would be **most** appropriate?
 	
  1. "I understand and will leave you alone for now."
  2. "Why are you angry with me?"
  3. "Are you upset because you do not feel better?"
  4. "You seem upset this morning."	

2. A client with a fractured arm tells the nurse, "I'm afraid to have the cast removed." Which response by the LPN/LVN is the **most** appropriate?
 	
  1. "I know it is unpleasant. Try not to be afraid. I will help you."
  2. "You seem very anxious. I will stay with you while the cast is removed."
  3. "I don't blame you. I'd be afraid also."
  4. "My aunt just had a cast removed and she's just fine."	

Questions	Reason the Option is Correct/Incorrect

3. A client comes to the clinic for a suspected pregnancy. The client tells the LPN/LVN, "I want to terminate this pregnancy because my spouse and I don't want to have children," and then begins to cry. Which statement by the LPN/LVN is the **most** appropriate?
 	
  1. "Are you upset because you forgot to use birth control?"
 	
  2. "Why are you so upset? You're married. There's no reason not to have the baby."
 	
  3. "If you're so upset, why don't you have the baby and put it up for adoption?"
 	
  4. "You seem upset. Let's talk about how you're feeling."	

4. A client is in the terminal stages of carcinoma of the lung. A family member asks the LPN/LVN, "How much longer will it be?" Which response by the LPN/LVN would be **most** appropriate?
 	
  1. "I cannot say exactly. What are your concerns at this time?"
 	
  2. "I don't know. I'll call your family member's oncologist."
 	
  3. "This must be a terrible situation for you."
 	
  4. "Don't worry, it will be very soon."	

Questions	Reason the Option is Correct/Incorrect

5. A client is admitted to the hospital with a diagnosis of bipolar disorder. The client approaches the nurse and says, "Hi, baby," and opens the robe, under which the client is naked. Which comment by the LPN/LVN would be **most** appropriate?

1. "This is inappropriate behavior. Please close your robe and return to your room."
2. "Please dress in your clothes and then join us for lunch in the dining room."
3. "I am offended by your behavior and will have to report you."
4. "Do you need some assistance dressing today?"

6. The LPN/LVN prepares to assist the client placed in Buck's traction with a bath. The client tells the nurse, "You're too young to know how to do this. Get me somebody who knows what they're doing." Which response by the LPN/LVN would be **most** appropriate?

1. "I am young, but I graduated from nursing school."
2. "If I don't bathe you now, you'll have to wait until I'm finished with my other clients."
3. "Can you be more specific about your concerns?"
4. "Your concerns are unnecessary. I know what I'm doing."

Questions	Reason the Option is Correct/Incorrect
7. A client with an abdominal mass is admitted to the hospital and scheduled for an exploratory laparotomy. The client asks the LPN/LVN, "Do you think I have cancer?" Which response by the LPN/LVN would be **most** appropriate? 1. "Would you like me to call your doctor so that you can discuss your specific concerns?" 2. "Your tests show a mass. It must be hard not knowing what is wrong." 3. "It sounds like you are afraid that you are going to die from cancer." 4. "Don't worry about it now; I'm sure you have many healthy years ahead of you."	
8. A client is admitted to the postpartum unit following a miscarriage. The next day the LPN/LVN finds the client crying while looking at the babies in the newborn nursery. Which approach by the LPN/LVN would be **most** appropriate? 1. "There is a reason for everything. The miscarriage was for the best." 2. "Don't cry, it will be okay. You are young enough to have more children." 3. "Why are you looking at the babies in the nursery?" 4. "You seem to be grieving the loss of your baby. Please share what you're feeling."	

Questions	Reason the Option is Correct/Incorrect
9. An older adult client is hospitalized with major neurocognitive disorder (NCD) due to Alzheimer disease. The client's adult daughter tells the LPN/LVN that caring for him is too hard, but that she feels guilty placing him in a nursing home. Which statement by the LPN/LVN is **most** appropriate? 1. "It is hard to be caught between taking care of your needs and your father's needs." 2. "Would you like me to help you find a nursing home?" 3. "Don't feel guilty. The only solution is to place your father in a nursing home." 4. "I think I would feel guilty too if I had to place my father in a nursing home."	

Read the explanations to these questions and make sure that the American approach to these communications questions is understandable to you. It will help you to choose the right answer on the NCLEX-PN® exam.

Answers to Sample Questions

1. The answer is 4

(4) "You seem upset this morning." This is the correct answer choice because the LPN/LVN seeks to verbally validate the client's behavior rather than simply responding to the behavior. This promotes the nurse-client relationship by encouraging the client to share feelings with the LPN/LVN.

(1) "I understand and will leave you alone for now." This is not the best approach because it does not promote further communication between the LPN/LVN and the client about how the client is feeling. In order to interpret this client's behavior, the LPN/LVN must first validate it with the client.

(2) "Why are you angry with me?" This response is incorrect. The LPN/LVN is drawing a conclusion about the client's behavior. This type of response is too confrontational. "Why" questions are considered nontherapeutic.

(3) "Are you upset because you do not feel better?" This response is not the best choice. The LPN/LVN is drawing a conclusion about the client's behavior without validating it first. This question may also belittle the client's actual concerns.

2. The answer is 2

(2) "You seem very anxious. I will stay with you while the cast is removed." This is the best choice because the LPN/LVN responds to the client's feelings of fear. Doing so is consistent with therapeutic communication used in American nursing. This response also provides an additional opportunity for the LPN/LVN to remain with the client in a supportive capacity enhancing the nurse-client relationship.

(1) "I know it is unpleasant. Try not to be afraid. I will help you." It is not clear what concerns the client has about this procedure. The LPN/LVN should establish what they are before responding. The LPN/LVN falsely reassures the client by saying, "I will help you." Because you do not know the nature of the client's concerns, you cannot honestly offer help.

(3) "I don't blame you. I'd be afraid also." This answer is incorrect because it shifts the focus of the conversation from the client to the LPN/LVN. This sets up a barrier to further communication. The LPN/LVN concedes the issue too quickly, leaving the source of the client's fear unknown.

(4) "My aunt just had a cast removed and she's just fine." This choice shifts the focus of the conversation from the client to the LPN/LVN's aunt, who is of no concern to the client. It fails to explore the source of the client's anxiety and sets up a block to further communication.

3. The answer is 4

(4) "You seem upset. Let's talk about how you're feeling." This the best answer to this question. It promotes the nurse-client relationship and illustrates therapeutic communication used in American nursing. The LPN/LVN responds to the client's feelings in a nonjudgmental, empathetic way.

(1) "Are you upset because you forgot to use birth control?" This response is inappropriate because it places blame on the client. The LPN/LVN should not assume that the client "forgot" to do something. It also fails to respond to the client's feelings and does not encourage the client to discuss concerns.

(2) "Why are you so upset? You're married. There's no reason not to have the baby." This response is inappropriate in terms of American therapeutic communication. It is harsh and presumptive, and assumes that the purpose of every marriage is to have children. This is not always the case in American culture. With this response, the LPN/LVN does not attempt to verify the reason for the client's tears, thereby discouraging further conversation about what the client is actually experiencing.

(3) "If you're so upset, why don't you have the baby and put it up for adoption?" This response is also inappropriate because it is a value-laden assumption placing positive value on adoption. Again, the

LPN/LVN fails to explore with the client the reason for the client's tears, thereby discouraging further communication. The LPN/LVN is also offering advice.

4. The answer is 1

(1) **"I cannot say exactly. What are your concerns at this time?"** This is the most appropriate response because it is unclear why the family member has approached the LPN/LVN at this point. Perhaps the client is in pain and the family member wants to discuss it with the LPN/LVN. This response allows for that possibility. It is also direct and factually correct.

(2) "I don't know. I'll call your family member's oncologist." This is not the most appropriate response. It shifts the focus of responsibility from the LPN/LVN to the physician, which prevents a nurse–family member relationship from developing.

(3) "This must be a terrible situation for you." This is not the most appropriate response. It is a value-laden statement that fails to explore the family member's reason for approaching the LPN/LVN.

(4) "Don't worry, it will be very soon." This answer is inappropriate because it offers the family member false reassurance. It also offers advice by telling the family member not to worry. This statement is demeaning and may sound as if the nurse is too busy to discuss the family member's concerns.

5. The answer is 1

(1) **"This is inappropriate behavior. Please close your robe and return to your room."** This statement by the LPN/LVN is the correct answer choice. It responds to the client's behavior, sets limits on the behavior, and directs the client toward more appropriate social behavior in the milieu. This statement rejects the client's behavior, not the client as a person.

(2) "Please dress in your clothes and then join us for lunch in the dining room." This answer is incorrect because it ignores the behavior of the client

improperly exposing the naked body. Instead it directs the client to dress and report to the dining room for lunch as though nothing has happened. This is inappropriate and nontherapeutic.

(3) "I am offended by your behavior and will have to report you." This response is incorrect because it shifts the focus from the client to the LPN/LVN and the LPN/LVN's feelings. The LPN/LVN's personal feelings are irrelevant. Threatening to report the client is also punitive, which is nontherapeutic.

(4) "Do you need some assistance dressing today?" This response is incorrect because it fails to respond to the client's behavior. It is also a yes/no question, which is nontherapeutic.

6. The answer is 3

(3) **"Can you be more specific about your concerns?"** This is the best answer choice because it seeks to validate the client's message. It is direct, is not defensive, and allows the client to express their point of view.

(1) "I am young, but I graduated from nursing school." This choice responds to only part of the message that the client sent to the LPN/LVN. It assumes that the LPN/LVN knows what the client's concerns are and agrees that there is some problem associated with being too young. Further clarification is necessary in this situation.

(2) "If I don't bathe you now, you'll have to wait until I'm finished with my other clients." This response is nontherapeutic. It fails to explore the client's concerns about the LPN/LVN. It is an uncaring and punitive statement by the LPN/LVN that is inappropriate in a nurse-client relationship.

(4) "Your concerns are unnecessary. I know what I'm doing." This response dismisses the client's feelings by saying the client shouldn't be concerned. The LPN/LVN should not tell a client how the client should be feeling. While a response asserting the LPN/LVN's competence may sound like reassurance, the LPN/LVN has yet to validate the concerns that underlie the client's statement.

7.   The answer is 2

(2)   **"Your tests show a mass. It must be hard not knowing what is wrong."** This is the best answer choice because it responds to the client's feelings. It allows the client to continue to identify and express concerns regarding surgery, hospitalization, and the possibility of having a potentially life-threatening illness. The LPN/LVN validates that the client has appropriate concerns and invites the client to elaborate on them.

(1)   "Would you like me to call your doctor so that you can discuss your specific concerns?" This response is incorrect because it shifts the focus of responsibility from the LPN/LVN to the doctor, thereby reducing the possibility of developing an ongoing nurse-client relationship.

(3)   "It sounds like you are afraid that you are going to die from cancer." This answer is inappropriate. It fails to validate with the client that "dying from cancer" is in fact the issue. The LPN/LVN reaches this conclusion on the basis of a brief question from the client without giving the client a chance to elaborate. This is inappropriate.

(4)   "Don't worry about it now; I'm sure that you have many healthy years ahead of you." The LPN/LVN is telling the client how the client should feel and then goes on to offer false reassurance. This response fails to address or explore the actual concerns of the client.

8.   The answer is 4

(4)   **"You seem to be grieving the loss of your baby. Please share what you're feeling."** This is the best answer choice. This response promotes the nurse-client relationship and allows for the identification of feelings and the expression of sadness. The client is in an acute stage of grief. Acknowledging the loss and offering support appropriately addresses this issue.

(1)   "There is a reason for everything. The miscarriage was for the best." This statement is insensitive to the client, offers false reassurance, and belittles the client's most immediate concerns.

(2)   "Don't cry, it will be okay. You are young enough to have more children." This statement it is insensitive to the grief that the client is experiencing. It also offers false reassurance by saying that the client can have other children.

(3)   "Why are you looking at the babies in the nursery?" This is a "why" question, which may cause the client to become defensive. This response by the LPN/LVN also fails to address the client's immediate grief.

9.   The answer is 1

(1)   **"It is hard to be caught between taking care of your needs and your father's needs."** This is the most therapeutic response as it allows for continued development of a relationship with the family member of the client. This response allows the LPN/LVN to explore and validate the daughter's feelings about the nursing home placement.

(2)   "Would you like me to help you find a nursing home?" This is not the best answer choice. It is a yes/no question and doesn't encourage discussion of the daughter's feelings.

(3)   "Don't feel guilty. The only solution is to place your father in a nursing home." Telling the adult daughter not to worry minimizes her concerns. While it may be true that the daughter has done all that she can, this is not the best therapeutic response because it cuts off an opportunity for further conversation with the LPN/LVN.

(4)   "I think I would feel guilty too if I had to place my father in a nursing home." This statement is value-laden and judgmental, and it blocks further communication between the LPN/LVN and the client's daughter. It is not important what the LPN/LVN thinks about the daughter's decision, nor is it the LPN/LVN's role to make the daughter feel more guilty about her decision.

Language

English is the predominant language spoken and written in the United States, and the NCLEX-PN® exam is administered only in English. With the exception of the medical terminology, the reading level of the NCLEX-PN® exam is that of a sophomore in an American high school. In order to be successful on the NCLEX-PN® exam, you must understand English—and the terminology—as it is used in the United States.

Vocabulary

Vocabulary can be a challenge for international nurses on the NCLEX-PN® exam. Not only must you know what each word means, but sometimes a word may have more than one meaning. You need to be able to correctly identify words as they are used in context. Refer to the NCLEX-PN® Exam Resources section in the back of this book for some of the commonly found words on the NCLEX-PN® exam. Some other ways to increase your vocabulary and learn how the words are used in everyday English include:

- Talking with Americans
- Watching American movies and television
- Reading American newspapers and magazines

Abbreviations

Many internationally educated nurses are unfamiliar with the abbreviations used in the United States. When studying, always look up unknown words in a medical dictionary. Consult Appendix C for a list of abbreviations used by nurses in American health care settings.

As an internationally educated nurse, you face special challenges in preparing for the NCLEX-PN® exam. Following the tips and guidelines outlined in this book will increase your chances of passing the NCLEX-PN® exam and will allow you to reach your career goals.

Kaplan Programs for International Nurses

Knowing something about U.S. culture and how U.S. nurses fit into the overall health care industry is important for nurses trained outside the United States. If you are not from the United States but are interested in learning more about U.S. nursing, wish to practice in the United States, or are exploring the possibilities of attending a U.S. nursing school for graduate study, Kaplan is able to help you.

CGFNS® (Commission on Graduates of Foreign Nursing Schools) Preparation for International Nurses

Many U.S. state boards of nursing require internationally educated nurses to obtain a CGFNS® certificate before applying for initial licensure as an LPN/LVN. The certification process requires that a candidate pass a two-part test of nursing knowledge and demonstrate English language proficiency on the TOEFL® exam. Kaplan offers a comprehensive course of study to help you pass this exam. To obtain information, please call 1-800-527-8378. Outside the United States, please call 1-212-997-5883 or log on to the website at **kaplannursing.com**.

Preparation for the NCLEX-PN® Examination for International Nurses

An internationally educated nurse must pass the NCLEX-PN® exam in order to obtain a license to practice as an LPN/LVN in the United States. Kaplan has a comprehensive course and review products to help international nurses pass this exam. To obtain information, please call 1-800-527-8378 (outside the United States: 1-212-997-5883) or log on to the website at **https://www.kaptest.com /ispn-cgfns/courses/ispn-cgfns-prep**.

Kaplan English Programs

In addition to Kaplan Nursing programs, Kaplan also offers English programs to help you improve your English skills and score on the TOEFL® exam. Kaplan's English programs are designed to help students and professionals from outside the United States meet their educational and career goals. At locations throughout the United States, international students take advantage of Kaplan's programs to help them improve their academic and conversational English skills, raise their scores on the TOEFL® and other standardized exams, and gain admission to the schools of their choice. Our staff and instructors give international students the individualized instruction they need to succeed. The following sections provide brief descriptions of some of Kaplan's programs for non-native English speakers.

English Language Programs

Kaplan offers a wide range of English language programs to help you improve your English quickly and effectively, regardless of your current level. Each of our programs has a special focus, allowing you to direct your study in a way that suits your particular language needs. All of the essential language skills are covered, and your fluency and confidence will increase rapidly thanks to Kaplan's communicative teaching method.

TOEFL® and Academic English

Kaplan has updated its world-famous TOEFL® course to prepare students for the TOEFL® iBT. Designed for high-intermediate to advanced-level English speakers, our course focuses on the academic English skills you will need to succeed on the test. The course includes TOEFL®-focused reading, writing, listening, and speaking instruction and hundreds of practice items similar to those on the exam. Kaplan's expert instructors help you prepare for the four sections of the TOEFL® iBT, including the Speaking section. Our simulated online TOEFL® tests help you monitor your progress and provide you with feedback on areas where you require improvement. We will teach you how to get a higher score!

Other Kaplan Programs

Since 1938, more than 3 million students have come to Kaplan to advance their studies, prepare for entry to American universities, and further their careers. In addition to the above programs, Kaplan offers courses to prepare for the SAT®, ACT®, GMAT®, GRE®, LSAT®, MCAT®, DAT®, USMLE®, and other standardized exams both online and at locations throughout the United States.

Applying to Kaplan English Programs*

To get more information, or to apply for admission to any of Kaplan's programs for non-native English speakers, contact us at:

Kaplan English Programs
Phone: 1-800-818-9128 (within the United States)
Phone: +44 (0) 20 7045 5000 (elsewhere)
Website: **kaplaninternational.com**

> ### FREE Services for International Students
>
> Kaplan now offers international students many services online—free of charge! Students may assess their TOEFL® skills and gain valuable feedback on their English language proficiency in just a few hours with Kaplan's TOEFL® Skills Assessment. Log on to **kaplaninternational.com today**.

---

*Kaplan is authorized under federal law to enroll nonimmigrant alien students.

Test names are registered trademarks of their respective owners.

THE PRACTICE TEST

PART FOUR

THE PROPHETS

PRACTICE TEST

Directions: This practice test consists of 150 exam-style questions. Allot 5 hours of uninterrupted time to take the practice test. For each fill-in-the-blank question, write in the correct answer. For each drag-and-drop ordered response question, write the number of each step in the sequence in which the steps should be performed. For each item of the remaining question types, HIGHLIGHT the option or options that best answer the question.

1. The LPN/LVN is gathering data from a client who is receiving treatment for obsessive-compulsive disorder (OCD). Which is the **most** important question the LPN/LVN should ask this client?

   1. "Do you find yourself forgetting simple things?"
   2. "Do you find it difficult to focus on a given task?"
   3. "Do you have trouble controlling upsetting thoughts?"
   4. "Do you experience feelings of panic in a closed area?"

2. A newly admitted client with a history of seizures suddenly says to the LPN/LVN, "I hear drums." Which should the LPN/LVN do **first**?

   1. Tell the client to ignore the drums.
   2. Place client in a darkened room away from nurses' station.
   3. Continue to question the client about the drum sound.
   4. Insert an oral airway in the client.

Refer to the Case Study to answer the next six questions.

The LPN/LVN is providing care in a medical surgical unit for an older adult client with a diagnosis of type 2 diabetes.

| Admission Notes | Nurse's Notes | Vital Signs | Medications |

The client is admitted from home three days ago for evaluation of progressive right lower limb ischemia related to peripheral artery disease. The client is experiencing intermittent claudication, paresthesia in toes and feet, increasing limb pain, and has an arterial ulcer on the right great toe. The client has a history of type 2 diabetes that is managed with PO metformin. The client reports limited exercise, poor eating habits, and infrequent self-monitoring of blood glucose.

The client is requiring insulin to manage glucose levels during this hospitalization. The client's regimen consists of sliding scale rapid-acting insulin (aspart) at mealtimes combined with an intermediate-acting (NPH) insulin twice daily for background metabolic needs.

| Admission Notes | Nurse's Notes | Vital Signs | Medications |

2330: On nursing rounds, observed the client sweating profusely around the face, neck, upper extremities, and torso. Pillow and bed linens are wet. The client is rousable to verbal stimuli, opens eyes, but is unable to answer questions appropriately and has slurred, incoherent speech. The client is not alert, unable to stay awake, and returns to sleep quickly. Pupils equal, round, reactive to light. Skin is pale, cool, extremely diaphoretic with elastic turgor. Apical heart rate 124, regular; 2+ radial pulses equal, bilaterally; capillary refill less than 2 seconds; no pedal edema. Chest expansion equal with soft, vesicular lung sounds throughout. Abdomen soft, non-tender, bowel sounds present. Moves all extremities spontaneously. Right lower leg: 1+ pedal pulses; skin is cool, thin, shiny, taut. Gauze dressing to right great toe intact, no drainage. Left leg: no edema, 2+ pedal pulses.

| Admission Notes | Nurse's Notes | Vital Signs | Medications |

Vital Signs	Results
Blood pressure	118/78 mmHg
Heart rate	124 beats/minute, regular
Respiratory rate	20, regular
Temperature (oral)	97.6° F (36.44° C)
Pulse oximetry	97% on room air
Body Mass Index (BMI)	31 kg/m^2 (obese)

| | Admission Notes | Nurse's Notes | Vital Signs | Medications |

Time	Blood Glucose	Insulin	Food/Snack
1700	240 mg/dL (13.32 mmol/L)	Intermediate acting (NPH) insulin 15 units with rapid-acting (aspart) insulin 4 units sliding scale subcutaneously to right upper abdomen	100% dinner meal eaten
2100			0% bedtime snack eaten

3. The LPN/LVN reviews the admission notes, 2330 nurse's notes, vital signs, and medications.

Highlight the client findings in the table that require **immediate** follow up. Highlight correct sections.

Assessment	Client Findings
Vital Signs	Heart rate 124 bpm, regular Blood pressure 118/78 BMI 31 kg/m^2 (obese)
Skin	Pale, cool Profuse sweating
Respiratory	Soft, vesicular lung sounds
Neurologic	Unable to answer questions appropriately Slurred, incoherent speech
Medications	Intermediate-acting NPH insulin at 1700 Uneaten bedtime snack at 2100

4. Complete the following sentence by choosing from the list of options.

   The LPN/LVN identifies the client is most likely experiencing symptoms of [Select from list 1] as a result of [Select from list 2], and [Select from list 3].

(1)	(2)	(3)
hypoglycemia	not enough exercise or activity	insulin administered subcutaneously instead of intramuscularly
insulin allergic reaction	current illness and the risk for infection	lack of food intake during peak action of NPH insulin
diabetic ketoacidosis	too much insulin relative to blood glucose	sliding scale aspart insulin at mealtime

5. The RN directs the LPN/LVN to obtain a capillary blood glucose. The LPN/LVN reports a result of 39 mg/dL (2.16 mmol/L) to the RN immediately.

   Due to the client's low blood glucose, the LPN/LVN's priority consideration is the client's risk to develop which complication?

   1. Osmotic diuresis.
   2. Hypokalemia.
   3. Hypovolemia.
   4. Seizures.

6. The LPN/LVN and the RN collaborate on the primary goal of treating the client's low blood glucose. Select **2** interventions appropriate for the client.

   1. Oral administration of 15 grams of a fast-acting carbohydrate.
   2. Intravenous administration of a short-acting insulin.
   3. Subcutaneous or intramuscular injection of 1 mg glucagon.
   4. Administer potassium chloride 20 mEq orally.
   5. 50 mL of 50% dextrose intravenously.
   6. Intravenous fluids with 0.9% sodium chloride.

7. Following treatment, the client is alert and verbally responding appropriately. The client's blood glucose is 60 mg/dL (3.33 mmol/L). The LPN/LVN continues to provide care.

Complete the following sentences by choosing from the list of options.

It is now appropriate for the LPN/LVN to provide [Select from list 1]. Next, the LPN/LVN will [Select from list 2]. If the client's blood glucose is less than 70 mg/dL (3.9 mmol/L), the LPN/LVN will [Select from list 3].

(1)	(2)	(3)
oral carbohydrates with fat, such as whole milk or ice cream	obtain a urine sample and check for ketones	provide 15 grams of fast-acting carbohydrates
four to six ounces regular soda or orange juice	consider the client's blood glucose as corrected	give a snack of peanut butter and crackers
a drink or food containing at least 15 grams of protein	wait 15 minutes and recheck the client's blood glucose	prepare to administer a continuous insulin infusion intravenously

8. The LPN/LVN continues to monitor the client. Which finding indicates that the nursing actions have been effective? **(Select all that apply.)**

1. Heart rate 88, regular.

2. Shakiness.

3. Blood glucose 115 mg/dL (6.38 mmol/L).

4. Dizziness when standing.

5. Coherent thoughts with smooth flow to speech.

6. Fruity odor to breath.

7. Respirations 28, rapid and deep.

9. A client diagnosed with multiple myeloma is admitted to the unit after developing pneumonia. When the LPN/LVN enters the client's room wearing a mask, the client says, in an irritated tone of voice, "Why are you wearing that mask?" Which response by the LPN/LVN is **best**?

   1. "The chest x-ray taken this morning indicates you have pneumonia."
   2. "What have you been told about the x-rays that were taken this morning?"
   3. "You have been placed on contact precautions due to your infection."
   4. "I am trying to protect you from the germs in the hospital."

10. A nursing team consists of an RN, an LPN/LVN, and an unlicensed assistive personnel (UAP). The LPN/LVN should be assigned to which client?

    1. A client with a diabetic ulcer that requires a dressing change.
    2. A client with cancer who is reporting bone pain.
    3. A client with terminal cancer being transferred to hospice home care.
    4. A client with a fracture of the right leg who asks to use the urinal.

11. The LPN/LVN is caring for a client receiving paroxetine. It is **most** important for the LPN/LVN to report which information to the primary health care provider?

    1. The client reports no appetite change.
    2. The client reports recently being started on digoxin.
    3. The client reports applying sunscreen to go outdoors.
    4. The client reports driving the car to work.

12. A client with a "do not resuscitate" order experiences a cardiac arrest. Which is the **first** action the LPN/LVN should take?

    1. Administer lifesaving medications.
    2. Assess the client for signs of death.
    3. Open the airway and give 2 breaths.
    4. Summon the emergency code team.

13. An LPN/LVN is working in the newborn nursery. Which client-care assignment should the LPN/LVN question?

    1. A 2-day-old client lying quietly alert with a heart rate of 185 beats/minute.
    2. A 1-day-old client who is crying and has a bulging anterior fontanel.
    3. A 12-hour-old client whose respirations are 45 breaths/minute and irregular while being held.
    4. A 5-hour-old client whose hands and feet appear blue bilaterally while sleeping.

Refer to the Case Study to answer the next six questions.

The LPN/LVN is caring for a 66-year-old client on the medical-surgical unit.

| Nurse's Notes | Vital Signs | History and Physical |

1500: Client is alert and oriented ×3. Coarse crackles noted to bilateral lung bases. S1 and S2 heart sounds heard, no murmur or gallop noted. Skin is warm to the touch and appears flushed; capillary refill >3 seconds.

| Nurse's Notes | Vital Signs | History and Physical |

Vital Signs	Results
HR	114
BP	98/56 mmHg
RR	24
Pulse oximetry	89% on room air
Temperature	101.6° F (38.7° C) (temporal)

| Nurse's Notes | Vital Signs | History and Physical |

History: Client admitted with cough, headache, and shortness of breath. Was treated at home for an upper respiratory tract infection (URI) approximately 5 days ago. Started antibiotic therapy at home but reports "not feeling well" the last 2 days and inability to take anything by mouth, including antibiotics.

Body System	Findings
Neurological	Alert and oriented ×3.
Eye, Ear, Nose, and Throat (EENT)	Admitted for worsening upper respiratory infection. Reports sore throat, nasal drainage, and headache.
Pulmonary	Reports cough and shortness of breath. Coarse crackles to bilateral lung bases.
Cardiovascular	S1 and S2 heart sounds heard, no murmur or gallop noted. Skin is warm to the touch and appears flushed, capillary refill >3 seconds. Peripheral pulses bounding and equal bilaterally.
Gastrointestinal	Reports inability to take anything by mouth the last 2 days due to nausea.
Genitourinary	Has not voided all day, prior to admission. Voided 20 mL clear, dark urine, when prompted.
Musculoskeletal	Full range of motion against resistance.

14. The LPN/LVN reviews the nurse's notes, vital signs, and history and physical.

    Which finding requires follow-up by the LPN/LVN? **(Select all that apply.)**

    1. Coarse crackles to bilateral lung bases.
    2. Skin is warm to the touch and appears flushed.
    3. Capillary refill >3 seconds.
    4. Alert and oriented ×3.
    5. No murmur or gallop noted.
    6. Unable to finish antibiotic therapy.

15. For each assessment finding, specify if the finding is consistent with pneumonia or sepsis. **Each column must have at least 1 response option selected.**

Assessment Finding	Pneumonia	Sepsis
Shortness of breath.	☐	☐
BP 98/56 mmHg.	☐	☐
Capillary refill >3 seconds.	☐	☐
Temperature 101.6° F (38.7° C).	☐	☐
Coarse crackles to lung bases.	☐	☐
Decreased urine output.	☐	☐

16. Based on the client's symptoms, which complication of URI is the client **most likely** experiencing?

    1. Sepsis.
    2. Pneumonia.
    3. Angina.
    4. Urinary tract infection (UTI).

17. The LPN/LVN and RN discuss potential nursing interventions needed in order to plan care for the client.

For each body system below, specify the potential nursing intervention that is appropriate for the care of the client. Each body system supports 1 potential nursing intervention.

Body System	Potential Nursing Interventions
Respiratory	Select... ▾
	Apply supplemental oxygen via nasal cannula.
	Perform nasotracheal suctioning.
	Obtain ventilation/perfusion (V/Q) scan.
Cardiovascular	Select... ▾
	Infuse 0.45% sodium chloride 500 mL IV bolus.
	Infuse 5% dextrose in water 500 mL IV bolus.
	Infuse Lactated Ringer (LR) 500 mL IV bolus.
Genitourinary	Select... ▾
	Obtain urine specific gravity.
	Encourage toileting every 2 hours.
	Perform a bladder ultrasound.

Nurse's Notes | Vital Signs | History and Physical | Orders

Physician's Orders

- Vital signs every 1 hour.
- Insert indwelling urinary catheter.
- Monitor intake and output. Notify physician for urine output < 30 mL per hour.
- Lactated Ringer (LR) bolus 500 mL IV over one hour.
- Following bolus, infuse LR at 75 mL IV per hour.
- Initiate oxygen therapy and titrate to maintain pulse oximetry $>92\%$.
- Obtain laboratory tests: Serum lactate, complete blood count (CBC), blood culture and sensitivity (C&S), and sputum C&S.
- Administer piperacillin/tazobactam 3.375 g IV every 6 hours.
- Acetaminophen 325 mg PO every 4 hours PRN temperature $>100.5°$ F ($38.1°$ C).

18. The LPN/LVN and RN review the physician's orders.

Complete the following sentence by choosing from the list of options.

The LPN/LVN understands that before the antibiotics can be administered,
_____ [Select from the list] .

the client will receive acetaminophen
the laboratory tests need to be drawn
the RN will infuse the IV fluid bolus
the LPN/LVN will insert the indwelling urinary catheter

19. The LPN/LVN speaks with the client and reinforces the measures to prevent and treat infection.

For each statement made by the client, specify whether the statement indicates understanding or no understanding of instructions.

Client Statement	Understanding	No Understanding
"I will make sure to finish the course of antibiotics."	○	○
"If I start feeling cold and clammy, I will notify the nurse."	○	○
"Acetaminophen will help prevent further inflammation."	○	○
"This urinary catheter is convenient and should stay in as long as possible."	○	○

20. The LPN/LVN is inserting a nasogastric (NG) tube. The LPN/LVN should use which personal protective equipment during NG tube insertion?

    1. Gloves, gown, goggles, and surgical cap.
    2. Sterile gloves, mask, and gown.
    3. Gloves, gown, mask, and goggles.
    4. Double gloves, goggles, mask, and surgical cap.

21. The LPN/LVN is caring for clients in the outpatient clinic. Which client should the LPN/LVN see **first**?

    1. A client with hepatitis A who states, "My arms and legs are itching."
    2. A client with a cast on the right leg who states, "I have a funny feeling in my right leg."
    3. A client with osteomyelitis of the spine who states, "I am so nauseous that I can't eat."
    4. A client with rheumatoid arthritis who states, "I am having trouble sleeping."

22. Which client assignment should an LPN/LVN question?

    1. A client with a chest tube who is ambulating in the hallway.
    2. A client with a colostomy who requires colostomy irrigation assistance.
    3. A client with a right-sided stroke who requires assistance with bathing.
    4. A client who is refusing medication to treat cancer of the colon.

23. The LPN/LVN is caring for a client with hepatitis B. The client is to be discharged the next day. The LPN/LVN would be **most** concerned if the client made which statement?

    1. "I must not share eating utensils with my family members."
    2. "I must use my own bath towel."
    3. "I'm glad I can have intimate relations with my partner."
    4. "I must eat small, frequent meals."

24. The LPN/LVN is carrying out the plan for care of a client with anemia who reports weakness. Which task could be assigned to the unlicensed assistive personnel (UAP)?

    1. Auscultate the client's breath sounds.
    2. Set up the client's lunch tray.
    3. Obtain client's dietary history.
    4. Instruct client how to balance rest and activity.

25. A client scheduled for a cardiac catheterization says to the LPN/LVN, "I know you were in here when I signed the consent form for the test. I thought I understood everything, but now I'm not so sure." Which response by the LPN/LVN is **best**?

    1. "Why didn't you listen more closely to the explanation?"
    2. "You sound as if you would like to ask more questions."
    3. "I'll get you a pamphlet about cardiac catheterization."
    4. "That often happens during explanation of this procedure."

26. A 1-day-old client diagnosed with intrauterine growth restriction has a high-pitched shrill cry and appears restless and irritable. The LPN/LVN also observes fist-sucking behavior. Based on this data, which action should the LPN/LVN take **first**?

    1. Gently massage the client's back every 2 hours.
    2. Tightly swaddle the client in a flexed position.
    3. Schedule feeding times every 3 to 4 hours.
    4. Encourage eye contact with the client during feedings.

27. The LPN/LVN notes that a client newly admitted to the pediatric unit is scratching the head almost constantly. It would be **most** important for the LPN/LVN to take which action?

    1. Discuss basic hygiene with the parents.
    2. Instruct the child not to sleep with the dog.
    3. Advise parents to contact an exterminator.
    4. Observe the scalp for small white specks.

28. The client diagnosed with major depressive disorder who was admitted to the psychiatric unit for treatment and observation a week ago suddenly appears cheerful and motivated. The LPN/LVN should be aware of which potential cause of the client's change in behavior?

    1. The client is likely sleeping well because of the medication.
    2. The client has made new friends and has a support group.
    3. The client may have finalized a suicide plan.
    4. The client is no longer depressed due to treatment.

29. The LPN/LVN is caring for clients in the GYN clinic. A client reports an off-white vaginal discharge with a curdlike appearance and vulvar itching. The LPN/LVN observes the discharge and vulvular erythema. It would be **most** important for the LPN/LVN to ask which question?

    1. "Do you routinely douche?"
    2. "Are you sexually active?"
    3. "What kind of birth control do you use?"
    4. "Have you taken any cough medicine?"

30. The primary health care provider orders application of an elastic wrap bandage for a client's left leg from toes to mid-thigh. The LPN/LVN should take which action?

    1. Increase friction between skin and bandage surfaces.
    2. Leave a small distal portion of the extremity exposed.
    3. Use multiple pins to secure the bandage.
    4. Position the left leg in abduction.

31. A client recovering from a laparoscopic laser cholecystectomy says to the LPN/LVN, "I hate the thought of eating a low-fat diet for the rest of my life." Which response by the LPN/LVN is **most** appropriate?

    1. "I will ask the dietician to come speak with you."
    2. "What do you think is so bad about following a low-fat diet?"
    3. "It may not be necessary for you to follow a low-fat diet for that long."
    4. "At least you will be alive and not suffering that pain."

32. A client begins to breathe very rapidly. Which action by the LPN/LVN would be the **most** appropriate?

    1. Auscultate the client's apical pulse rate.
    2. Measure client's blood pressure and pulse.
    3. Notify the primary health care provider.
    4. Obtain the client's oxygen saturation level.

33. The LPN/LVN is planning morning care for a client hospitalized after a stroke resulting in left-sided paralysis and homonymous hemianopia. During morning care, the LPN/LVN should take which action?

    1. Provide morning care from the right side of the client.
    2. Speak loudly and distinctly when talking with the client.
    3. Reduce the level of lighting in the client's room to prevent glare.
    4. Provide the client's care to reduce the client's energy expenditure.

Refer to the Case Study to answer the next six questions.

The LPN/LVN is caring for an older adult client in the intermediate care unit.

| Nurse's Notes | Vital Signs |

1100: Client admitted with a diagnosis of chronic obstructive pulmonary disease (COPD) exacerbation. Client has used home oxygen at 3 L/minute by nasal cannula for 3 years but reports increased dyspnea over the last several days. Client increased portable oxygen to 6L/minute (O_2 6L/min). At this time, the client is lethargic but alert and oriented × 3. Client reports having shortness of breath at rest and expectorating copious amounts of thick, tan sputum. Visual assessment reveals labored breathing and tripod positioning. Lung sounds with wheezes bilaterally. S1 and S2 heart sounds heard, no murmur or gallop noted. Vital signs obtained and physician notified.

| Nurse's Notes | Vital Signs |

Vital Sign	Result 1100
HR	108
BP	146/82
RR	22
Pulse oximetry	84% (O_2 6 L/minute by nasal cannula)
Temperature (temporal)	98.6° F (38° C)

34. The LPN/LVN reviews the nurse's notes and vital signs.

    Which finding requires follow-up? **(Select all that apply.)**

    1. Client uses home oxygen.
    2. Expectorating copious amounts of thick, tan sputum.
    3. S1 and S2 heart sounds.
    4. Wheezes to bilateral lungs.
    5. Shortness of breath at rest.
    6. BP 146/82 mmHg.

35. For which **3** complications of COPD exacerbation is the client at risk?

    1. Hypercapnia.
    2. Mania.
    3. Hypoxemia.
    4. Leukopenia.
    5. Lethargy.
    6. Thrombocytopenia.

36. Complete the following sentence by choosing from the list of options.

The client is at risk for developing [Select from list 1] due to [Select from list 2].

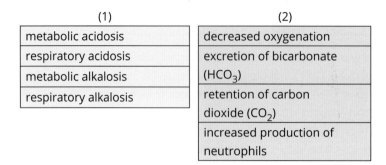

(1)	(2)
metabolic acidosis	decreased oxygenation
respiratory acidosis	excretion of bicarbonate (HCO$_3$)
metabolic alkalosis	retention of carbon dioxide (CO$_2$)
respiratory alkalosis	increased production of neutrophils

37. For each finding below, specify the potential nursing interventions that are appropriate for the care of the client. **Each finding may support more than 1 potential nursing intervention.**

Finding	Potential Nursing Interventions
Shortness of breath at rest	☐ Elevate head of bed (HOB) 45 degrees. ☐ Encourage pursed-lip breathing.
Wheezes to bilateral lung fields	☐ Administer a long-acting beta2 agonist (LABA). ☐ Prepare client for computed tomography (CT) scan of the chest.
Pulse oximetry 84% on 6 L/ minute by nasal cannula	☐ Place client on continuous pulse oximetry. ☐ Instruct client to breathe into a paper bag.
Copious amounts of thick, tan sputum	☐ Administer an expectorant. ☐ Obtain sputum culture and sensitivity (C&S).

| Nurse's Notes | Vital Signs | Orders |

Physician's Orders

- Continuous pulse oximetry monitoring.

- Oxygen via Venturi face mask, titrate to maintain pulse oximetry > 88%.

- Computed tomography (CT) of chest today.

- Laboratory tests: arterial blood gas (ABG), complete blood count (CBC), and sputum culture and sensitivity (C&S).

- Medication therapy:

    - Salmeterol 50 mcg via inhaler twice daily.

    - Fluticasone 88 mcg via inhaler twice daily.

    - Guaifenesin 400 mg PO every 4 hours.

    - Prednisone 20 mg PO once daily.

38. The LPN/LVN receives and reviews the latest physician's orders.

    Which medication is given **first**?

    1. Salmeterol 50 mcg via inhaler twice daily.
    2. Fluticasone 88 mcg via inhaler twice daily.
    3. Guaifenesin 400 mg PO every 4 hours.
    4. Prednisone 20 mg PO once daily.

39. The LPN/LVN obtains vital signs after implementation of physician's orders.

    Highlight the finding(s) that indicate **improvement.**

Vital Sign	Result 1300
HR	98 beats/minute
BP	136/72 mmHg
RR	18
Pulse oximetry	92% (O_2 per 50% Venturi mask)
Temperature (temporal)	99.8° F (37.6° C)

40. A primigravid client at 32 weeks' gestation comes to the clinic for her initial prenatal visit. The client reports periodic headaches and continually bumping into things. The LPN/LVN observes numerous bruises in various stages of healing around the client's breasts and abdomen. Vital signs are: BP 120/80, pulse 72 beats/minute, respirations 18 breaths/minute, and fetal heart tones 142 beats/minute. Which response by the LPN/LVN is **best**?

    1. "Are you battered by your partner?"
    2. "How do you feel about being pregnant?"
    3. "Tell me about your headaches."
    4. "You may be more clumsy due to your size."

41. The LPN/LVN is providing care for a client with chronic obstructive pulmonary disease (COPD) who is receiving oxygen through a nasal cannula. The LPN/LVN should expect which implementation in the client's plan of care?

    1. Arterial blood gases will be analyzed every 2 hours.
    2. The client's oral intake will be restricted.
    3. The client will be maintained on bed rest.
    4. The oxygen flow rate will be set at 3 L/minute or less.

42. The LPN/LVN is caring for a pediatric client in a leg cast for treatment of a right ankle fracture. It is **most** important for the LPN/LVN to reinforce which activity after discharge?

    1. The client performs isometric exercises of the right leg.
    2. The parent massages the client's right foot with moisturizer.
    3. The parent cleans the leg cast with mild soap and water.
    4. The parent elevates the right leg on several pillows.

43. The LPN/LVN is caring for a client who had a thyroidectomy 12 hours ago for treatment of Graves disease. The LPN/LVN would be **most** concerned if which were observed?

    1. The client's vital signs include: blood pressure 138/82 mmHg, pulse 84 beats/minute, and respirations 16 breaths/minute.
    2. The client supports the head and neck to turn head to right.
    3. The client spontaneously flexes the wrist when the blood pressure cuff is inflated during blood pressure measurement.
    4. The client becomes drowsy and reports a sore throat.

44. A client is admitted who reports severe pain in the right lower quadrant of the abdomen. Which action should the LPN/LVN take to assist the client with pain relief?

    1. Encourage rhythmic, shallow breathing.
    2. Massage the right lower quadrant of the abdomen.
    3. Apply a warm heating pad to the client's abdomen.
    4. Position client for comfort using pillows.

45. Which action by the LPN/LVN would be considered negligence?

    1. Administering heparin subcutaneously into a client's abdomen without first aspirating for blood.
    2. Crushing furosemide and adding to a teaspoon of applesauce for an elderly client.
    3. Lowering the bed side rails after administering meperidine and hydroxyzine to a client preoperatively.
    4. Placing a used syringe and needle in a sharps container in a client's room.

46. The LPN/LVN is teaching an elderly client with right-sided weakness how to use a cane. Which behavior by the client indicates that the teaching was effective?

    1. The client holds the cane with the right hand, moves the cane forward followed by the right leg, and then moves the left leg.
    2. The client holds the cane with the right hand, moves the cane forward followed by the left leg, and then moves the right leg.
    3. The client holds the cane with the left hand, moves the cane forward followed by the right leg, and then moves the left leg.
    4. The client holds the cane with the left hand, moves the cane forward followed by the left leg, and then moves the right leg.

47. The LPN/LVN is caring for client whose vital signs have been within normal limits. Now vital signs include: tympanic temperature 103.6° F (39.7° C), pulse 82 beats/minute, regular and strong, respirations 14 breaths/minute, shallow and unlabored, and blood pressure 134/88 mmHg. What should the LPN/LVN's next action be?

    1. Notify primary health care provider immediately.
    2. Proceed with the client's care.
    3. Record vital signs in medical record.
    4. Retake the temperature with different thermometer.

48. The LPN/LVN is helping an unlicensed assistive personnel (UAP) provide a bed bath to a comatose client who is incontinent. The LPN/LVN should intervene if which action is noted?

    1. The UAP answers the phone while wearing gloves.
    2. The UAP log-rolls the client to provide back care.
    3. The UAP places an incontinence pad under the client.
    4. The UAP positions client on the left side, head elevated.

49. A client is brought to the emergency department for treatment after being found on the floor by a family member. When comparing the legs, the LPN/LVN would most likely make which observation?

    1. The client's left leg is longer than the right leg and externally rotated.
    2. The client's left leg is shorter than the right leg and internally rotated.
    3. The client's left leg is shorter than the right leg and adducted.
    4. The client's left leg is longer than the right leg and is abducted.

50. The LPN/LVN is caring for a client with a cast on the left leg. The LPN/LVN would be **most** concerned if which is observed?

    1. Capillary refill time is less than 3 seconds.
    2. Client reports discomfort and itching.
    3. Client reports tightness and pain.
    4. Client's foot is elevated on a pillow.

51. The LPN/LVN is assisting with discharging a client from an inpatient alcohol treatment unit. Which statement by the client's wife indicates that the family is coping adaptively?

    1. "My husband will do well as long as I keep him engaged in activities that he likes."
    2. "My focus is learning how to live my life."
    3. "I am so glad that our problems are behind us."
    4. "I'll make sure that the children don't give my husband any problems."

52. A client with a history of alcohol use disorder is transferred to the unit in an agitated state. The client is vomiting and diaphoretic, and states that it has been 5 hours since the last drink. The LPN/LVN would expect to administer which medication?

    1. Chlordiazepoxide.
    2. Disulfiram.
    3. Methadone.
    4. Naloxone.

53. The LPN/LVN is caring for a client diagnosed with end-stage colon cancer. The spouse of the client says, "We have been married for so long. I am not sure how I can go on now." What is the **most** appropriate response by the LPN/LVN?

    1. "It sounds like your children will be there to help during your time of grieving."
    2. "I know this is difficult. Tell me more about what you are feeling now."
    3. "Think about the pain and suffering your spouse has endured lately."
    4. "I will call the hospice nurse to discuss to your spouse's condition with you."

54. The LPN/LVN is reinforcing teaching with an elderly client about how to use a standard aluminum walker. Which behavior by the client indicates that the reinforcement of teaching was effective?

    1. The client slowly pushes the walker forward 12 inches (30 cm), then takes small steps forward while leaning on the walker.
    2. The client lifts the walker, moves it forward 10 inches (25 cm), and then takes several small steps forward.
    3. The client supports weight on the walker while advancing it forward, then takes small steps while balancing on the walker.
    4. The client slides the walker 18 inches (46 cm) forward, then takes small steps while holding onto the walker for balance.

55. The LPN/LVN would expect which client to be able to sign a consent form for nonemergent medical treatment?

    1. A school-age child with a right tibia and fibula fracture.
    2. A client requiring surgery for acute appendicitis.
    3. A client who is confused after a motor vehicle accident.
    4. A client who has been legally declared incompetent.

56. An LPN/LVN is assisting with the discharge of a client with a diagnosis of hepatitis of unknown etiology. The LPN/LVN knows that teaching has been successful if the client makes which statement?

    1. "I am so sad that I am not able to hold my baby."
    2. "I will eat my meal after my family finishes eating."
    3. "I will make sure that my children don't use my eating utensils."
    4. "I'm glad that I don't have to get help taking care of my children."

57. The LPN/LVN checks the IV flow rate for a postoperative client. The client is to receive 3,000 mL of lactated Ringer's lactate solution IV infused over 24 hours. The IV administration set has a drop factor of 10 drops per milliliter. The LPN/LVN would expect the client's IV to infuse at how many drops per minute?

    1. 18.
    2. 21.
    3. 35.
    4. 40.

58. A client diagnosed with emphysema becomes restless and confused. Which action should the LPN/LVN take next?

1. Encourage pursed-lip breathing.
2. Measure the client's temperature.
3. Assess the client's potassium level.
4. Increase oxygen flow rate to 5 L/minute.

59. The LPN/LVN is caring for a client following cataract surgery on the right eye. The client reports severe eye pain in the right eye. Which activity should the LPN/LVN do **first**?

1. Administer an analgesic to the client.
2. Recheck the client's condition in 30 minutes.
3. Document finding in client's medical record.
4. Report the finding to the supervising RN.

60. The LPN/LVN is caring for a client 4 hours after intracranial surgery. Which action should the LPN/LVN take immediately?

1. Instruct the client to deep breathe, cough, and expectorate into a tissue.
2. Position the client in a left lateral position with neck flexed.
3. Perform passive range-of-motion exercises every two hours.
4. Use a turning sheet under the client's head to midthigh to reposition in bed.

Refer to the Case Study to answer the next six questions.

The LPN/LVN is caring for a pregnant client who was admitted 2 hours ago to the labor/delivery (L/D) unit.

History

Client is a 43-year-old primigravida at 34 weeks gestation. The client has been diagnosed with mild pre-eclampsia. Client presented for a routine obstetric appointment today and reported daily headaches unresolved with the use of acetaminophen. Evaluation by provider revealed a BP of 158/92, a weight gain of 12 lb (5.4 kg) since previous office visit 2 weeks ago with 2+ pretibial edema. Reflexes 2+ and without clonus. Urine sample evaluated in provider's office revealed 2+ protein via dipstick. Client admits to intermittently using cocaine, smoking 5–6 cigarettes daily, and consuming 3–4 servings of decaffeinated soda daily throughout pregnancy. Remainder of past medical history and obstetric history are unremarkable.

61. The LPN/LVN reviews the client's history.

Highlight the information in the client's history that **most** concerns the LPN/LVN.

Client is a 43-year-old primigravida at 34 weeks gestation with mild pre-eclampsia. Client presented for a routine obstetric appointment today and reported daily headaches unresolved with the use of acetaminophen. Evaluation by provider revealed a BP of 158/92, a weight gain of 12 lb (5.4 kg) since previous office visit 2 weeks prior with 2+ pretibial edema. Reflexes 2+ without clonus. Urine sample evaluated in provider's office revealed 2+ protein via dipstick. Client admits to intermittent use of cocaine, smoking 5–6 cigarettes daily and consuming 3–4 servings of decaffeinated soda daily throughout pregnancy. Remainder of past medical history and obstetric history are unremarkable.

History	Admission Notes

1030:

Client reports frontal headache 6/10 on 10-point pain scale with some photophobia and scotomas. Reports intermittent nausea with vague, generalized abdominal discomfort. BP 160/90, pulse 82, respirations 18, oral temperature 97.9°F (36.6°C). IV lactated Ringer (LR) infusing to left forearm at 100 mL/hour. Client on continuous external fetal monitor, which shows mild uterine irritability and fetal heart rate (FHR) ranging 120–150 bpm with moderate variability and no decelerations noted. Blood drawn for lab evaluation shortly after admission. Results called to physician.

Laboratory Test	Result	Range
Red Blood Cells (RBCs)	4.2 million/mm^3 (4.2 × 10^{12}/L)	normal
White Blood Cells (WBCs)	6300/mm^3 (6.3 × 10^9/L)	normal
Hemoglobin	11.1 g/dL (111 g/L)	low
Hematocrit	32% (0.32)	low
Platelets	99,000/mm^3 (99 × 10^9/L)	low
Glucose	112 mg/dL (6.22 mmol/L)	normal
BUN	22 mg/dL (8.2 mmol/L)	high
Uric Acid	6.3 mg/dL (374.7 mmol/L)	high

62. The LPN/LVN reviews the client's admission notes and laboratory results.

    The LPN/LVN recognizes that the client is at **increased** risk for which complication of pregnancy? **(Select all that apply.)**

    1. Low birth weight.
    2. Gestational diabetes.
    3. Placental abruption.
    4. Preterm birth.
    5. Birth defects.
    6. Hyperemesis gravidarum.
    7. Stillbirth.
    8. Placenta previa.

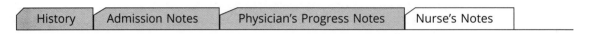

| History | Admission Notes | Physician's Progress Notes | Nurse's Notes |

1230:

Lab results discussed with client and significant other. BP remains elevated, and labs indicate desirability of delivering fetus in the near future. Decision made to induce labor with IV oxytocin and manage blood pressure with IV magnesium sulfate. Cervix 1 centimeter dilated, 30% effaced, firm consistency with vertex presenting at −3 station and membranes intact. Vital signs relatively unchanged from admission. Magnesium sulfate 4 g/100 mL 0.9% normal saline (NS) at 1 g/hour (25 mL/hr) ordered. FHR baseline 120–140 bpm with moderate variability and no decelerations noted.

| History | Admission Notes | Physician's Progress Notes | Nurse's Notes |

1300:

IV oxytocin initiated per protocol at 3 milliunits/minute.

1330:

FHR monitor strip displays mild uterine contractions every 6 minutes. Client's blood pressure now 172/98 mmHg with heart rate 88 bpm. Spontaneous rupture of membranes and blood-tinged fluid observed. Client reporting sudden left upper quadrant abdominal pain and back discomfort. IV oxytocin rate at 6 milliunits/minute. FHR baseline at 100–110 bpm, and variability is now minimal with intermittent late decelerations.

63. The LPN/LVN reviews the physician's progress notes and assists the RN with the client's care.

Complete the following sentence by choosing from the list of options.

The client is at high risk for [Select from list 1] as evidenced by [Select from list 2] and [Select from list 3].

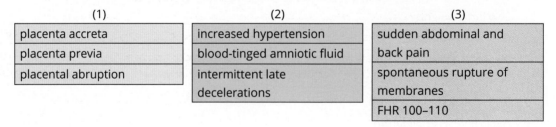

(1)	(2)	(3)
placenta accreta	increased hypertension	sudden abdominal and back pain
placenta previa	blood-tinged amniotic fluid	spontaneous rupture of membranes
placental abruption	intermittent late decelerations	FHR 100–110

64. The LPN/LVN and RN work together to plan and provide the client's immediate care.

    Complete the following sentences by choosing from the list of options.

    The LPN/LVN should anticipate the nurse would [Select from list 1]. It would be a priority for
    the LPN/LVN to [Select from list 2]. The LPN/LVN recognizes that the client should be positioned
    [Select from list 3].

(1)	(2)	(3)
discontinue the IV oxytocin infusion	insert an indwelling urinary catheter	on the left side
increase the client's magnesium infusion	apply antiembolism stockings	in semi-Fowler
discontinue the primary IV	apply oxygen by mask	in Trendelenburg

65. The RN and LPN/LVN prepare the client for an emergency cesarean birth to deliver the infant.

    Which nursing intervention will the RN delegate to the LPN/LVN?

    1. Notifying the blood bank.
    2. Inserting an indwelling urinary catheter.
    3. Explaining the procedure to the client's family.
    4. Providing report to the neonatal intensive care nurse.

66. The client undergoes an emergency cesarean birth under general anesthesia and has
    delivered a viable newborn. The LPN/LVN is caring for the client 2 hours after the procedure.

    For each finding below, specify whether the finding indicates the client's condition has
    improved, not changed, or declined.

Finding	Improved	No Change	Declined
Blood pressure 158/90 mmHg	○	○	○
Pulse 78 beats/minute	○	○	○
Respirations 16 breaths/minute	○	○	○
Hematocrit 28% (0.28)	○	○	○
Platelets 93,000/mm^3 (93×10^9/L)	○	○	○
Serum uric acid 6.1 mg/dL (362.8 mmol/L)	○	○	○
Headache mild, 2/10 on pain scale	○	○	○

67. A pediatric client with a congenital heart disorder is admitted with heart failure. Digoxin 0.12 mg by mouth daily is ordered for the client. The bottle contains 0.05 mg of digoxin in 1 mL of solution. Which amount should the LPN/LVN administer to the client after validating the dose with the RN?

1. 1.2 mL.
2. 2.4 mL.
3. 3.5 mL.
4. 4.2 mL.

68. The LPN/LVN is caring for a client diagnosed with chronic lymphocytic leukemia, hospitalized for treatment of hemolytic anemia. The LPN/LVN should expect to implement which action?

1. Encourage activities with other clients in the day room.
2. Isolate the client from visitors and clients to avoid infection.
3. Provide a diet that contains foods that are high in vitamin C.
4. Maintain a quiet environment to promote adequate rest.

69. The LPN/LVN is caring for a client with cervical cancer. The LPN/LVN notes that the radium implant has become dislodged. Which action should the LPN/LVN take **first**?

1. Grasp the implant with a sterile hemostat and carefully reinsert it into the client.
2. Wrap the implant in a blanket and place it behind a lead shield until reimplantation.
3. Ensure the implant is picked up with long-handled forceps and placed in a lead container.
4. Obtain a dosimeter reading on the client and report it to the primary health care provider.

70. The LPN/LVN comes to the home of a client with cellulitis of the left leg to perform a daily dressing change. The client tells the LPN/LVN that the unlicensed assistive personnel (UAP) changed the dressing earlier that morning. Which action by the LPN/LVN is **best**?

1. Tell client that the new dressing looks fine.
2. Notify the RN supervisor of the situation.
3. Ask the client to describe the dressing change.
4. Report the UAP to the home care agency.

71. The LPN/LVN is caring for a client with pernicious anemia. The LPN/LVN reinforces teaching about the plan of care. The LPN/LVN should report which statement to the RN?

1. "In order to get better, I will take iron pills."
2. "I will attend smoking cessation classes."
3. "I will learn how to perform IM injections."
4. "I will make sure to eat a well-balanced diet."

72. The LPN/LVN is caring for clients on a general medical/surgical unit of an acute care facility. Four clients have been admitted in the last 20 minutes. Which admission should the LPN/LVN see **first**?

1. A client reporting vomiting and diarrhea.
2. A client with third-degree burns to face.
3. A client with a fractured left hip.
4. A client reporting epigastric pain.

73. The LPN/LVN is caring for a client with a diagnosis of chronic bronchitis. The client has audible wheezing, and an oxygen saturation of 85%. Four hours ago, the oxygen saturation was 88%. It is **most** important for the LPN/LVN to take which action?

    1. Give beclomethasone, 2 puffs via metered-dose inhaler.
    2. Auscultate the client's bilateral breath sounds.
    3. Increase oxygen flow rate to 4 L/minute via mask.
    4. Administer albuterol, 2 puffs via metered-dose inhaler.

74. The LPN/LVN is caring for a client hospitalized for observation following a fall. The client states, "My friend fell last year, and no one thought anything was wrong. She died 2 days later!" Which response by the LPN/LVN is **best**?

    1. "This happens to quite a few people."
    2. "We are monitoring you, so you'll be okay."
    3. "Don't you think I'm taking good care of you?"
    4. "You're concerned that it might happen to you?"

75. The LPN/LVN is caring for clients on the pediatric unit. A client with second- and third-degree burns on the right thigh is being admitted. The LPN/LVN should expect the new client to be placed with which roommate?

    1. A client with chickenpox.
    2. A client with asthma.
    3. A client who developed acute diarrhea after antibiotic.
    4. A client with methicillin-resistant *Staphylococcus aureus*.

76. The LPN/LVN is performing chest physiotherapy on a client with chronic airflow limitations (CAL). Which action should the nurse take **first**?

    1. Perform chest physiotherapy prior to meals.
    2. Auscultate breath sounds before the procedure.
    3. Administer bronchodilators after the procedure.
    4. Percuss each lobe prior to asking client to cough.

77. In which situation would it be **most** appropriate for the LPN/LVN to wear a gown and gloves?

    1. Administering oral medications to client with human immunodeficiency virus disease.
    2. Assisting in the care of a motor vehicle accident victim who continues to bleed.
    3. Bathing a client with an abdominal wound infection.
    4. Changing the linen of a client with sickle-cell anemia.

78. A client is receiving 1,000 mL of 5% dextrose in half normal saline solution IV to infuse over 8 hours. The IV administration set tubing delivers 15 drops per milliliter. The LPN/LVN should expect the flow rate to be how many drops per minute?

    1. 15.
    2. 31.
    3. 45.
    4. 60.

79. A client is admitted to the hospital reporting seizures and a high fever. A positron emission tomography (PET) brain scan is ordered. Before the PET brain scan, the client asks the LPN/LVN what position is necessary for the test. Which statement by the LPN/LVN is **most** accurate?

    1. "You will be in a side-lying position, with the foot of the bed elevated."
    2. "You will be in a semi-upright sitting position, with your knees flexed."
    3. "You will be lying on your back with a small pillow under your head."
    4. "You will be flat on your back, with your feet higher than your head."

80. A client is to receive 3,000 mL of normal saline solution IV to infuse over 24 hours. The IV administration set delivers 15 drops per milliliter. The LPN/LVN would expect the flow rate to be how many drops of fluid per minute?

    1. 21.
    2. 28.
    3. 31.
    4. 42.

81. The LPN/LVN is caring for a client diagnosed with asthma. The primary health care provider prescribes neostigmine IM. Which action by the LPN/LVN is **most** appropriate?

    1. Administer medication, as prescribed.
    2. Obtain the client's blood pressure and pulse.
    3. Ask pharmacist if medication can be given orally.
    4. Notify the primary health care provider.

82. The LPN/LVN is caring for a client with a history of Addison disease who has received steroid therapy for several years. The LPN/LVN would expect the client to exhibit which change in appearance?

    1. Buffalo hump, girdle-obesity, gaunt facial appearance.
    2. Skin tanning, mucous membrane discoloration, weight loss.
    3. Emaciation, nervousness, breast engorgement, hirsutism.
    4. Truncal obesity, purple striations on the skin, moon face.

83. The LPN/LVN is caring for a client with a history of pancreatic cancer who appears jaundiced. The LPN/LVN should give the **highest** priority to which need?

    1. Nutrition.
    2. Self-image.
    3. Skin integrity.
    4. Urinary elimination.

84. The client diagnosed with anorexia nervosa is admitted to the hospital. Which statement by the client requires immediate follow-up by the LPN/LVN?

    1. "My gums bled this morning."
    2. "I'm getting fatter every day."
    3. "Nobody likes me, I'm so ugly."
    4. "I feel dizzy and weak today."

85. A client is admitted to the hospital for treatment of *Pneumocystis jiroveci* pneumonia and Kaposi's sarcoma. The client informs the LPN/LVN about a personal decision to become an organ donor. Which response by the LPN/LVN is **best**?

1. "What does your family think about your decision?"
2. "You will help many people by donating your organs."
3. "Would you like to speak to an organ donor coordinator?"
4. "Your illness prevents you from becoming an organ donor."

86. The LPN/LVN is caring for a client 2 days after a pancreatectomy for cancer of the pancreas. The LPN/LVN observes minimal drainage from the nasogastric (NG) tube. It is **most** important for the LPN/LVN to take which action?

1. Notify primary health care provider.
2. Monitor vital signs every 15 minutes.
3. Check the NG tube for kinking.
4. Replace the NG tube immediately.

Refer to the Case Study to answer the next question.

The LPN/LVN in the inpatient rehabilitation facility is caring for an adult client with a diagnosis of a right middle cerebral artery stroke.

History	Nurse's Notes

Client admitted to hospital 10 days ago after waking with loss of use of the left arm and hand, dizziness, difficulty speaking, loss of balance, and double vision in the right eye. The client underwent a computed tomography (CT) of the brain and was diagnosed with a right middle cerebral artery ischemic stroke. Unfortunately, the client and the client's family could not be sure about the beginning of the client's symptoms; therefore, the client was not eligible for t-PA infusion.

Client is 70 inches (177.8 cm) tall and weighs 248 pounds (112.5 kg). Client's body mass index (BMI) is 35.6 kg/m^2. Client smokes 1 pack of cigarettes per day for the past 18 years (18 pack years). Client also has diagnoses of hypercholesterolemia and hypertension. Per the client's family, the client has not been taking the prescribed medications due to difficulty affording the prescriptions. The client is right-handed and has no known allergies.

Client was initially admitted to the neurologic intensive care unit due to a declining level of consciousness, hypertension, and worsening aphasia. The client stabilized after 5 days and was transferred to the step-down unit, where the client was evaluated for physical therapy, occupational therapy, and speech therapy for treatment of right upper extremity hemiparesis, complete right hemianopsia, dysphagia, and expressive aphasia. The client was transferred to the inpatient rehabilitation facility for further evaluation and treatment.

History | Nurse's Notes

Entered client's room to obtain vital signs. Client is in semi-Fowler position in bed. Note unlicensed assistive personnel (UAP) has brought client's pureed diet breakfast tray into the room and is preparing to feed the client. The tray includes scrambled eggs, pureed fruit, oatmeal, milk, and orange juice.

87. The LPN/LVN reviews the client's history and prepares to care for the client.

Complete the diagram by dragging from the choices below to specify which potential condition concerns the LPN/LVN, 2 actions the LPN/LVN takes to prevent that condition, and 2 parameters the LPN/LVN monitors to ensure the client remains free from harm.

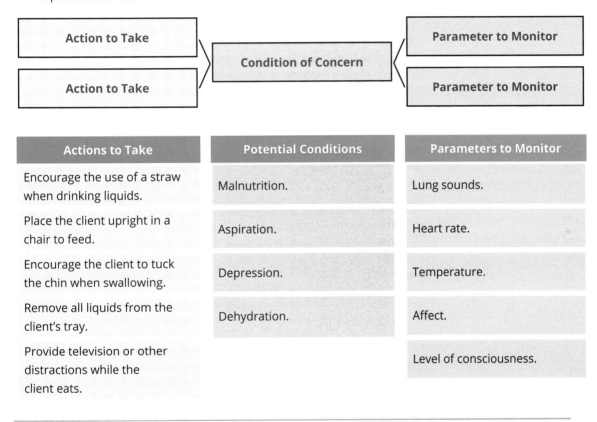

Actions to Take	Potential Conditions	Parameters to Monitor
Encourage the use of a straw when drinking liquids.	Malnutrition.	Lung sounds.
Place the client upright in a chair to feed.	Aspiration.	Heart rate.
Encourage the client to tuck the chin when swallowing.	Depression.	Temperature.
Remove all liquids from the client's tray.	Dehydration.	Affect.
Provide television or other distractions while the client eats.		Level of consciousness.

88. The LPN/LVN is planning to administer furosemide 20 mg PO to a client diagnosed with chronic kidney disease. The client asks the LPN/LVN the reason for receiving this medication. Which response by the LPN/LVN is **best**?

1. "To increase the blood flow to your kidney."
2. "To decrease your circulating blood volume."
3. "To increase excretion of sodium and water."
4. "To decrease the workload on your heart."

89. The LPN/LVN is reinforcing discharge teaching for a client with chronic pancreatitis. Which statement by the client indicates that further teaching is necessary?

1. "I do not have to restrict physical activity."
2. "I should take pancrelipase before meals."
3. "I will eat three large meals every day."
4. "I must not drink any alcoholic beverages."

90. Following a laparoscopic cholecystectomy, the client reports abdominal pain and bloating. Which response by the LPN/LVN is **best**?

1. "Increase intake of fresh fruits and vegetables."
2. "I'll give you the prescribed pain medication."
3. "Why don't you take a walk down the hallway?"
4. "You may need an indwelling urinary catheter."

Refer to the Case Study to answer the next question.

The LPN/LVN is making a home visit to an older adult client who is undergoing outpatient chemotherapy.

| Nurse's Notes | Flow Sheet |

RN Assessment Visit 1:

The client is being referred for ongoing home healthcare related to bone cancer chemotherapy treatment at the outpatient cancer center. Past history includes hypertension, coronary artery disease, hyperlipidemia, and obesity. The plan of care includes monitoring and evaluating treatment effects of chemotherapy, including monthly hemoglobin and hematocrit results. Findings recorded on the flow sheet. Client is oriented × 4, cheerful, and states, "I feel pretty good, considering all the treatment I'm getting." Skin warm, pink, elastic turgor. Lung sounds clear bilaterally. Apical pulse regular, 2 + radial pulses. Abdomen, rounded with active bowel sounds × 4. No nausea or vomiting, appetite is healthy. Muscle strength 5/5, no joint pain or tenderness.

RN Assessment Visit 2:

Client reports no new concerns or problems. Clinical findings are unchanged from the previous assessment. Vital signs are stable. Blood drawn for hemoglobin and hematocrit.

RN Assessment Visit 3:

Client seems lethargic and is not as talkative as usual. Client's spouse states, "My spouse has little interest in daily living activities and seems very tired all the time." Client is oriented × 4, skin and oral mucous membranes are pale, skin turgor is decreased. No petechiae, ecchymoses, or gingival bleeding noted. Lung sounds are clear bilaterally, non labored breathing. Client states, "Sometimes, I get a little short-winded when I get up and walk." Apical pulse regular, radial pulses are 3+, increased. Abdomen soft, with active bowel sounds × 4. Muscle strength 4/5 bilaterally. Client's clinical findings and laboratory results reported to the physician. The client has an oncology clinic visit next week. PRN LPN/LVN visit scheduled for follow-up later this week.

| Nurse's Notes | Flow Sheet |

RN Visit	Hemoglobin	Interpretation	Hematocrit	Interpretation
1	14 g/dL (140 g/L)	Normal	42% (0.42)	Normal
2	11.5 g/dL (115 g/L)	Low	35% (0.35)	Low
3	7.5 g/dL (75 g/L)	Low	22% (0.22)	Low

Vital Signs	Visit 1	Visit 2	Visit 3
BP	118/76 mmHg	113/80 mmHg	116/78 mmHg
Pulse	82, regular	80, regular	90, regular
Respiratory rate	16, regular	16, regular	20, regular
Temperature (oral)	98° F (36.66° C)	98.4° F (36.88° C)	98.9° F (37.16° C)
Pulse Oximetry	97% (room air)	96% (room air)	94% (room air)

91. The LPN/LVN makes a PRN follow up visit to the client's home and reviews the nurse's notes and the flow sheet.

Complete the following sentences by choosing from the list of options.

The LPN/LVN identifies the client findings are consistent with [Select from list 1]. The LPN/LVN will [Select from list 2]. The LPN/LVN anticipates the client may need [Select from list 3]. On future home visits, the LPN/LVN recognizes further decline in the hemoglobin and hematocrit may be indicated by [Select from list 4].

(1)	(2)	(3)	(4)
leukopenia	encourage alternating activities with frequent rest breaks	meticulous skin care and oral hygiene	bleeding from nose and gums
pancytopenia		supplemental oxygen	oral temperature $\geq$ 100.4° F (38° C)
anemia	provide examples of foods high in potassium	correction of vitamin B_{12} deficiency	heart palpitations
	promote complete bedrest until the client's next oncology visit		

92. The nursing team consists of an RN, an unlicensed assistive personnel (UAP), and an LPN/LVN. The LPN/LVN would expect to be assigned to which client?

    1. A client scheduled for MRI of the brain.

    2. An unconscious client who requires a bed bath.

    3. A client in balanced suspension traction.

    4. A client with diabetes who needs help bathing.

93. The primary health care provider prescribes 1 L dextrose 5% in half normal saline solution IV to infuse over 8 hours. The drip factor stated on the IV administration set tubing is 15 gtt/mL. How many milliliters should the LPN/LVN expect to be infused every hour?

_____ mL

Refer to the Case Study to answer the next question.

The nurse is caring for a 74-year-old client in the intensive care unit (ICU).

Nurse's Notes	Client Data

0900: Client admitted 2 days ago to the ICU with acute decompensated heart failure (ADHF). Extubated this morning and placed on 50% Venturi mask. 40 mg furosemide IV push administered.

1200: Coarse crackles noted to bilateral lower lung bases upon auscultation. 2+ bilateral lower extremity edema noted. Repeat dose of 40 mg furosemide IV push administered.

1500: Client reports thirst and weakness. Oral mucous membranes are dry and lips are chapped. Oral care performed and ice chips offered.

Vital Sign	Result 0900	Result 1200	Result 1500
HR	88	90	96
RR	16	16	18
BP	138/84	134/80	122/76
CVP	10 mmHg	8 mmHg	4 mmHg

1800: Client reports dizziness. Intake and output calculated. Sitting and standing blood pressures obtained.

Nurse's Notes	Client Data

Vital Sign	Result 1800
Sitting: HR	90
Sitting: BP	108/54
Standing: HR	116
Standing: BP	84/48

Shift Total:	
Intake 0600–1800	Output 0600–1800
540 mL	2400 mL

94. The nurse reviews the nurse's notes, vital signs, and intake and output record.

    Which action does the nurse take to provide for client safety? **(Select all that apply.)**

    1. Offer PO fluids every 1 to 2 hours.
    2. Educate the client on limiting potassium intake.
    3. Monitor BP and HR hourly.
    4. Obtain blood for electrolyte levels.
    5. Encourage the client to change positions slowly.
    6. Teach client to measure body weight every week.
    7. Instruct the client to increase sodium intake.

95. A client underwent vagotomy with antrectomy for treatment of a duodenal ulcer. Postoperatively, the client develops dumping syndrome. Which statement by the client indicates to the LPN/LVN that further dietary teaching is necessary?

1. "I should eat bread with each meal."
2. "I should eat smaller meals more frequently."
3. "I should lie down right after eating."
4. "I should avoid drinking fluids with my meals."

96. The LPN/LVN reinforces discharge teaching with a client with emphysema. Which statement by the client indicates that teaching was successful?

1. "Cold weather should help my breathing problems."
2. "I'll eat three balanced meals daily but limit my fluid intake."
3. "I'll limit outside activity when polution levels are high."
4. "Intensive exercise should help me regain strength."

97. The LPN/LVN is hearing a client call for help. The LPN/LVN enters the room and finds a client in bilateral wrist restraints with a cool, pale right hand and no palpable radial pulse. Which would be the most appropriate action for the LPN/LVN to take **first**?

1. Leave to find the client's nurse.
2. Massage the client's wrist and hand.
3. Remove the right wrist restraint.
4. Reposition the client to reduce pressure.

98. The LPN/LVN is reinforcing discharge teaching for a client with a new colostomy. The LPN/LVN knows teaching was successful when the client chooses which menu option?

1. Sausage, sauerkraut, baked potato, and fresh fruit.
2. Cheese omelet with bran muffin and fresh pineapple.
3. Pork chop, mashed potatoes, turnips, and salad.
4. Baked chicken, boiled potato, cooked carrots, and yogurt.

99. The LPN/LVN is implementing the protocol for teaching a new mother how to breastfeed her newborn. The LPN/LVN knows that teaching has been successful if the client makes which statement?

1. "My baby's weight should equal the birthweight in 5 to 7 days."
2. "My baby should have at least 6 to 8 wet diapers per day."
3. "My baby will sleep at least 6 hours between feedings."
4. "My baby will feed for about 10 minutes per feeding."

100. A client is admitted to the telemetry unit for evaluation of reported chest pain. Eight hours after admission, the client's cardiac monitor shows ventricular fibrillation. The primary health care provider defibrillates the client. The LPN/LVN understands that the purpose of defibrillation is to do which of these?

1. Increase cardiac contractility, preload, and cardiac output.
2. Depolarize cells allowing SA node to recapture pacing node
3. Reduce the degree of cardiac ischemia and acidosis.
4. Provide electrical energy for depleted myocardial cells.

101. The LPN/LVN is caring for a client who suddenly reports chest pain. The LPN/LVN knows that which symptom would be **most** characteristic of an acute myocardial infarction (MI)?

1. Intermittent, localized epigastric pain.
2. Sharp, localized, unilateral chest pain.
3. Severe substernal pain radiating down the left arm.
4. Sharp, burning chest pain moving from place to place.

102. The primary health care provider prescribes packing for a nonhealing open surgical wound. Which is the **first** action by the LPN/LVN?

1. Identify wound size, shape, and depth.
2. Observe for wound drainage or discharge.
3. Plan to set up for clean technique.
4. Select the proper dressing material.

103. A client returns to the clinic 2 weeks after hospital discharge. The client is taking warfarin sodium 2 mg PO daily. Which statement by the client to the LPN/LVN indicates that further teaching is necessary?

1. "I take an antihistamine before bedtime."
2. "I take aspirin whenever I have a headache."
3. "I put on sunscreen whenever I go outside."
4. "I take an antacid if my stomach gets upset."

104. To enhance the percutaneous absorption of nitroglycerin ointment, which characteristic of the administration site selected by the LPN/LVN would be **most** important?

1. Muscular.
2. Near the heart.
3. Non-hairy.
4. Bony prominence.

105. When assisting the RN in planning care for a postoperative client, which should be the **first** choice of the LPN/LVN to reduce the client's risk for pooled airway secretions and decreased chest wall expansion?

1. Chest percussion.
2. Incentive spirometry.
3. Position changes.
4. Postural drainage.

106. Which action by the LPN/LVN would be **most** helpful in preventing injury to elderly clients in a health care facility?

1. Closely monitor the temperature of hot oral fluids.
2. Keep unnecessary furniture out of the way.
3. Maintain the safe function of all electrical equipment.
4. Use safety protection caps on all medications.

107. Which statement by a client during a group therapy session requires immediate follow-up by the LPN/LVN?

1. "I know I'm a chronically compulsive liar, but I can't help it."
2. "I don't ever want to go home; I feel safer here."
3. "I don't really care if I ever see my girlfriend again."
4. "I'll make sure that doctor is sorry for what he said."

108. A female client visits the clinic reporting right calf tenderness and pain. It would be **most** important for the LPN/LVN to ask which question?

1. "Do you exercise excessively?"
2. "Have you had any recent fractures?"
3. "What type of birth control do you use?"
4. "Are you under a lot of stress?"

109. Which should be the LPN/LVN's **first** priority in providing care for a client who has end-stage ovarian cancer and has been weakened by chemotherapy?

1. Collect data to see if client has pain.
2. Determine if the client is hungry or thirsty.
3. Explore client's feelings about dying.
4. Observe the client's self-care abilities.

110. The LPN/LVN in the postpartum unit is caring for a client who delivered her first child the previous day. The LPN/LVN notes multiple varicosities on the client's lower extremities. Which action should the LPN/LVN perform?

1. Teach the client to rest in bed when the baby sleeps.
2. Encourage early and frequent ambulation.
3. Apply warm soaks for 20 minutes every 4 hours.
4. Perform passive range-of-motion exercises 3 times daily.

111. The LPN/LVN is caring for a client who sustained a left femur fracture in a bicycle accident. A cast is applied. The nurse knows that which exercise would be **most** beneficial for this client?

1. Passive exercise of the affected limb.
2. Quadriceps setting of the affected limb.
3. Active range-of-motion exercises of the unaffected limb.
4. Passive exercise of the upper extremities.

112. In preparation for a dressing change, the LPN/LVN puts on sterile gloves. Where should the LPN/LVN initially grip the first sterile glove?

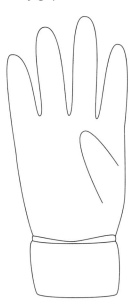

113. A client is being discharged from the hospital following a right total hip arthroplasty. The LPN/LVN reinforces discharge teaching. Which statement by the client indicates that teaching was successful?

1. "I can bend over to pick up something on the floor."
2. "I should not cross my ankles when sitting in a chair."
3. "I need to lie on my stomach when sleeping in bed."
4. "I should spread my knees apart to put on my shoes."

114. The LPN/LVN is caring for a client with continuous bladder irrigation. At 7 A.M., the LPN/LVN notes 4,200 mL of normal saline solution left in the irrigation bags. During the next shift (7 A.M. to 3 P.M.), the LPN/LVN hangs another 3,000 mL and empties a total of 5,625 mL from the urine drainage bag. At 3 P.M., there are 2,300 mL of irrigant left hanging. What is the actual urine output for the client from 7 A.M. to 3 P.M.?

_____ mL

115. A client with a history of type 1 diabetes mellitus is admitted to the unit reporting nausea, vomiting, and abdominal pain. The client reduced the insulin dose four days ago when influenza symptoms prevented eating. The LPN/LVN observes poor skin turgor, dry mucous membranes, and fruity breath odor. The LPN/LVN should be alert for which problem?

1. Rebound hypoglycemia.
2. Viral gastrointestingal illness.
3. Diabetic ketoacidosis.
4. Hyperglycemic hyperosmolar nonketotic coma.

116. The LPN/LVN is caring for a group of clients. The nurse knows that it is **most** important for which client to receive scheduled medications on time?

1. A client diagnosed with myasthenia gravis receiving pyridostigmine bromide.
2. A client diagnosed with bipolar disorder receiving lithium carbonate.
3. A client diagnosed with tuberculosis receiving isonicotinic acid hydrazide.
4. A client diagnosed with Parkinson disease receiving levodopa.

Refer to the Case Study to answer the next question.

The LPN/LVN is monitoring an adult client in the labor/delivery unit.

| Maternal History | Nurse's Notes | Newborn Apgar Scores |

Client is a GTPAL 65005 (Gravida 6 / Term 5 / Preterm 0 / Abortion, Miscarriage 0 / Living 5) admitted directly to the labor and delivery unit at 0600. Client received intermittent prenatal care in the home by the community midwife. Client estimates gestational age of infant at 34 weeks, although unable to confirm last menstrual period because was still breastfeeding a 14-month-old child. Client notes that all previous children have weighed > 10 lbs (4500 grams) at birth. Community midwife estimated current fetal weight at > 9 lbs (4100 grams) at onset of labor per client report.

Client planned a home birth, but due to prolonged labor of > 24 hours duration and spontaneous rupture of membranes > 36 hours was encouraged to seek further labor management in a hospital setting. No prenatal blood testing completed; denies history of diabetes, hypertension, preterm birth, or excessive bleeding postpartum in previous pregnancies.

| Maternal History | Nurse's Notes | Newborn Apgar Scores |

0600: Client notes irregular mild contractions on admission. Also voices generalized malaise and vague headache. Baby active with fetal heart rate (FHR) 164 and intermittent variable decelerations. Cervix 3 cm dilated and 40% effaced with head at −2 station. Client leaking clear amniotic fluid. IV oxytocin augmentation of labor initiated at 3 milliunits/minute by RN.

0800: Contractions now every 5–7 minutes and of moderate intensity with IV oxytocin at 9 milliunits/minute. Client becoming more uncomfortable but declines analgesia now. Client notes occasional chills and continued headache. Cervix not reassessed at this time. FHR baseline 170 beats/min with persistent occasional late decelerations. Encouraged client to reposition to left side.

1100: Client now rates contraction discomfort as 7/10 on a pain scale. Contractions every 3–5 minutes, palpably strong intensity with IV oxytocin infusing at 12 milliunits/minute. Cervix now 5–6 centimeters dilated, 75% effaced with head at −1 station during a contraction per RN exam. Foul-smelling, green-tinged amniotic fluid noted. FHR baseline 182 beats/min with variable decelerations to 100–110 bpm with most contractions. Oxygen by mask at 5L/minute applied. Client encouraged to reposition to right side. Preparing room for delivery per RN request.

1200: Client beginning to note involuntary urge to push. Client nauseated and shivering, reporting increasing headache and body aches. RN notified of client's change in status.

Maternal Vital Signs	0600	0800	1100	1200
Pulse (beats/minute)	82	90	94	96
Blood Pressure (mmHg)	140/90	144/90	146/92	150/100
Respirations (breaths/minute)	16	18	20	24
Oral Temperature	99.4° F (37.4° C)	100.5° F (38.1° C)	100.8° F (38.2° C)	101.5° F (38.6° C)

| Maternal History | Nurse's Notes | Newborn Apgar Scores |

Apgar Score	1 minute	5 minutes	10 minutes
Heart rate	2	2	2
Respirations	1	2	1
Color	0	1	1
Muscle Tone	1	1	1
Reflexes	1	1	2

117. At 1208, the client spontaneously delivers an infant weighing 9 lbs 11 ounces (4,394 grams). The LPN/LVN provides supportive care to the newborn.

Which maternal history or labor factor can **negatively** impact the infant's Apgar score? **(Select all that apply.)**

1. Prolonged rupture of membranes.
2. Elevated maternal blood pressure of uncertain duration.
3. Presence of foul smelling, meconium-stained amniotic fluid.
4. Elevated maternal temperature.
5. Maternal history of large-for-gestational age infants.
6. Uncertain current gestational age.
7. Prolonged labor with multiple cervical assessments.
8. Persistent late decelerations of fetal heart rate.

118. An school-age client is admitted to the hospital for evaluation for a kidney transplant. The LPN/LVN learns that the client received hemodialysis for 3 years due to stage 5 kidney disease. The LPN/LVN knows that the illness can interfere with this client's achievement of which stage of personality development?

1. Intimacy.
2. Trust.
3. Industry.
4. Identity.

119. The LPN/LVN notes that a client has an unsteady gait. The LPN/LVN should take which action? **(Select all that apply.)**

1. Apply a chest or vest restraint at night.
2. Help the client put on nonskid shoes for walking.
3. Keep the call light within the client's reach.
4. Lower the bed and raise all 4 side rails.
5. Provide adequate lighting in room and bathroom.
6. Remove obstacles and room clutter.

120. Haloperidol 5 mg PO tid is prescribed for a client with schizophrenia. Two days later, the client reports "tight jaws and a stiff neck." What does the LPN/LVN recognize these complaints to be?

1. Common side effects of therapy that will diminish over time.
2. Early symptoms of extrapyramidal reactions to the medication.
3. Psychosomatic symptoms resulting from a delusional system.
4. Permanent side effects associated with haloperidol therapy.

121. A client is receiving a continuous gastric tube feeding at 100 mL per hour. The LPN/LVN checks for gastric residual volume and finds 90 mL in the client's stomach. Which action should the LPN/LVN take?

1. Discard the gastric residual volume and continue the tube feeding.
2. Discard the gastric residual volume and stop the tube feeding.
3. Return the gastric residual volume and continue the tube feeding.
4. Return the gastric residual volume and stop the tube feeding.

122. The LPN/LVN is opening several sterile gauze dressings on the client's over-the-bed table. The LPN/LVN knows that taking which action will contaminate the sterile dressings?

1. Preventing prolonged exposure of the dressings to the air.
2. Keeping sterile dressings inside border of the sterile packaging.
3. Positioning the top of the over-the-bed table at or above waist level.
4. Pouring sterile saline onto the opened sterile dressing on table.

123. The LPN/LVN is caring for a client in labor. The primary health care provider palpates a firm, round form in the uterine fundus, small parts on the client's right side, and a long, smooth, curved section on the left side. Based on these findings, where should the LPN/LVN anticipate auscultating the fetal heart tones?

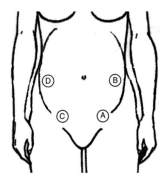

1. A
2. B
3. C
4. D

124. When completing data collection of an immobilized client, the LPN/LVN knows that edema is commonly observed in which location?

1. Abdomen.
2. Feet and ankles.
3. Fingers and wrists.
4. Sacrum.

125. A client is preparing to take her 1-day-old infant home from the hospital. The LPN/LVN discusses the test for phenylketonuria (PKU) with the client. The LPN/LVN's reinforcement of teaching should be based on an understanding that the test is **most** reliable in which circumstance?

1. After source of protein has been ingested.
2. After the meconium has been excreted.
3. After the danger of hyperbilirubinemia has passed.
4. After the effects of delivery have subsided.

Refer to the Case Study to answer the next question.

The LPN/LVN is caring for a 65-year-old client in the cardiac care unit.

| Nurse's Notes | Nursing Assessment |

0900: Client admitted yesterday for diagnosis of atrial fibrillation with rapid ventricular response (RVR). Later in the day, the client's heart rhythm was converted to normal sinus rhythm using intravenous medication therapy. History of persistent atrial fibrillation, hypertension, hyperlipidemia, and osteoarthritis. Client is sitting in the bedside recliner. Reports "racing" heartbeat and feeling "like I can't take a good deep breath." Irregular heart rhythm auscultated.

| Nurse's Notes | Nursing Assessment |

Body system	Findings 0900
Neurological	Alert and oriented × 4.
Eye, Ear, Nose, and Throat (EENT)	Normocephalic, denies sore throat, nasal congestion, or vision changes. No swelling or drainage visualized
Pulmonary	Reports some shortness of breath (SOB), no cough. Lung sounds clear throughout.
Cardiovascular	Irregular heart rhythm auscultated. Denies chest pain. Skin is warm and dry to the touch. Capillary refill > 3 seconds. 2+ bilateral lower extremity edema and peripheral pulses 1+, equal bilaterally. Jugular vein distention (JVD) noted.
Gastrointestinal	Abdomen protuberant and firm. Reports slight nausea, bowel sounds hypoactive × 4 quadrants. Reports bowel movement (BM) prior to admission.
Genitourinary	Voiding clear yellow urine per self without complications.
Musculoskeletal	Full range of motion against resistance.

126. The LPN/LVN is reviewing the client's assessment data and medications to collaborate with the RN to prepare the client's plan of care.

Complete the diagram by dragging from the choices below to specify what condition the client is most likely experiencing, 2 actions the LPN/LVN takes to address that condition, and 2 findings the LPN/LVN reports to the RN for follow-up.

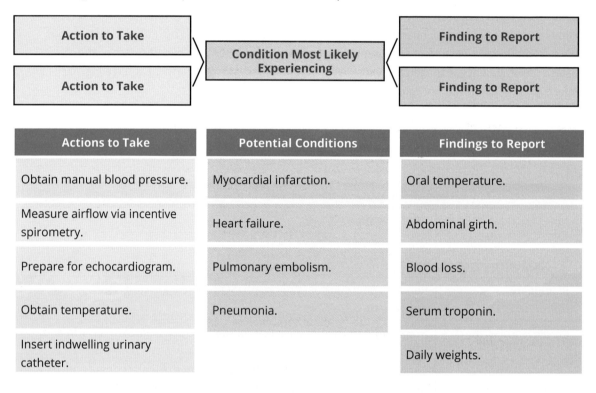

Actions to Take	Potential Conditions	Findings to Report
Obtain manual blood pressure.	Myocardial infarction.	Oral temperature.
Measure airflow via incentive spirometry.	Heart failure.	Abdominal girth.
Prepare for echocardiogram.	Pulmonary embolism.	Blood loss.
Obtain temperature.	Pneumonia.	Serum troponin.
Insert indwelling urinary catheter.		Daily weights.

---

127. The LPN/LVN is caring for an Rh-negative client who has delivered an Rh-positive child. The client states, "The doctor told me about RhoGAM, but I'm still a little confused." Which response by the LPN/LVN is **most** appropriate?

1. "RhoGAM is given to your child to prevent the development of antibodies."
2. "RhoGAM is given to your child to supply the necessary antibodies."
3. "RhoGAM is given to you to prevent the formation of antibodies."
4. "RhoGAM is given to you to encourage the production of antibodies."

128. A client is hospitalized with a diagnosis of bipolar disorder. While in the activities room on the psychiatric unit, the client flirts with other clients and disrupts unit activities. Which approach would be **most** appropriate for the LPN/LVN to take at this time?

1. Set limits on the behavior and remind the client of the rules.
2. Distract the client and escort the client back to the room.
3. Instruct the other clients to ignore this client's behavior.
4. Inform client of negative behavior and return client to room.

Refer to the Case Study to answer the next question.

The LPN/LVN on the surgical floor is caring for an older adult client following abdominal surgery.

| Transfer Summary | Medications | Nurse's Notes |

Client admitted two days ago due to increasing abdominal pain with vomiting and abdominal swelling. The client was diagnosed with a small bowel obstruction and underwent an exploratory laparotomy with small bowel resection and lysis of adhesions. This morning, the client's nasogastric tube was removed and the client is taking sips of clear liquids. Lung sounds are diminished in the bases bilaterally, but otherwise clear. Bowel sounds are hypoactive throughout and surgical incision is well approximated with sutures intact and no drainage noted. Client is getting up to the chair and bedside commode with assistance. Voiding clear yellow urine. Plan to move from the surgical intensive care unit to the surgical floor this afternoon, advance diet as tolerated, resume home medications, and ambulate in halls. Discharge is anticipated once the client is eating a regular diet and is passing flatus.

Client has previous history of colon cancer which was successfully resected 10 years ago. The client also has a history of hypothyroidism, hypertension, coronary artery disease, Parkinson disease, and mild dementia. Home medications include carbidopa/levodopa, amlodipine, lisinopril, quetiapine, furosemide, and levothyroxine. No known allergies.

| Transfer Summary | Medications | Nurse's Notes |

Medication Administration Record (MAR)

Time Given	Medication	Dose	Route	Frequency
0830	Carbidopa/levodopa	25 mg/100 mg	PO	Three times daily
0830	Amlodipine	10 mg	PO	Daily
0830	Lisinopril	20 mg	PO	Daily
0830	Quetiapine	50 mg	PO	Three times daily
0830	Furosemide	20 mg	PO	Twice daily
0700	Levothyroxine	125 mcg	PO	Daily
0715	Hydrocodone/acetaminophen	7.5 mg/325 mg	PO	Every 4 hours PRN pain

| Transfer Summary | Medications | Nurse's Notes |

0700: Client awake and alert. IV 0.9% normal saline infusing to right arm at 75 mL/hr. Lungs clear, clear S1 S2. Dressing intact, site without redness or edema. Abdominal dressing dry and intact. Reports slept fairly well last night. Using urinal and voiding clear yellow urine. States having some abdominal incision pain when using incentive spirometer and requests pain medication. Pain rated 6/10.

0830: Client states has rested well since pain medication received. Sitting up in chair, ate 70% of soft diet for breakfast and is tolerating well. Would like to get bath after breakfast. Vital signs: BP 156/82; HR 78, regular; RR 16; SpO$_2$ 96% on room air; Temperature 99.2° F (37.3° C). Morning medications given.

0915: Client requested to ambulate to toilet, then complete bath at sink. Unlicensed assistive personnel (UAP) walked with client to bathroom. Client became pale and diaphoretic, reported feeling lightheaded and nauseated, then slid down to floor. UAP called for assistance.

129. The LPN/LVN responds to a call for assistance from the UAP. Client is awake, but appears dazed and states, "Everything went dark for a second."

Complete the following sentences by choosing from the list of options.

The LPN/LVN believes it is likely the client [Select from list 1]. It is a **priority** for the LPN/LVN to [Select from list 2]. The LPN/LVN understands the cause of the client's condition is **most** likely [Select from list 3]. The LPN/LVN will [Select from list 4].

(1)	(2)	(3)	(4)
is having a myocardial infarction	measure the client's vital signs	a complication of surgery	discuss altering the client's medication schedule with the RN
has become hypoglycemic	give the client some orange juice	related to fluid volume deficit	encourage the client to increase oral intake of fluid
is experiencing postural hypotension	administer oxygen by face mask	due to effects of the client's medications	discontinue the lisinopril

130. A client is brought to the emergency department bleeding profusely from a stab wound in the left chest area. Vital signs include: blood pressure 80/50 mmHg, pulse 110 beats/minute, and respiratory rate 28 breaths/minute. The LPN/LVN should expect which potential problem?

1. Hypovolemic shock.
2. Cardiogenic shock.
3. Neurogenic shock.
4. Septic shock.

Refer to the Case Study to answer the next question.

The LPN/LVN is caring for a 12-year-old client in the walk-in clinic.

History and Physical

Client presents with shortness of breath. Parent at the bedside and reports the client was running around in the backyard with a sibling when client became short of breath. Client denies injury or insect sting. History of allergic rhinitis and frequent sinus infections. Focused assessment completed.

Body system	Finding
Neurological	Client alert and oriented × 4.
Pulmonary	Reports severe shortness of breath, wheezing heard. Lung sounds diminished to bilateral bases, wheezes auscultated throughout all lung fields.
Cardiovascular	S1 and S2 heart sounds auscultated. Denies chest pain. Skin is warm to the touch, capillary refill < 3 seconds. No edema and peripheral pulses 2+, equal bilaterally.

131. The LPN/LVN is reviewing the client's history and physical before providing the client's care.

Complete the diagram by dragging from the choices below to specify what condition the client is most likely experiencing, 2 medications the LPN/LVN administers to address that condition, and 2 parameters the LPN/LVN monitors to assess the client's progress.

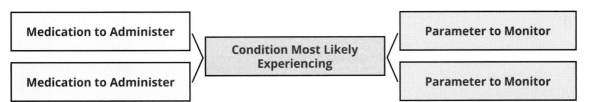

Medications to Administer	Potential Conditions	Parameters to Monitor
Intramuscular (IM) epinephrine.	Anaphylactic reaction.	Peak expiratory flow rate (PEFR).
Albuterol nebulizer.	Asthma attack.	Sputum culture.
Beclomethasone nebulizer.	Pericarditis.	C-reactive protein (CRP).
Oral (PO) metoprolol.	Upper respiratory tract infection (URI).	Pulse oximetry.
Acetylcysteine nebulizer.		Transesophageal echocardiogram (TEE).

132. A client is admitted to the hospital for surgical repair of a detached retina in the right eye. In implementing the plan of care for this client postoperatively, the LPN/LVN should encourage the client to take which action?

1. Perform self-care activities.
2. Maintain patches over both eyes.
3. Limit movement of both eyes.
4. Refrain from excessive talking.

133. The LPN/LVN is caring for a client who receives a balanced complete formula through an enteral feeding tube. The LPN/LVN knows that the **most** common complication of an enteral tube feeding is which of these?

1. Edema.
2. Diarrhea.
3. Hypokalemia.
4. Vomiting.

134. The LPN/LVN is caring for a preschool-age client diagnosed with a fractured pelvis caused by a motor vehicle accident. The LPN/LVN prepares the child for the application of a hip spica cast. It is **most** important for the LPN/LVN to take which action?

1. Obtain a doll for the client with a hip spica cast in place.
2. Tell the client that the cast will feel cold when applied.
3. Reassure the client that cast application is painless.
4. Introduce the client to another client who has a hip spica cast.

135. An infant is brought to the pediatrician's office for a well-baby visit. During the examination, congenital subluxation of the left hip is suspected. The LPN/LVN would expect to see which symptom?

1. Lengthening of the limb on the affected side.
2. Deformities of the foot and ankle.
3. Asymmetry of the gluteal and thigh folds.
4. Plantarflexion of the foot.

136. A client comes to the clinic because for suspected pregnancy. Tests confirm pregnancy. The client's last menstrual period began on September 8 and lasted for 6 days. The LPN/LVN calculates which expected date of confinement (EDC) for this client?

1. May 15.
2. June 15.
3. June 21.
4. July 8.

137. After completing data collection, the LPN/LVN observes that a client is exhibiting early symptoms of a dystonic reaction related to the use of an antipsychotic medication. Which action by the LPN/LVN would be **most** appropriate?

1. Reality-test with the client and assure the client that physical symptoms are not real.
2. Teach the client about common side effects of antipsychotic medications.
3. Explain to the client that there is no treatment that will relieve these symptoms.
4. Notify the primary health care provider to obtain a prescription for IM diphenhydramine.

138. As a client nears death, the client's family member says, "I wish I could do something for her." Which response by the LPN/LVN is **most** appropriate?

1. "It may be comforting if you talk to her calmly and clearly."
2. "She does not know that you are here, but you can sit here."
3. "Unfortunately, there is little that you can do at this point."
4. "Why don't you take a break? It is just a matter of time now."

139. The LPN/LVN is providing care to clients in a long-term care facility. Four meal choices are available to the clients. The LPN/LVN should ensure that a client on a low-cholesterol diet receives which meal?

　1. Egg custard and boiled liver.

　2. Fried chicken and potatoes.

　3. Hamburger and french fries.

　4. Grilled flounder and green beans.

140. The LPN/LVN is removing a client's breakfast tray and notes that the client consumed 4 oz of pudding, 4 oz of gelatin, 6½ oz of tea, and 5 oz of apple juice. How many milliliters should the LPN/LVN record for the client's oral fluid intake?

　_____ mL

141. A client comes to the clinic at 32 weeks' gestation. A diagnosis of pregnancy-induced hypertension (PIH) is made. The LPN/LVN is reinforcing teaching performed by the RN. Which statement by the client indicates that further teaching is required?

　1. "Lying in bed on my left side is likely to increase my urinary output."

　2. "If the bed rest works, I may lose a pound or two in the next few days."

　3. "I should be sure to maintain a diet that has a good amount of protein."

　4. "I will have to keep my room darkened and not watch much television."

142. The LPN/LVN is collecting data about a client's fluid balance. Which finding **most** accurately indicates to the LPN/LVN that the client has retained fluid during the previous 24 hours?

　1. Edema is found in both ankles.

　2. Fluid intake is equal to fluid output.

　3. Intake of fluid exceeds output by 200 mL.

　4. Weight gain of 4 lb (1.8 kg) is noted.

143. The LPN/LVN is caring for a client diagnosed with bipolar disorder. Which behavior by the client indicates that a manic episode is subsiding?

　1. The client tells several jokes during a group meeting.

　2. The client sits and talks with other clients at mealtimes.

　3. The client begins to write a book about personal story.

　4. The client initiates a unit effort to start a radio station.

144. A parent brings a child to the pediatrician for treatment of chronic otitis media. The parent asks the LPN/LVN how to prevent the child from getting ear infections. The LPN/LVN's response should be based on an understanding that the recurrence of otitis media can be decreased by which of the following?

　1. "Cover your child's ears during baths."

　2. "Treat upper respiratory infections quickly."

　3. "Administer nose drops at bedtime."

　4. "Isolate your child from other children."

145. A client is calling the suicide prevention hotline to report a personal suicide plan. Which question should the LPN/LVN ask **first**?

　1. "What happened to cause you to want to end your life?"

　2. "Tell me the details of the plan you developed to kill yourself?"

　3. "When did you start to feel as though you wanted to die?"

　4. "Do you want me to prevent you from killing yourself?"

146. Prior to the client undergoing a scheduled intravenous pyelogram (IVP), it would be **most** important for the LPN/LVN to ask which question?

1. "Do you have any difficulty voiding?"
2. "Do you have any allergies to shellfish or iodine?"
3. "Do you have a history of constipation?"
4. "Do you have a history of frequent headaches?"

147. A client observes the LPN/LVN in the delivery room place drops in her newborn's eyes. The client asks the LPN/LVN why this was done. Which response by the LPN/LVN is **best**?

1. "The drops constrict your baby's pupils to prevent injury."
2. "The drops will remove mucus from your baby's eyes."
3. "The drops will prevent infections that might cause blindness."
4. "The drops will prevent neonatal conjunctivitis."

148. The LPN/LVN is caring for a client admitted for a possible herniated intervertebral disk. The primary health care provider prescribed ibuprofen, propoxyphene hydrochloride, and cyclobenzaprine hydrochloride to be given as needed for pain. Several hours after admission, the client reports increased discomfort. Which action should the LPN/LVN take **first**?

1. Give the client ibuprofen to promptly manage the pain.
2. Ask the primary health care provider which drug to give first.
3. Gather more information from the client about the complaint.
4. Allow the client some time to rest to see if the pain subsides.

149. A client is transferred to a long-term care facility after a stroke. The client has right-sided paralysis and dysphagia. The LPN/LVN observes an unlicensed assistive personnel (UAP) preparing the client to eat lunch. Which situation would require an intervention by the LPN/LVN?

1. The client remains in bed in the high Fowler position.
2. The client's head and neck are positioned slightly forward.
3. The UAP places food in back of the mouth of unaffected side.
4. The UAP adds tap water to the pudding to help client swallow.

150. The LPN/LVNs is collecting data and a client's blood pressure is 146/92 mmHg with labored respirations at a rate of of 24 breaths/minute. Bloody drainage appears on the client's IV dressing. The client reports pain in the left hip, depression, and hunger. The LPN/LVN identifies which of these as subjective data? **(Select all that apply.)**

1. Blood pressure.
2. Depression.
3. Hip pain.
4. Hunger.
5. IV drainage.
6. Respirations.

YOUR PRACTICE TEST SCORES

The test included in this book is designed to provide practice answering exam-style questions along with a review of nursing content. Your results on this test indicate where you are NOW. It is NOT designed to predict your ability to pass the NCLEX-PN® exam.

- If you scored 70 percent or better, you have a good understanding of essential nursing content and you are able to utilize the critical thinking skills required to answer exam-style questions.

- If you scored 60 to 69 percent, you have areas of essential nursing content that need further review, or you may need continued work to master the critical thinking skills needed to correctly answer exam-style questions.

- If you scored 59 percent or less, you need concentrated study of nursing content and continued practice utilizing the critical thinking skills required to be successful on the NCLEX-PN® exam.

If you are looking for additional preparation materials for the NCLEX-PN® exam, Kaplan's NCLEX-PN® Question Bank provides access to more than 1,100 exam-like practice questions. This resource is designed to develop both your knowledge of the nursing content as well as your critical thinking skills. Learn more at: **kaptest.com/nclex-pn/practice/nclex-pn-qbank**

ANSWER KEY

1. **3**	39. **See explanation**	77. **2**	115. **3**
2. **4**	40. **1**	78. **2**	116. **1**
3. **See explanation**	41. **4**	79. **3**	117. **1, 2, 3, 4, 6, 7,**
4. **See explanation**	42. **1**	80. **3**	**and 8**
5. **4**	43. **3**	81. **4**	118. **3**
6. **3 and 5**	44. **4**	82. **4**	119. **2, 3, 5, and 6**
7. **See explanation**	45. **3**	83. **1**	120. **2**
8. **1, 3, and 5**	46. **3**	84. **4**	121. **4**
9. **2**	47. **4**	85. **4**	122. **4**
10. **1**	48. **1**	86. **3**	123. **1**
11. **2**	49. **3**	87. **See explanation**	124. **4**
12. **2**	50. **3**	88. **3**	125. **1**
13. **1**	51. **2**	89. **3**	126. **See explanation**
14. **1, 2, 3, and 6**	52. **1**	90. **3**	127. **3**
15. **See explanation**	53. **2**	91. **See explanation**	128. **2**
16. **1**	54. **2**	92. **3**	129. **See explanation**
17. **See explanation**	55. **2**	93. **125**	130. **1**
18. **See explanation**	56. **3**	94. **1, 3, 4, and 5**	131. **See explanation**
19. **See explanation**	57. **2**	95. **1**	132. **3**
20. **3**	58. **1**	96. **3**	133. **2**
21. **2**	59. **4**	97. **3**	134. **1**
22. **4**	60. **4**	98. **4**	135. **3**
23. **3**	61. **See explanation**	99. **2**	136. **2**
24. **2**	62. **1, 3, 4, 5, 7, and 8**	100. **2**	137. **4**
25. **2**	63. **See explanation**	101. **3**	138. **1**
26. **2**	64. **See explanation**	102. **1**	139. **4**
27. **4**	65. **2**	103. **2**	140. **465**
28. **3**	66. **See explanation**	104. **3**	141. **4**
29. **3**	67. **2**	105. **3**	142. **4**
30. **2**	68. **4**	106. **2**	143. **2**
31. **3**	69. **3**	107. **4**	144. **2**
32. **4**	70. **2**	108. **3**	145. **2**
33. **1**	71. **1**	109. **1**	146. **2**
34. **2, 4, and 5**	72. **2**	110. **2**	147. **3**
35. **1, 3, and 5**	73. **4**	111. **2**	148. **3**
36. **See explanation**	74. **4**	112. **See explanation**	149. **4**
37. **See explanation**	75. **2**	113. **2**	150. **2, 3, and 4**
38. **1**	76. **2**	114. **725**	

PRACTICE TEST ANSWERS AND EXPLANATIONS

1. The answer is 3

The LPN/LVN is gathering data from a client who is receiving treatment for obsessive-compulsive disorder (OCD). Which is the **most** important question the LPN/LVN should ask this client?

Reworded Question: What are the signs and symptoms of obsessive-compulsive disorder?

Strategy: "*Most* important" indicates there may be more than one correct response.

Needed Info: Obsessive-compulsive disorder is characterized by a history of obsessions and compulsions. Obsessions are recurrent and persistent thoughts, ideas, impulses, or images that are experienced as intrusive and senseless. The client may know that the thoughts are ridiculous or morbid but cannot stop, forget, or control them. Compulsions are repetitive behaviors performed in a certain way to prevent discomfort and neutralize anxiety.

Category: Data Collection/Psychosocial Integrity

(1) "Do you find yourself forgetting simple things?"—should be used to collect data for a client with suspected cognitive disorder

(2) "Do you find it difficult to focus on a given task?"—collects data for disorders that disrupt the ability to concentrate, such as depression

(3) "Do you have trouble controlling upsetting thoughts?"—CORRECT: one feature of obsessive-compulsive disorder is the client's inability to control intrusive thoughts that repeat over and over

(4) "Do you experience feelings of panic in a closed area?"—appropriate for client with suspected panic disorder related to closed spaces or claustrophobia

2. The answer is 4

A newly admitted client with a history of seizures suddenly says to the LPN/LVN, "I hear drums." Which should the LPN/LVN do **first**?

Reworded Question: What does a sudden visual, olfactory, or auditory sensation often signal in a client with a history of seizures?

Strategy: Quickly review the most likely causes of the client's unusual perception.

Needed Info: Aura: brief sensory alteration often preceding seizure or migraine, likely for client with history of seizures. Petit mal seizures: usually occur in children, not associated with an aura. Grand mal seizures: involve loss of consciousness and convulsions.

Category: Evaluation/Physiological Integrity/Physiological Adaptation

(1) Tell the client to ignore the drums—client is experiencing an auditory sensation that may signal the start of a seizure

(2) Place the client in a darkened room away from the nurses' station—the client needs continued observation

(3) Continue to question the client—many adult clients experience unusual sensory perceptions (an aura) before the onset of a seizure; this client has a history of seizures

(4) Insert an oral airway in the client—CORRECT: an oral airway prevents the client from biting cheek or tongue during a seizure

3. See explanation for answers

Assessment	Client Findings
Vital Signs	Heart rate 124 bpm, regular
	Blood pressure 118/78
	BMI 31 kg/m^2 (obese)
Skin	Pale, cool
	Profuse sweating
Respiratory	Soft, vesicular lung sounds
Neurologic	Unable to answer questions appropriately
	Slurred, incoherent speech
Medications	Intermediate-acting NPH insulin at 1700
	Uneaten bedtime snack at 2100

CORRECT OPTIONS: The LPN/LVN recognizes the client findings that require immediate follow up are **heart rate 124** beats/minute, regular; skin **pale and cool** with **profuse sweating**; **unable to answer questions appropriately**; and **slurred, incoherent speech.** The LPN/LVN is also concerned the **client received NPH insulin at 1700 and did not eat a bedtime snack at 2100.**

INCORRECT OPTIONS: A blood pressure of 118/78 is within an acceptable adult range. Obesity decreases insulin effectiveness and is one of many risk factors contributing to the development of type 2 diabetes. However, the LPN/LVN does not identify the client's BMI as requiring immediate follow up. Soft, vesicular lung sounds are normal clinical findings.

4. See explanation for answers

The LPN/LVN identifies the client is most likely experiencing symptoms of **hypoglycemia**. When blood glucose falls below 70 mg/dL (3.9 mmol/L), the release of epinephrine and norepinephrine produces symptoms (e.g., tachycardia and sweating). A deficit of glucose impairs the central nervous system, deprives the brain of glucose, and can produce symptoms of confusion, difficulty speaking, and stupor. INCORRECT OPTIONS: An insulin allergic reaction can produce local inflammatory effects such as itching, erythema, and burning at the injection site; systemic effects occur rarely. Diabetic ketoacidosis, acute insulin deficiency, is identified by hyperglycemia, ketosis, and acidosis, not hypoglycemia.

The LPN/LVN recognizes the client may have received **too much insulin relative to the blood glucose** level, which could lower the blood glucose to less than 70 mg/dL (3.9 mmol/L), causing hypoglycemia. INCORRECT OPTIONS: In clients with diabetes, exercise has blood glucose lowering effects. Inactivity and lack of exercise can contribute to hyperglycemia, not hypoglycemia. Illness and infection can produce counterregulatory hormone effects that increase the blood glucose level resulting in hyperglycemia, not hypoglycemia.

Lack of food intake during peak action of an intermediate-acting insulin (NPH) may also be causing the client's hypoglycemia. The peak action of an intermediate-acting insulin ranges from 4–12 hours. NPH insulin given before the dinner meal may be peaking (i.e., exerting its strongest effect, around midnight). This can cause hypoglycemia, particularly in clients who have not eaten a bedtime snack. INCORRECT OPTIONS: Subcutaneous injection is the appropriate route to deliver routine doses of insulin; intramuscular injection can result in rapid and unpredictable absorption. Because of a rapid effect and shorter duration, sliding scale aspart insulin is for management of postprandial blood glucose. The client had mealtime aspart insulin coverage by eating 100% of the dinner meal.

5. The answer is 4

CORRECT OPTION: Due to the client's low blood glucose, the LPN/LVN's priority consideration is the risk for the client to develop **seizures**. The brain needs sufficient quantities of glucose and seizures may occur in untreated hypoglycemia due to significant impairment in function of the central nervous system.

INCORRECT OPTIONS: Osmotic diuresis, hypokalemia, and hypovolemia are manifestations that may occur in clients with diabetic ketoacidosis when there is insulin deficiency and improper utilization of glucose.

6. The answer is 3 and 5

CORRECT OPTIONS: The LPN/LVN includes **subcutaneous or intramuscular administration of 1 mg glucagon** and **intravenous 50 mL of 50% dextrose** as appropriate interventions to treat the client's low blood glucose, especially in clients who are unconscious, cannot swallow, or have no intravenous access. Glucagon will stimulate a hepatic response to make glucose quickly available. In acute care settings, for clients who cannot swallow or are unconscious, 25–50 mL of 50% dextrose may be given to rapidly reverse low blood glucose.

INCORRECT OPTIONS: The client is not alert, has difficulty speaking, and may not be able to swallow; giving 15 grams of a fast-acting carbohydrate orally is inappropriate until the client can safely swallow. Intravenous administration of a short-acting insulin is treatment for insulin deficiency and hyperglycemia, not hypoglycemia. Potassium chloride supplementation is an appropriate intervention for electrolyte replacement. The client with diabetes who is experiencing acute hypoglycemia needs glucose. Additionally, potassium chloride by oral route would be inappropriate in a client who is not alert.

7. See explanation for answers

A concentrated source of carbohydrates is needed to reverse low blood glucose of less than 70 mg/dL (3.9 mmol/L). The LPN/LVN recognizes it is appropriate to give fast-acting carbohydrates (e.g. **4–6 ounces regular soda or orange juice**) because the client is awake and responding appropriately to ingest these orally. INCORRECT OPTIONS: It is not appropriate to give oral carbohydrates containing fat (e.g., whole milk or ice cream); treatment response is delayed because the fat in these foods slows absorption of the glucose. A drink or food with at least 15 grams of protein does not supply a concentrated source of carbohydrates that is needed to reverse low blood glucose.

Next, it is appropriate to **wait 15 minutes and recheck the client's blood glucose** after administering 15 grams of fast-acting carbohydrate to determine if it is still below 70 mg/dL (3.9 mmol/L). INCORRECT OPTIONS: A blood glucose less than 70 mg/dL (3.9 mmol/L) is termed hypoglycemia and needs continuing treatment. It is not appropriate to obtain a urine sample and check for ketones, byproducts of fat metabolism that are produced when a client has diabetic ketoacidosis, not hypoglycemia.

If the client's blood glucose is less than 70 mg/dL(3.9 mmol/L), it is appropriate to **provide 15 grams of fast-acting carbohydrates** (e.g., 4–6 ounces soda or orange juice). INCORRECT OPTIONS: A snack of peanut butter and crackers is not a fast-acting carbohydrate that is needed to correct low blood glucose; peanut butter contains fat, which slows absorption of glucose. It is not appropriate to prepare to administer a continuous insulin infusion intravenously; insulin treats hyperglycemia, not hypoglycemia.

8. The answer is 1, 3, and 5

CORRECT OPTIONS: The LPN/LVN identifies normal client findings that indicate effective treatment for low blood glucose as **heart rate 88, regular; blood glucose 115 mg/dL (6.38 mmol/L); and coherent thoughts with smooth flow to speech**.

INCORRECT OPTIONS: Client findings of shakiness and dizziness when standing are symptoms that can occur with low blood glucose and may indicate the nursing actions have not been effective. Fruity odor to breath is due to acetone, a byproduct of ketones that are produced when a client has diabetic ketoacidosis. In clients with diabetes, rapid and deep breathing can indicate Kussmaul respirations, a type of respirations associated with metabolic acidosis.

9. The answer is 2

A client diagnosed with multiple myeloma is admitted to the unit after developing pneumonia. When the LPN/LVN enters the client's room wearing a mask, the client says in an irritated tone of voice, "Why are you wearing that mask?" Which response by the LPN/LVN is **best**?

Reworded Question: What is the most therapeutic response?

Strategy: Remember therapeutic communication.

Needed Info: Multiple myeloma: a neoplastic disease that infiltrates bone and bone marrow, causes anemia, renal lesions, and high globulin levels in blood; pneumonia is inflammatory process resulting in edema of lung tissue and extravasion of fluid into alveoli, causing hypoxia.

Category: Data Collection/Safe and Effective Care Environment/Safety and Infection Control

(1) "The chest x-ray taken this morning indicates you have pneumonia."—does not help determine what client knows; primary health care provider is responsible for telling client the medical diagnosis

(2) "What have you been told about the x-rays that were taken this morning?"—CORRECT: data collection; determines what client knows before responding; allows client to verbalize

(3) "You have been placed on contact precautions due to your infection."—certain types of pneumonia require droplet precautions

(4) "I am trying to protect you from the germs in the hospital."—certain types of pneumonia require droplet precautions

10. The answer is 1

A nursing team consists of an RN, an LPN/LVN, and an unlicensed assistive personnel (UAP). The LPN/LVN should be assigned to which client?

Reworded Question: Which client is an appropriate assignment for the LPN/LVN?

Strategy: Think about the skill level involved in each client's care.

Needed Info: LPN/LVN: assists with implementation of care; performs procedures; differentiates normal from abnormal; cares for stable clients with predictable conditions; has knowledge of asepsis and dressing changes; administers medications (varies with educational background and state nurse practice act).

Category: Planning/Safe and Effective Care Environment/Coordinated Care

(1) A client with a diabetic ulcer that requires a dressing change—CORRECT: stable client with an expected outcome

(2) A client with cancer who is reporting bone pain—requires assessment; RN is the appropriate caregiver

(3) A client with terminal cancer being transferred to hospice home care—requires nursing judgment; RN is the appropriate caregiver

(4) A client with a fracture of the right leg who asks to use the urinal—standard unchanging procedure; would be assigned to the UAP

11. The answer is 2

The LPN/LVN is caring for a client receiving paroxetine. It is **most** important for the LPN/LVN to report which information to the physician?

Reworded Question: What is a potential drug interaction?

Strategy: "*Most* important" indicates priority.

Needed Info: Paroxetine (Paxil) is a selective serotonin reuptake inhibitor (SSRI) used to treat depression, panic disorder, obsessive-compulsive disorder; side effects include palpitations, bradycardia, nausea and vomiting, and decreased appetite.

Category: Evaluation/Physiological Integrity/Pharmacological Therapies

(1) The client reports no appetite change—causes anorexia; monitor weight and nutritional intake; report continued weight loss

(2) The client reports recently being started on digoxin—CORRECT: may decrease effectiveness of digoxin

(3) The client reports applying sunscreen to go outdoors—appropriate action; prevents photosensitivity reactions

(4) The client reports driving the car to work—driving is acceptable after determining client's response to drug

12. The answer is 2

A client with a "do not resuscitate" order experiences a cardiac arrest. Which is the **first** action the LPN/LVN should take?

Reworded Question: What actions are appropriate for a client with a do not resuscitate order who has no heartbeat?

Strategy: Determine which actions meet DNR standards.

Needed Info: "Do not resuscitate" requires a written primary health care provider order in the medical record: no extraordinary care given in the event of the client's death. Extraordinary care after cardiac or pulmonary cessation: cardiopulmonary resuscitation (CPR), medications, ventilators, defibrillation.

Category: Data Collection/Safe and Effective Care Environment/Coordinated Care

(1) Administer lifesaving medications—"Do not resuscitate" means these medications are not given

(2) Assess the client for signs of death—CORRECT: client has signs of death and requires further data collection to confirm death

(3) Open the airway and give 2 breaths—CPR should not be initiated for clients with a "do not resuscitate" order

(4) Summon the emergency code team—CPR should not be initiated for clients with a "do not resuscitate" order

13. The answer is 1

An LPN/LVN is working in the newborn nursery. Which client-care assignment should the LPN/LVN question?

Reworded Question: Which infant is outside the scope of practice for an LPN/LVN?

Strategy: Remember the ABCs (airway, breathing, circulation).

Needed Info: Need to meet client's needs. Physical stability of client is LPN/LVN's first concern. Most unstable client should be cared for by RN.

Category: Evaluation/Safe and Effective Care Environment/Coordinated Care

(1) A 2-day-old client lying quietly alert with a heart rate of 185 beats/minute—CORRECT: client has tachycardia; normal resting rate is 120–160 beats/minute; requires further investigation

(2) A 1-day-old client who is crying and has a bulging anterior fontanel—crying causes increased intracranial pressure, which normally causes fontanel to bulge

(3) A 12-hour-old client whose respirations are 45 breaths/minute and irregular while being held—normal respiratory rate is 30–60 breaths/minute with apneic episodes

(4) A 5-hour-old client whose hands and feet appear blue bilaterally while sleeping—acrocyanosis normally occurs for 2–6 hours after delivery due to poor peripheral circulation

14. The answer is 1, 2, 3, and 6

CORRECT OPTIONS: The LPN/LVN will be concerned about **coarse crackles, warm and flushed skin, and capillary refill > 3 seconds** in a client with an upper respiratory infection (URI). These symptoms indicate that the client's condition is worsening. Flushed skin that is warm to the touch is seen in early sepsis due to vasodilation and capillary refill >3 seconds indicates impaired perfusion. The LPN/LVN is also concerned that the client is **unable to take anything by mouth and finish the oral antibiotic**. The full course of the oral antibiotic must be taken in order to avoid the development of resistant bacteria.

INCORRECT OPTIONS: Alert and oriented ×3 means the client is able to accurately state name, location, and time; this is a normal finding. Distinct heart sounds are a positive finding and indicate normal pumping action of the heart.

15. See explanation for answers

Pneumonia and Sepsis: Inflammation in the lungs from pneumonia causes the client to feel **short of breath**. Sepsis causes a similar response as inflammation occurs throughout the body, including the lungs. **Fever** is commonly seen with any kind of infection. Pneumonia and sepsis both cause the inflammatory response that results in fever. Adventitious lung sounds, like **coarse crackles**, are caused by fluid in the lungs. The inflammation that occurs with both sepsis and pneumonia causes fluid in the lungs.

Sepsis only: The profound, systemic vasodilation which occurs with sepsis causes **hypotension**. Systemic inflammation that occurs with sepsis is characterized by vasodilation and leaky capillaries. This decreases peripheral tissue perfusion and **capillary refill would be slower**. Pneumonia is a localized infection in the lungs and does not have systemic effects that impact circulation. Progression of sepsis is marked by circulatory changes and poor organ perfusion. One of the first signs of poor organ perfusion is **decreased urine output**. This systemic symptom does not occur with pneumonia.

16. The answer is 1

The client is at risk for developing pneumonia, but the systemic symptoms the client is experiencing indicates further progression of the infection. An infection that has spread into the bloodstream and impacts perfusion is defined as **sepsis**, a life-threatening infection.

The client is not displaying any symptoms consistent with angina. The client has had minimal, dark urine output but no reports of burning, urgency, or frequency that are normally associated with a UTI.

17. See explanation for answers

Respiratory: **Titrating oxygen** to maintain SpO_2 greater than 92% is a crucial intervention. INCORRECT OPTIONS: Nasotracheal suctioning can be a helpful intervention for clients unable to clear their own airways, but there is no data that indicates the client is experiencing this problem. A V/Q scan gives detailed insight into lung function but takes time to perform/obtain results and does not help the client right now.

Cardiovascular: A crucial measure to increase BP in sepsis is fluid resuscitation; therefore, administration of an IV fluid bolus would be appropriate. The type of IV fluid is important as not all will adequately expand intravascular volume. **Lactated Ringer** solution is isotonic and will increase BP. INCORRECT OPTIONS: 0.45% sodium chloride and 5% dextrose in water are hypotonic solutions, which will cause fluid to shift out of the vessels.

Genitourinary: Performing an **ultrasound of the bladder** will determine if any urine remains in the bladder following voiding. This would be important to know in order to obtain accurate readings of the urine output. For this client, perfusion of the kidneys is likely impaired, and tracking the intake and output can help assess the effectiveness of interventions. INCORRECT OPTIONS: Urine specific gravity is a laboratory test that measures the kidneys' ability to concentrate urine, which is unnecessary at this time. Placing the client on a toileting schedule is not an appropriate intervention; this intervention is often used in clients who are confused and may forget to use the bathroom.

18. See explanation for answers

Immediate, one-hour management for sepsis includes the following: Measure serum lactate, obtain blood cultures, administer broad-spectrum antibiotics, and rapidly infuse crystalloid fluids for hypotension. In this case, the first action for the LPN/LVN to take is to **draw laboratory tests**. Administration of a broad-spectrum antibiotic prior to blood cultures will interfere with the results. Mortality rates rise with delay in administration of antibiotic therapy, making identifying causative organism and initiating antimicrobial therapy crucial.

19. See explanation for answers

Understanding: The client is correct that the **full course of the antibiotic must be taken** as this prevents development of resistant bacteria. If the client feels cold and clammy, this could indicate progression of sepsis to septic shock. In later stages, perfusion to extremities could be impaired and the **skin will be cool to the touch and pale in color**.

No Understanding: **Acetaminophen** does not prevent inflammation. It has analgesic and antipyretic properties. **Urinary catheter use should be limited** to the shortest possible duration of time to avoid catheter-associated urinary tract infection (CAUTI).

20. The answer is 3

The LPN/LVN is inserting a nasogastric (NG) tube. The LPN/LVN should use which personal protective equipment during NG tube insertion?

Reworded Question: What is the correct standard precaution?

Strategy: Think about each answer choice. How does each piece of equipment protect the LPN/LVN?

Needed Info: Mask, eye protection, and face shield protect against mucous membrane exposure; used if activities are likely to generate splashes or sprays. Gowns used if activities are likely to generate splashes or sprays.

Category: Planning/Safe and Effective Care Environment/Safety and Infection Control

(1) Gloves, gown, goggles, and surgical cap—surgical caps offer protection to hair but aren't required

(2) Sterile gloves, mask, and gown—sterile gloves are used to protect the client during sterile procedures

(3) Gloves, gown, mask, and goggles—CORRECT: must use standard precautions on all clients; prevent skin and mucous membrane exposure when contact with blood or other body fluids is anticipated

(4) Double gloves, goggles, mask, and surgical cap—surgical cap not required for standard precautions; unnecessary to double glove

21. The answer is 2

The LPN/LVN is caring for clients in the outpatient clinic. Which client should the LPN/LVN see **first**?

Reworded Question: Who is the priority client?

Strategy: Think ABCs.

Needed Info: Need to meet client's needs. Physical stability is LPN/LVN's first concern. Client with most serious problem should be seen first.

Category: Planning/Safe and Effective Care Environment/Coordinated Care

(1) A client with hepatitis A who states, "My arms and legs are itching."—caused by accumulation of bile salts under the skin; treat with calamine lotion and antihistamines

(2) A client with a cast on the right leg who states, "I have a funny feeling in my right leg."—CORRECT: may indicate neurovascular compromise; requires immediate data collection

(3) A client with osteomyelitis of the spine who states, "I am so nauseous that I can't eat."—requires follow-up, but not highest priority

(4) A client with rheumatoid arthritis who states, "I am having trouble sleeping."—requires data collection, but not a priority

22. The answer is 4

Which client assignment should an LPN/LVN question?

Reworded Question: Which client is an inappropriate assignment for an LPN/LVN?

Strategy: Think about the skill level involved in each client's care.

Needed Info: Determine nursing care required to meet clients' needs; take into account time required, complexity of activities, acuity of client, and infection control issues. Consider knowledge and abilities of staff members and decide which staff person is best able to provide care.

Category: Planning/Safe and Effective Care Environment/Coordinated Care

(1) A client with a chest tube who is ambulating in the hallway—LPN/LVN can care for client

(2) A client with a colostomy who requires colostomy irrigation assistance—LPN/LVN can care for client

(3) A client with a right-sided stroke who requires assistance with bathing—LPN/LVN can care for client

(4) A client who is refusing medication to treat cancer of the colon—CORRECT: requires the assessment skills of the RN

23. The answer is 3

The LPN/LVN is caring for a client with hepatitis B. The client is to be discharged the next day. The LPN/LVN would be **most** concerned if the client made which statement?

Reworded Question: What is an incorrect statement about care with hepatitis B?

Strategy: "*Most* concerned" indicates you are looking for an incorrect statement.

Needed Info: Hepatitis A (HAV): high-risk groups include young children, institutions for custodial care, international travelers; fecal/oral transmission, poor sanitation; nursing considerations include prevention, improved sanitation, treat with gammaglobulin early postexposure, no preparation of food. Hepatitis B (HBV): high-risk groups include drug addicts, fetuses from infected mothers, homosexually active men, transfusions, health care workers; transmission by parenteral, sexual contact, blood/body fluids; nursing considerations include hepatitis vaccine, immune globulin (HBIG) postexposure, chronic carriers (potential for chronicity 5–10%). Hepatitis C (HVC): high-risk groups include transfusions, international travelers; transmission by blood/body fluids; nursing considerations include great potential for chronicity. Delta hepatitis: high-risk groups same as for HBV; transmission coinfects with HBV, close personal contact.

Category: Evaluation/Safe and Effective Care Environment/Coordinated Care

(1) "I must not share eating utensils with my family members."—prevents transmission; handwashing before eating and after toileting very important

(2) "I must use my own bath towel."—prevents transmission; don't share bed linens

(3) "I'm glad that I can have intimate relations with my partner."—CORRECT: avoid sexual contact until serologic indicators return to normal

(4) "I must eat small, frequent meals."—easier to tolerate than three standard meals; diet should be high in carbohydrates and calories

24. The answer is 2

The LPN/LVN is carrying out the plan for care of a client with anemia who reports weakness. Which task could be assigned to the unlicensed assistive personnel (UAP)?

Reworded Question: What is an appropriate assignment for the UAP?

Strategy: Think about the skill level involved in each task.

Needed Info: Unlicensed assistive personnel (UAPs): assist with direct client care activities (bathing, transferring, ambulating, feeding, toileting, obtaining vital signs/height/weight/intake/output, housekeeping, transporting, stocking supplies); includes nurse aides, assistants, technicians, orderlies, nurse extenders; scope of nursing practice is limited.

Category: Evaluation/Safe and Effective Care Environment/Coordinated Care

(1) Auscultate the client's breath sounds—requires data collection; could be performed by LPN/LVN and reported to RN

(2) Set up the client's lunch tray—CORRECT: standard, unchanging procedure; decreases cardiac workload

(3) Obtain client's dietary history—involves data collection; could be performed by LPN/LVN and reported to RN

(4) Instruct client how to balance rest and activity—instruction required; could be performed by LPN/LVN following established plan of care

25. The answer is 2

A client scheduled for a cardiac catheterization says to the LPN/LVN, "I know you were in here when I signed the consent form for the test. I thought I understood everything, but now I'm not so sure." Which response by the LPN/LVN is **best**?

Reworded Question: Which response is most therapeutic?

Strategy: "*Best*" indicates that discrimination is required to answer the question.

Needed Info: Informed consent is obtained by the individual who will perform the test; explanation of the test and expected results, anticipated risks and discomforts, potential benefits, possible alternatives are discussed; consent can be withdrawn at any time.

Category: Evaluation/Safe and Effective Care Environment/Coordinated Care

(1) "Why didn't you listen more closely to the explanation?"—"why" questions are nontherapeutic; does not respond to the client's feelings or concerns

(2) "You sound as if you would like to ask more questions."—CORRECT: directly responds to client's statement by paraphrasing; implies encouragement of expression of client's concern

(3) "I'll get you a pamphlet about cardiac catheterization."—may be helpful, but first the nurse needs to clarify the client's concerns through discussion

(4) "That often happens during explanation of this procedure."—does convey acceptance and lets the client know that the response is not abnormal; response is closed and does not allow client to express feelings or concerns

26. The answer is 2

A 1-day-old client diagnosed with intrauterine growth restriction has a high-pitched shrill cry and appears restless and irritable. The LPN/LVN also observes fist-sucking behavior. Based on this data, which action should the LPN/LVN take **first**?

Reworded Question: What do you do for a newborn client experiencing withdrawal?

Strategy: Determine the outcome of each answer.

Needed Info: Drug withdrawal may manifest from as early as 12 hours after birth up to 10 days after delivery. Symptoms: high-pitched cry, hyperreflexia, decreased sleep, diaphoresis, tachypnea, excessive mucus, vomiting, uncoordinated sucking. Nursing care: assess muscle tone, irritability, vital signs; administer phenobarbital as ordered; report symptoms of respiratory distress; reduce stimulation; provide adequate nutrition/fluids; monitor mother and newborn interactions.

Category: Implementation/Health Promotion and Maintenance

(1) Gently massage the client's back every 2 hours—may result in overstimulation of the client

(2) Tightly swaddle the client in a flexed position—CORRECT: promotes client's comfort and security

(3) Schedule feeding times every 3 to 4 hours—small, frequent feedings are preferable

(4) Encourage eye contact with the client during feedings—may result in overstimulation of client

27. The answer is 4

The LPN/LVN notes that a client newly admitted to the pediatric unit is scratching the head almost constantly. It would be **most** important for the LPN/LVN to take which action?

Reworded Question: What might head scratching indicate?

Strategy: Determine if data collection or implementation is appropriate.

Needed Info: Pediculosis (lice). Data collection: scalp—white eggs (nits) on hair shafts, itchy; body—macules and papules; pubis—red macules.

Category: Data Collection/Health Promotion and Maintenance

(1) Discuss basic hygiene with the parents—makes an assumption; must collect data first

(2) Instruct the child not to sleep with the dog—must first collect data to determine the problem

(3) Advise parents to contact an exterminator—not enough information to make this determination

(4) Observe the scalp for small white specks—CORRECT: nits (eggs) appear as small, white, oval flakes attached to hair shaft

28. The answer is 3

The client diagnosed with major depressive disorder who was admitted to the psychiatric unit for treatment and observation a week ago suddenly appears cheerful and motivated. The LPN/LVN should be aware of which potential cause of the client's change in behavior?

Reworded Question: What is the significance of sudden mood changes in a depressed client?

Strategy: Know the signs of impending suicide.

Needed Info: Data collection for suicidal ideation, suicidal gestures, suicidal threats, and actual suicidal attempt. Clients who have developed a suicide plan are more serious about following through, and are at grave risk. Clients emerging from severe depression have more energy with which to formulate and carry out a suicide plan (for which they had no energy before

treatment). The LPN/LVN should determine risk for suicide; suspect suicidal ideation in depressed client; ask the client if he is thinking about suicide; ask the client about the advantages and disadvantages of suicide to determine how client sees his situation; evaluate client's access to a method of suicide; and support the client's reason to live.

Category: Planning/Psychosocial Integrity

(1) The client is likely sleeping well because of the medication—improved sleep patterns would not explain the client's sudden mood change

(2) The client has made new friends and has a support group—support on the nursing unit would not explain the mood change

(3) The client may have finalized a suicide plan—CORRECT: as depressed clients improve, their risk for suicide is greater because they are able to mobilize more energy to plan and execute suicide

(4) The client is no longer depressed due to treatment—sudden cheerful and energetic mood does not indicate resolution of depression

29. The answer is 3

The LPN/LVN is caring for clients in the GYN clinic. A client reports an off-white vaginal discharge with a curdlike appearance and vulvar itching. It would be **most** important for the LPN/LVN to ask which question?

Reworded Question: What is a predisposing factor to developing candidiasis?

Strategy: "*Most* important" indicates there may be more than one correct response.

Needed Info: *Candida albicans.* Symptoms: odorless, cheesy white discharge; itching, inflames vagina and perineum. Treatment: topical clotrimazole, nystatin.

Category: Data Collection/Health Promotion and Maintenance

(1) "Do you routinely douche?"—not a factor in the development of candidiasis

(2) "Are you sexually active?"—candidiasis not usually sexually transmitted; predisposing factors include glycosuria, pregnancy, and oral contraceptives

(3) "What kind of birth control do you use?"—CORRECT: oral contraceptives predispose individuals to candidiasis

(4) "Have you taken any cough medicine?"—no relationship between cough medicine and candidiasis

30. The answer is 2

The primary health care provider orders application of an elastic wrap bandage for a client's left leg from toes to mid-thigh. The LPN/LVN should take which action?

Reworded Question: What should an LPN/LVN do for a bandaged extremity?

Strategy: Think of what is most important for a bandaged extremity.

Needed Info: Quality of circulation: determined by observing the color, motion, and sensitivity of an affected body part, particularly distal to the bandage.

Category: Data Collection/Safe and Effective Care Environment/Safety and Infection Control

(1) Increase friction between skin and bandage surfaces—would cause skin breakdown

(2) Leave a small distal portion of the extremity exposed—CORRECT: enables the LPN/LVN to determine the color, motion, and sensitivity of a distal body part

(3) Use multiple pins to secure the bandage—unnecessary

(4) Position the left leg in abduction—unnecessary

31. The answer is 3

A client recovering from a laparoscopic laser cholecystectomy says to the LPN/LVN, "I hate the thought of eating a low-fat diet for the rest of my life." Which response by the LPN/LVN is **most** appropriate?

Reworded Question: Is a low-fat diet required indefinitely?

Strategy: "*Most* appropriate" indicates discrimination may be required to answer the question.

Needed Info: Laparoscopic laser cholecystectomy is removal of the gallbladder by laser through a laparoscope; monitor T-tube if present; observe for jaundice; monitor intake and output; monitor for pain and encourage early ambulation to rid the body of carbon dioxide.

Category: Implementation/Physiological Integrity/Physiological Adaptation

(1) "I will ask the dietician to come speak with you."—passing the reponsibility; LPN/LVN should respond to the client

(2) "What do you think is so bad about following a low-fat diet?"—does not respond directly to the client's statement

(3) "It may not be necessary for you to follow a low-fat diet for that long."—CORRECT: fat restriction is usually lifted as the client tolerates fat; biliary ducts dilate sufficiently to accommodate bile volume that was held by the gallbladder

(4) "At least you will be alive and not suffering that pain."—nontherapeutic and judgmental

32. The answer is 4

A client begins to breathe very rapidly. Which action by the LPN/LVN would be the **most** appropriate?

Reworded Question: What is the most appropriate action for a client experiencing tachypnea?

Strategy: "*Most* appropriate" indicates priority.

Needed Info: Tachypnea: rapid respirations, respirations greater than 20 breaths/minute. Changes in respiratory rate: gather additional data in order to provide complete information to the RN and primary health care provider.

Category: Data Collection/Safe and Effective Care Environment/Coordinated Care

(1) Auscultate the client's apical pulse rate—initial data collection should be directed at respiratory data

(2) Measure client's blood pressure and pulse—initial data collection should be directed at respiratory data

(3) Notify the primary health care provider—the primary health care provider will need more data to respond to client's condition change

(4) Obtain the client's oxygen saturation level—CORRECT: provides the LPN/LVN with data about the client's oxygen saturation

33. The answer is 1

The LPN/LVN is planning morning care for a client hospitalized after a stroke resulting in left-sided paralysis and homonymous hemianopia. During morning care, the LPN/LVN should take which action?

Reworded Question: What should you do for morning care for this client?

Strategy: Think about the consequences of each answer choice.

Needed Info: Homonymous hemianopia: blindness in half of each visual field caused by damage to brain. Client cannot see past midline toward the side opposite the lesion without turning the head toward that side. Approach client from side that is not visually impaired. Reduce noise and complexity of decision making.

Category: Implementation/Physiological Integrity/Physiological Adaptation

(1) Provide morning care from the right side of the client—CORRECT: approach from side with intact vision

(2) Speak loudly and distinctly when talking with the client—no hearing loss

(3) Reduce the level of lighting in the client's room to prevent glare—increase light to assist with vision

(4) Provide client's care to reduce the client's energy expenditure—encourage independence

34. The answer is 2, 4, and 5

CORRECT OPTIONS: The LPN/LVN will be concerned about **copious amounts of thick, tan sputum**; **wheezes** to bilateral lungs; and **shortness of breath at rest**. These findings are consistent with a COPD exacerbation but require follow up. New onset of altered sputum production may mean an infection is causing the exacerbation of symptoms. Wheezes and shortness of breath indicate poor respiratory function.

INCORRECT OPTIONS: The client has used home oxygen for 3 years, so this does not require follow-up. S1 and S2 heart sounds are normal findings that indicate adequate cardiovascular function. The BP is slightly elevated, which is consistent with stress, and not the most pressing concern at this time.

35. The answer is 1, 3, and 5

CORRECT OPTIONS: COPD causes clients to retain CO_2 (**hypercapnia**) and have poor oxygenation (**hypoxemia**). The buildup of CO_2 shifts the acid-base balance to more acidic and makes the client **lethargic**. Poor oxygenation leads to less oxygen available for perfusion at the capillary level; decreased perfusion to the brain causes lethargy, as well.

INCORRECT OPTIONS: Mania is not routinely seen with poor oxygenation because the client does not have the oxygen reserves for rapid activity. Leukopenia and thrombocytopenia are seen with bone marrow suppression but not with COPD exacerbation. If an infection is causing the exacerbation, it is more likely the client would display leukocytosis.

36. See explanation for answers

CORRECT OPTIONS: **Buildup of acidic CO_2** in the client's bloodstream will cause the pH to become acidic. To determine if the acidosis is respiratory or metabolic, the nurse will evaluate the pCO_2. The alveoli control the amount of CO_2, and if this value is high, then the **cause of the acidosis is respiratory.**

INCORRECT OPTIONS: Metabolic acidosis would be indicated by a low pH and a low HCO_3 level, but normal or even low pCO_2. Metabolic and respiratory alkalosis are evidenced by an elevated pH. In metabolic alkalosis, the HCO_3 level is elevated. In respiratory alkalosis, the pCO_2 level is low. An increased production of neutrophils does not affect arterial blood pH.

37. See explanation for answers

CORRECT OPTIONS: A quick intervention to improve ease of breathing in any client is **raising the HOB.** In clients with COPD, **pursed-lip breathing** prolongs exhalation and gives them more voluntary control over their breath. Wheezes are caused by the squeezing of air through narrowed pathways. This indicates constriction of the lung tissue. **LABAs** dilate the bronchioles. A **CT scan of the chest** will help to visualize exactly what is happening in the airway. **Continuously monitoring pulse oximetry** is a non-invasive technique that will alert the nurse of changes in oxygenation. Clients experiencing a COPD exacerbation often see changes in sputum amount and consistency. **Expectorants** reduce viscosity of secretions so they are more easily expectorated. Obtaining a **sputum C&S** can help identify if there is an infection causing the exacerbation.

INCORRECT OPTION: Breathing into a paper bag will not improve oxygenation but will cause further CO_2 retention.

38. The answer is 1

CORRECT OPTION: Administering **salmeterol** prior to fluticasone allows bronchodilation prior to steroid absorption within the airway.

INCORRECT OPTIONS: An inhaled steroid, like fluticasone, should be administered after the client has received an inhaled bronchodilator. Guaifenesin and prednisone, as oral medications, will take longer to have noticeable effects on the client. Inhalation medications will be more quickly absorbed and provide breathing ease.

39. See explanation for answers

Vital Sign	Result 1300
HR	98 beats/minute
BP	136/72 mmHg
RR	18
Pulse oximetry	92% (O2 per 50% Venturi mask)
Temperature (temporal)	99.8° F (37.6° C)

CORRECT OPTIONS: Adequate oxygen administration will improve the client's **pulse oximetry**. As the client feels less stressed by lack of oxygen, the **respiratory rate and pulse will decrease.** The client's **BP is closer to normal range.**

INCORRECT OPTION: The temperature is slightly elevated, which does not indicate improvement.

40. The answer is 1

A primigravid client at 32 weeks' gestation comes to the clinic for her initial prenatal visit. The client reports periodic headaches and continually bumping into things. The LPN/LVN observes numerous bruises in various stages of healing around the client's breasts and abdomen. Vital signs are: BP 120/80, pulse 72 beats/minute, respirations 18 breaths/minute, and fetal heart tones 142 beats/minute. Which of the following responses by the LPN/LVN is **best**?

Reworded Question: What might bruising indicate?

Strategy: Determine if it is appropriate to collect data or implement.

Needed Info: Symptoms of domestic abuse: frequent visits to physician's office or emergency room for unexplained trauma; client being cued, silenced, or threatened by an accompanying family member; evidence of multiple old injuries, scars, healed fractures seen on x-ray; fearful, evasive, or inconsistent replies, or nonverbal behaviors such as flinching when approached or touched. Nursing care: provide privacy during initial interview to ensure perpetrator of violence does not remain with client; carefully document all injuries (with consent); determine safety of client by asking specific questions about weapons, substance abuse, extreme jealousy; develop with client a safety or escape plan; refer client to community resources.

Category: Data Collection/Health Promotion and Maintenance

(1) "Are you battered by your partner?"—CORRECT: evidence of injury should be investigated; assess head, neck, chest, abdomen, breasts, upper extremities

(2) "How do you feel about being pregnant?"—injuries take priority

(3) "Tell me about your headaches."—injuries take priority

(4) "You may be more clumsy due to your size."—assumption; need to collect data

41. The answer is 4

The LPN/LVN is providing care for a client with chronic obstructive pulmonary disease (COPD) who is receiving oxygen through a nasal cannula. The LPN/LVN should expect which implementation in the client's plan of care?

Reworded Question: What physiological changes occur with chronic obstructive pulmonary disease (COPD) that affect oxygen usage?

Strategy: Note the guidelines for oxygen use for clients with COPD.

Needed Info: Clients with COPD retain carbon dioxide. Client's respiratory drive may be controlled by the level of oxygen present in the arterial blood. Administration of oxygen at high-liter flows can suppress the respiratory drive. Humidification effective only for flow rates above 5 L.

Category: Planning/Physiological Integrity/Physiological Adaptation

(1) Arterial blood gases will be analyzed every 2 hours—blood gases are not drawn that often unless the client is in acute distress

(2) The client's oral intake will be restricted—fluids should be encouraged, not restricted

(3) The client will be maintained on bed rest—client should rest as needed: maintaining the client on bed rest is unnecessary

(4) The oxygen flow rate will be set at 3 L/minute or less—CORRECT: the respiratory drive for clients with COPD can be suppressed by high levels of oxygen

42. The answer is 1

The LPN/LVN is caring for a pediatric client in a leg cast for treatment of a right ankle fracture. It is **most** important for the LPN/LVN to reinforce which activity after discharge?

Reworded Question: What is the priority action for a client in a cast?

Strategy: Determine the outcome of each answer choice.

Needed Info: Immediate nursing care for plaster cast: don't cover cast until dry (48 hours), handle with palms not fingertips; don't rest on hard surfaces; elevate affected limb above heart on soft surface until dry; don't use head lamp; check for blueness or paleness, pain, numbness, tingling (if present, elevate area; if it persists, contact physician); client should remain inactive while cast dries. Intermediate nursing care: mobilize client, isometric exercises; check for break in cast or foul odor; tell client not to scratch skin under cast and not to put anything underneath cast; if fiberglass cast gets wet, dry with hair dryer on cool setting. After-cast nursing care: wash skin gently, apply baby powder/cornstarch/baby oil; have client gradually adjust to movement without support of cast; swelling is common, elevate limb and apply elastic bandage.

Category: Implementation/Physiological Integrity/ Reduction of Risk Potential

(1) The client performs isometric exercises of the right leg—CORRECT: contraction of muscle without moving joint; promotes venous return and circulation, prevents thrombi; quadriceps setting (push back knees into bed) and gluteal setting (push heels into bed)

(2) The parent massages the client's right foot with moisturizer—will help prevent dryness of foot but does not address skin under cast

(3) The parent cleans the leg cast with mild soap and water—unnecessary to clean cast

(4) The parent elevates the right leg on several pillows—unnecessary

43. The answer is 3

The LPN/LVN is caring for a client who had a thyroidectomy 12 hours ago for treatment of Graves disease. The LPN/LVN would be **most** concerned if which were observed?

Reworded Question: What is a complication after a thyroidectomy?

Strategy: "*Most* concerned" indicates a complication.

Needed Info: Nursing care for Graves disease/hyperthyroidism: limit activities and provide frequent rest periods; advise light, cool clothing; avoid stimulants; use calm, unhurried approach; administer antithyroid medication, irradiation with I^{131} PO. Post-thyroidectomy care: low or semi-Fowler position; support head, neck, and shoulders to prevent flexion or hyperextension of suture line; tracheostomy set at bedside; observe for complications—laryngeal nerve injury, thyroid storm, hemorrhage, respiratory obstruction, tetany (decreased calcium from parathyroid involvement), check Chvostek and Trousseau signs.

Category: Data Collection/Physiological Integrity/ Reduction of Risk Potential

(1) The client's vital signs include: blood pressure 138/82 mmHg, pulse 84 beats/minute, and respirations 16 breaths/minute—vital signs within normal limits

(2) The client supports the head and neck to turn head to right—prevents stress on the incision

(3) The client spontaneously flexes the wrist when the blood pressure is inflated during blood pressure measurement—CORRECT: carpal spasms indicate hypocalcemia

(4) The client becomes drowsy and reports a sore throat—expected outcome after surgery

44. The answer is 4

A client is admitted who reports severe pain in the right lower quadrant of the abdomen. Which action should the LPN/LVN take to assist the client with pain relief?

Reworded Question: What is an appropriate nonpharmacological method for pain relief?

Strategy: Determine the outcome of each answer choice.

Needed Info: Establish a 24-hour pain profile. Teach client about pain and its relief: explain quality and location of impending pain; slow, rhythmic breathing to promote relaxation; effects of analgesics and benefits of preventative approach; splinting techniques to reduce pain. Reduce anxiety and fears. Provide comfort measures: proper positioning; cool, well-ventilated, quiet room; back rub; allow for rest.

Category: Implementation/Physiological Integrity/ Basic Care and Comfort

(1) Encourage rhythmic, shallow breathing—slow, rhythmic deep breathing promotes relaxation

(2) Massage the right lower quadrant of the abdomen— if appendicitis is suspected, massage or palpation should never be performed as these actions may cause the appendix to rupture

(3) Apply a warm heating pad to the client's abdomen—if pain is caused by appendicitis, increased circulation from heat may cause appendix to rupture

(4) Position the client for comfort using pillows— CORRECT: nonpharmacological methods of pain relief

45. The answer is 3

Which action by the LPN/LVN would be considered negligence?

Reworded Question: What is incorrect behavior?

Strategy: Think about the consequences of each action.

Needed Info: Negligence is the unintentional action or failure to act of an LPN/LVN that a reasonable person would or would not perform in similar circumstances; can be an act of commission or omission. Standards of care: the actions that other LPN/LVNs would take in the same or similar circumstances that provide for quality care. Nurse practice acts: state laws that determine the scope of the practice of nursing.

Category: Implementation/Safe and Effective Care Environment/Safety and Infection Control

(1) Administering heparin subcutaneously into a client's abdomen without first aspirating for blood—correct procedure

(2) Crushing furosemide and adding to a teaspoon of applesauce for an elderly client—correct procedure

(3) Lowering the bed side rails after administering meperidine and hydroxyzine to a client preoperatively—CORRECT: bed side rails should be raised after administering preoperative medication

(4) Placing a used syringe and needle in a sharps container in a client's room—correct procedure

46. The answer is 3

The LPN/LVN is teaching an elderly client with right-sided weakness how to use a cane. Which behavior by the client indicates that the teaching was effective?

Reworded Question: What is the appropriate technique used to ambulate with a cane?

Strategy: Determine the outcome of each answer choice.

Needed Info: Cane tip should have concentric rings (shock absorber for stability). Flex elbow 30 degrees and hold handle up; tip of cane should be 15 cm lateral to base of the fifth toe. Hold cane in hand opposite affected extremity; advance cane and affected leg; lean on cane when moving good leg. To manage stairs, step up on good leg, place the cane and affected leg on step; reverse when going down ("up with the good, down with the bad"); same sequence used with crutches.

Category: Evaluation/Physiological Integrity/Basic Care and Comfort

(1) The client holds the cane with the right hand, moves the cane forward followed by the right leg, and then moves the left leg—should hold cane with the stronger (left) hand

(2) The client holds the cane with the right hand, moves the cane forward followed by the left leg, and then moves the right leg—should hold cane with the stronger (left) hand

(3) The client holds the cane with the left hand, moves the cane forward followed by the right leg, and then moves the left leg—CORRECT: the cane acts as a support and aids in weight-bearing for the weaker right leg

(4) The client holds the cane with the left hand, moves the cane forward followed by the left leg, and then moves the right leg—cane needs to be a support and aid in weight-bearing for the weaker right leg

47. The answer is 4

The LPN/LVN is caring for client whose vital signs have been within normal limits. Now vital signs include: tympanic temperature 103.6° F (39.7° C), pulse 82≈beats/minute, regular and strong, respirations 14 breaths/minute, shallow and unlabored, and blood pressure 134/88 mmHg. What should the LPN/LVN's next action be?

Reworded Question: What do you do first when you obtain a vital sign that represents a significant change in the client's status and conflicts with other data?

Strategy: Think about what other vital sign changes occur with a significant temperature elevation.

Needed Info: Vitals in normal range: pulse 82 beats/minute, respirations 14 breaths/minute, BP 134/88 (slightly elevated likely due to age). Temperature significantly elevated: should result in a more rapid pulse rate and an increased respiratory rate due to increased cellular metabolism. Validation of the temperature reading with another thermometer is required to determine the accuracy of the initial temperature reading.

Category: Planning/Physiological Integrity/Physiological Adaptation

(1) Notify primary health care provider immediately—the LPN/LVN should take responsibility for gathering additional data before calling the physician

(2) Proceed with the client's care—a temperature elevation to 103.6° F (39.7° C) is abnormal

(3) Record vital signs in medical record—the LPN/LVN should ensure the accuracy of reading before documenting them in a legal document

(4) Retake the temperature with a different thermometer—CORRECT: a temperature of 103.6° F (39.7° C) is abnormal without a corresponding increase in pulse and respiratory rate, the thermometer may be defective

48. The answer is 1

The LPN/LVN is helping an unlicensed assistive personnel (UAP) provide a bed bath to a comatose client who is incontinent. The LPN/LVN should intervene if which of the following actions is noted?

Reworded Question: What is an incorrect action?

Strategy: "Should intervene" indicates that you are looking for something wrong.

Needed Info: Standard precautions used with all clients: primary strategy for preventing exposure to blood or body fluids. Gloves are worn when exposure to blood, body fluids, secretions, excretions, or contaminated articles is likely; remove and discard promptly after use, and perform hand hygiene, before touching items and environmental surfaces to reduce the risk for pathogen transmission.

Category: Evaluation/Safe and Effective Care Environment/Safety and Infection Control

(1) The UAP answers the phone while wearing gloves—CORRECT: contaminated gloves should be removed and discarded, and then hand hygiene performed before answering the phone.
(2) The UAP log-rolls the client to provide back care—appropriate action, maintains proper body alignment
(3) The UAP places an incontinence pad under the client—appropriate for a client with incontinence
(4) The UAP positions the client on the left side, with the head of bed elevated—appropriate position to prevent aspiration and protect the client's airway

49. The answer is 3

A client is brought to the emergency department for treatment after being found on the floor by a family member. When comparing the legs, the LPN/LVN would most likely make which observation?

Reworded Question: What is a symptom of a hip fracture?

Strategy: Think about each answer choice.

Needed Info: Symptoms of fracture: swelling, pallor, ecchymosis; loss of sensation to other body parts; deformity; pain, acute tenderness, or both; muscle spasms; loss of function, abnormal mobility; crepitus (grating sound on movement); shortening of affected limb; decreased or absent pulses distal to injury; affected extremity colder than contralateral part. Emergency nursing care: immobilize joint above and below fracture using splints before moving client; in open fracture, cover the wound with sterile dressings or cleanest material available, control bleeding by direct pressure; check temperature, color, sensation, capillary refill time distal to fracture; in emergency department, manage pain.

Category: Data Collection/Physiological Integrity/Physiological Adaptation

(1) The client's left leg is longer than the right leg and externally rotated—affected leg shortens due to contraction of muscles attached above and below fracture site
(2) The client's left leg is shorter than the right leg and internally rotated—affected leg is usually externally rotated
(3) The client's left leg is shorter than the right leg and adducted—CORRECT: affected leg shortens due to contraction of muscles attached above and below fracture site, fragments overlap by 1–2 inches (2.5 to 5 cm)
(4) The client's left leg is longer than the right leg and is abducted—affected leg shortens and externally rotates

50. The answer is 3

The LPN/LVN is caring for a client with a cast on the left leg. The LPN/LVN would be **most** concerned if which is observed?

Reworded Question: What is a complication of a cast?

Strategy: "*Most* concerned" indicates a complication.

Needed Info: Immediate nursing care for plaster cast: Don't cover cast until dry (48 hours), handle with palms not fingertips; don't rest on hard surfaces; elevate affected limb above heart on soft surface until dry; don't use head lamp; check for blueness or paleness, pain, numbness, tingling (if present, elevate area; if it persists, contact primary health care provider); client should remain inactive while cast dries. Intermediate nursing care: mobilize client, isometric exercises; check for break in cast or foul odor; tell client not to scratch skin under cast and not to put anything underneath cast; if fiberglass cast gets wet, dry with hair dryer on cool setting. After-cast nursing care: Wash skin gently; have client gradually adjust to movement without support of cast; swelling is common, elevate limb.

Category: Data Collection/Physiological Integrity/Physiological Adaptation

(1) Capillary refill time is less than 3 seconds—capillary refill time is within normal limits

(2) Client reports discomfort and itching—a casted extremity may itch or feel uncomfortable due to prolonged immobility

(3) Client reports of tightness and pain—CORRECT: pain and tightness may develop if swelling occurs and the cast becomes too tight; if left untreated compartment syndrome may develop

(4) Client's foot is elevated on a pillow—newly casted extremity may be slightly elevated to help relieve edema; it should remain in correct anatomical position and below heart level to allow sufficient arterial perfusion

51. The answer is 2

The LPN/LVN is assisting with discharging a client from an inpatient alcohol treatment unit. Which statement by the client's wife indicates that the family is coping adaptively?

Reworded Question: What indicates that the client's family is coping with the client's alcoholism?

Strategy: Think about what each statement means.

Needed Info: Nursing care for alcohol use disorder: safety; monitor for withdrawal; reality orientation; increase self-esteem and coping skills; balanced diet; abstinence from alcohol; identify problems related to drinking in family relationships, work, etc.; help client to see/admit problem; confront denial with slow persistence; maintain relationship with client; establish control of problem drinking; provide support; Alcoholics Anonymous; disulfiram (Antabuse): drug used to maintain sobriety, based on behavioral therapy.

Category: Evaluation/Psychosocial Integrity

(1) "My husband will do well as long as I keep him engaged in activities that he likes."—wife is accepting responsibility; codependent behavior

(2) "My focus is learning how to live my life."—CORRECT: wife is working to change codependent patterns

(3) "I am so glad that our problems are behind us."—unrealistic; discharge is not the final step of treatment

(4) "I'll make sure that the children don't give my husband any problems."—wife is accepting responsibility; codependent behavior

52. The answer is 1

A client with a history of alcohol use disorder is transferred to the unit in an agitated state. The client is vomiting and diaphoretic, and states that it has been 5 hours since the last drink. The LPN/LVN would expect to administer which medication?

Reworded Question: What is the best medication to treat acute alcohol withdrawal?

Strategy: Think about the action of each drug.

Needed Info: Alcohol sedates the central nervous system (CNS); rebound during withdrawal. Early symptoms occur 4–6 hours after last drink. Symptoms: tremors; easily startled; insomnia; anxiety; anorexia; alcoholic hallucinosis (48 hours after last drink). Nursing care: administer sedation as needed, usually benzodiazepines; monitor vital signs, particularly pulse; institute seizure precautions; provide a quiet, well-lit environment; orient client frequently; don't leave hallucinating, confused client alone; administer anticonvulsants as needed, thiamine IV or IM, and IV dextrose.

Category: Planning/Psychosocial Integrity

(1) Chlordiazepoxide—CORRECT: antianxiety; used to treat symptoms of acute alcohol withdrawal; side effects (S/E): lethargy, hangover effect, agranulocytosis

(2) Disulfiram—used as a deterrent to compulsive drinking; contraindicated within 12 hours of alcohol consumption

(3) Methadone—opioid agonist; used to treat opioid withdrawal syndrome; S/E: respiratory depression, hyptension, dizziness, lightheadedness

(4) Naloxone—opioid antagonist used to reverse opioid-induced respiratory depression; S/E: ventricular fibrillation, seizures, pulmonary edema

53. The answer is 2

The LPN/LVN is caring for a client diagnosed with end-stage colon cancer. The spouse of the client says, "We have been married for so long. I am not sure how I can go on now." What is the **most** appropriate response by the LPN/LVN?

Reworded Question: What is the most therapeutic response to the spouse of the person diagnosed with terminal colon cancer?

Strategy: Remember therapeutic communication.

Needed Info: The client in this interaction is the spouse of the client diagnosed with end-stage colon cancer; focus on the present; encourage verbalization of feelings; provide support.

Category: Implementation/Psychosocial Integrity

(1) "It sounds like your children will be there to help during your time of grieving."—dismisses client's concern; keep focus on client

(2) "I know this is difficult. Tell me more about what you are feeling now."—CORRECT: acknowledges client's feelings; allows client to express feelings

(3) "Think about the pain and suffering your spouse has endured lately."—gives advice; discourages verbalization

(4) "I will call the hospice nurse to discuss to your spouse's condition with you." —passes responsibility to the hospice nurse; instead the LPN/LVN should encourage the spouse to express feelings

54. The answer is 2

The LPN/LVN is reinforcing teaching with an elderly client about how to use a standard aluminum walker. Which behavior by the client indicates that the reinforcement of teaching was effective?

Reworded Question: What is the correct technique when ambulating with a walker?

Strategy: Determine the outcome of each answer choice.

Needed Info: Elbows flexed at 20- to 30-degree angle when standing with hands on grips. Lift and move walker forward 8–10 inches (20–25 cm). With partial or non-weight-bearing, put weight on wrists and arms and step forward with affected leg, supporting self on arms, and follow with good leg. Nurse should stand behind client, hold onto gait belt at waist as needed for balance. Sit down by grasping armrest on affected side, shift weight to good leg and hand, lower self into chair. Client should wear sturdy shoes.

Category: Evaluation/Physiological Integrity/Basic Care and Comfort

(1) The client slowly pushes the walker forward 12 inches (30 cm), then takes small steps forward while leaning on the walker—should not push the walker

(2) The client lifts the walker, moves it forward 10 inches (25 cm), and then takes several small steps forward—CORRECT: the client should pick up the walker, and then place it down on all legs

(3) The client supports weight on the walker while advancing it forward, then takes small steps while balancing on the walker—the client should not support weight on walker while trying to move it

(4) The client slides the walker 18 inches (46 cm) forward, then takes small steps while holding onto the walker for balance—client should pick up the walker, not slide it forward

55. The answer is 2

The LPN/LVN would expect which client to be able to sign a consent form for nonemergent medical treatment?

Reworded Question: Which of these clients can give consent for own medical treatment?

Strategy: Think about the requirements for informed consent in nonemergent medical situations.

Needed Info: Clients requiring consent by an agent: under 18 years of age unless emancipated, declared legally incompetent, under the influence of drugs or alcohol, unable to understand or respond to information. In emergency situations: assumption that clients would want to be treated.

Category: Planning/Safe and Effective Care Environment/Coordinated Care

(1) A school-age child with a right tibia and fibula fracture—this client requires the consent of the legal guardian in this nonemergent situation

(2) A client requiring surgery for acute appendicitis—CORRECT: this client can provide own informed consent

(3) A client who is confused after a motor vehicle accident —informed consent would be required from designate health care agent in this nonemergent situation

(4) A client who has been legally declared incompetent—consent is required from the designate health care agent in this nonemergent situation

56. The answer is 3

An LPN/LVN is assisting with the discharge of a client with a diagnosis of hepatitis of unknown etiology. The LPN/LVN knows that teaching has been successful if the client makes which statement?

Reworded Question: What is a correct statement about hepatitis?

Strategy: Determine the outcome of each statement.

Needed Info: Hepatitis A (HAV): high-risk groups include young children, residents of institutions for custodial care, international travelers; transmission by fecal/oral route, poor sanitation; nursing considerations include prevention, improved sanitation, treat with gammaglobulin early postexposure, no preparation of food. Hepatitis B (HBV): high-risk groups include drug addicts, fetuses from infected mothers, homosexually active men, transfusions, health care workers; transmission by parenteral, sexual contact, blood/body fluids; nursing considerations include hepatitis vaccine, immune globulin (HBIG) postexposure, chronic carriers (potential for chronicity 5–10%). Hepatitis C (HVC): high-risk groups include transfusions, international travelers; transmission by blood or body fluids. Delta hepatitis: high-risk groups same as for HBV; transmission coinfects with HBV, transmitted through close personal contact.

Category: Evaluation/Physiological Integrity/Reduction of Risk Potential

(1) "I am so sad that I am not able to hold my baby."—hepatitis not spread by casual contact

(2) "I will eat my meal after my family finishes eating."—client can eat with family; cannot share eating utensils

(3) "I will make sure that my children don't use my eating utensils—CORRECT: to avoid hepatitis transmission, the client should not share eating utensils or drinking glasses, and should wash hands before eating and after using the toilet

(4) "I'm glad that I don't have to get help taking care of my children."—need to alternate rest and activity to promote hepatic healing; caregivers of young children will need help

57. The answer is 2

The LPN/LVN checks the IV flow rate for a postoperative client. The client is to receive 3,000 mL of lactated Ringer's lactate solution IV infused over 24 hours. The IV administration set has a drop factor of 10 drops per milliliter. The LPN/LVN would expect the client's IV to infuse at how many drops per minute?

Reworded Question: What is the IV flow rate?

Strategy: Remember the formula to calculate IV flow rate: total volume × drop factor divided by the time in minutes.

Needed Info: Lactated Ringer's: electrolyte solution used to expand extracellular fluid volume, and reduce blood viscosity.

Category: Implementation/Physiological Integrity/Pharmacological Therapies

(1) 18—incorrect

(2) 21—CORRECT: $(3{,}000 \times 10)$ divided by (24×60) = 30,000 divided by 1,440 = 20.8 = 21

(3) 35—incorrect

(4) 40—incorrect

58. The answer is 1

A client diagnosed with emphysema becomes restless and confused. Which action should the LPN/LVN take next?

Reworded Question: What should the LPN/LVN do to raise the oxygen levels of a client with emphysema?

Strategy: Determine the outcome of each answer choice.

Needed Info: Emphysema: overinflation of alveoli resulting in destruction of alveoli walls; predisposing factors include smoking, chronic infections, environmental pollution. Teaching includes breathing exercises; stop smoking; avoid hot and cold air or allergens; instructions regarding medications; avoid crowds or close contact with persons who have colds or influenza; adequate rest and nutrition; oral hygiene; influenza vaccines; observe sputum for indications of infection.

Category: Implementation/Physiological Integrity/ Reduction of Risk Potential

(1) Encourage pursed-lip breathing—CORRECT: purse-lipped breathing helps the client control the rate and depth of breathing

(2) Measure the client's temperature—confusion is probably due to decreased oxygenation

(3) Assess the client's potassium level—confusion is most likely caused by poor oxygenation, not electrolyte imbalance

(4) Increase the client's oxygen flow rate to 5 L/ minute—should receive low flow oxygen to prevent carbon dioxide narcosis

59. The answer is 4

The LPN/LVN is caring for a client following cataract surgery on the right eye. The client reports severe eye pain in the right eye. Which action should the LPN/ LVN take **first**?

Reworded Question: Is pain after cataract surgery normal?

Strategy: Remember what you know about cataract removal.

Needed Info: Cataract: change in the transparency of crystalline lens of eye. Causes: aging, trauma, congenital, systemic disease. S/S: blurred vision, decrease in color perception, photophobia. Treated by removal of lens under local anesthesia with sedation. Intraocular lens implantation, eyeglasses, or contact lenses after surgery. Complications: glaucoma, infection, bleeding, retinal detachment.

Category: Planning/Physiological Integrity/Reduction of Risk Potential

(1) Administer an analgesic to the client—mild discomfort treated with analgesics

(2) Recheck the client's condition in 30 minutes— action should be taken immediately

(3) Document finding in client's medical record— action should be taken immediately

(4) Report the finding to the supervising RN— CORRECT: ruptured blood vessel or suture causing hemorrhage or increased intraocular pressure; notify primary health care provider for restlessness, increased pulse rate, drainage on dressing

60. The answer is 4

The LPN/LVN is caring for a client 4 hours after intra-cranial surgery. Which action should the LPN/LVN take immediately?

Reworded Question: What is a priority after intracra-nial surgery?

Strategy: Determine the outcome of each answer choice.

Needed Info: Monitor vital signs hourly. Elevate head 30 to 45 degrees (as ordered) to promote venous return from brain, and prevent increased intracranial pressure (ICP). Avoid neck flexion and head rotation. Reduce environmental stimuli. Prevent the Valsalva maneuver by teaching the client to exhale when turning or moving in bed. Administer stool softeners. Restrict fluids to 1,200–1,500 mL/day. Administer medications: an osmotic diuretic, corticosteroid and anticonvulsant.

Category: Implementation/Physiological Integrity/ Reduction of Risk Potential

(1) Instruct the client to deep breathe, cough, and expectorate into a tissue—coughing should be avoided because it increases ICP

(2) Position the client in a left lateral position with neck flexed—the head should be maintained in a neutral position to promote venous return and reduce risk for increased ICP

(3) Perform passive range-of-motion exercises every two hours—position changes required during range-of-motion exercises can increase ICP

(4) Use a turning sheet under the client's head to midthigh to reposition in bed—CORRECT: using a turning sheet under the client's head to midthigh helps move the client as a unit maintaining body alignment, and reducing the risk for increased ICP

61. See explanation for answers

Client is a 43-year-old primigravida at 34 weeks gestation with mild pre-eclampsia. Client presented for a routine obstetric appointment today and reported daily headaches unresolved with the use of acetaminophen. Evaluation by provider revealed a BP of 158/92, a weight gain of 12 lb (5.4 kg) since previous office visit 2 weeks prior with 2+ pretibial edema. Reflexes 2+ without clonus. Urine sample evaluated in provider's office revealed 2+ protein via dipstick. Client admits to intermittent use of cocaine, smoking 5–6 cigarettes daily and consuming 3–4 servings of decaffeinated soda daily throughout pregnancy. Remainder of past medical history and obstetric history are unremarkable.

CORRECT OPTIONS: Risk factors for chromosomal abnormalities, as well as pathophysiological pregnancy challenges, are statistically increased in **women aged** >35. A diagnosis of **pre-eclampsia** increases the risk of maternal morbidity and adverse fetal outcomes. The client is demonstrating signs and symptoms of worsening pre-eclampsia with **daily headaches, elevated blood pressure, peripheral edema**, and **proteinuria**. Use of stimulants such as **cocaine** during pregnancy increases the risk for severe adverse effects for both the mother and fetus. **Smoking** during pregnancy also increases the risk of health problems for developing fetuses and increases the risk of sudden infant death syndrome (SIDS).

INCORRECT OPTIONS: Reflexes are within normal limits. Consumption of non-nutritive, sugar-laden beverages during pregnancy is not recommended but is less concerning if the beverages are decaffeinated.

62. The answer is 1, 3, 4, 5, 7, and 8

CORRECT OPTIONS: Historical factors of cigarette and cocaine use, as well as maternal age >35, are statistically documented risks for the development of numerous complications, including **low birth weight, placental abruption, preterm birth, birth defects, stillbirth,** and **placenta previa**.

INCORRECT OPTIONS: There is no indication the client is at risk for gestational diabetes. The client's lab work does not demonstrate an elevated blood glucose. There is no indication the client is obese nor is there mention of a medical history or family history of diabetes mellitus. Hyperemesis gravidarum refers to a complication of early pregnancy in which severe, persistent nausea, vomiting, and weight loss occur during pregnancy.

63. See explanation for answers

CORRECT OPTIONS: The LPN/LVN recognizes that the client is most likely experiencing a **placental abruption**. The client may or may not have vaginal bleeding with an abruption, may have **blood-tinged amniotic fluid**, or may have a large amount of vaginal bleeding, depending on where the abruption occurs. **Sudden abdominal/back pain** and uterine tenderness are also consistent with placental abruption.

INCORRECT OPTIONS: Placenta previa is the abnormal implantation of the placenta in the lower uterine segment. The location of the placenta causes painless vaginal bleeding when the cervix dilates or the lower uterine segment effaces. Placenta accreta is unusual adherence of the placenta, penetrating slightly into the myometrium. The sudden increase in blood pressure and the spontaneous rupture of membranes are not evidence of a placental abruption but may exacerbate the abruption. Intermittent late decelerations and a dropping FHR indicate poor perfusion to the fetus but are not of themselves evidence of placental abruption.

64. See explanation for answers

CORRECT OPTIONS: **Discontinuing the IV oxytocin** infusion diminishes uterine contractility, which potentiates the abruption process. **Applying oxygen by mask** and **positioning the client on the left side** enhances fetoplacental perfusion.

INCORRECT OPTIONS: Increasing the magnesium infusion, with its smooth muscle relaxant effect, would be used to suppress preterm labor. Increasing this medication, as well as discontinuation of the primary IV, will have little to no effect on the incidence or progression of the placental abruption. Insertion of an indwelling urinary catheter and the application of antiembolism stockings are standard cesarean birth preoperative care; however, they do not take precedence over the need for supplemental oxygen in this situation. Positioning the client in the Trendelenburg or semi-Fowler position does not directly enhance needed fetoplacental perfusion at this time.

65. The answer is 2

CORRECT OPTION: It is within the scope of practice for the LPN/LVN to **insert a urinary catheter** in order to prepare the client for an emergency cesarean birth.

INCORRECT OPTIONS: The RN will notify the blood bank that blood will likely be needed for the client. The physician will explain the situation and need for the procedure to the client's family. The RN should contact the NICU to provide needed information and the status of the client and fetus.

66. See explanation for answers

Improved: **Blood pressure, pulse, respirations**, and **uric acid** are all improved as a result of placental separation as the placenta is the root cause of pre-eclampsia. **Headache** likely improved due to decreased blood pressure and improved central nervous system irritability, again related to placental separation.

Declined: **Hematocrit** and **platelet count** have declined further following the cesarean birth. This is related to the likely accompanying blood loss of the placental abruption and resulting coagulation cascade. Hemodilution from fluid volume replacement can also impact the hematocrit at this time.

67. The answer is 2

A pediatric client with a congenital heart disorder is admitted with heart failure. Digoxin 0.12 mg by mouth daily is ordered for the client. The bottle contains 0.05 mg of digoxin in 1 mL of solution. Which amount should the LPN/LVN administer to the client after validating the dose with the RN?

Reworded Question: How much of the medication should you give?

Strategy: Remember how to calculate dosages. Be careful and don't make math errors.

Needed Info: Formula: dose on hand over 1 mL = dose desired.

Category: Implementation/Physiological Integrity/Pharmacological Therapies

(1) 1.2 mL—inaccurate

(2) 2.4 mL—CORRECT: $0.05 \text{ mg}/1 \text{ mL} = 0.12 \text{mg}/x$ mL, $0.05x = 0.12$, $x = 2.4$ mL

(3) 3.5 mL—inaccurate

(4) 4.2 mL—inaccurate

68. The answer is 4

The LPN/LVN is caring for a client diagnosed with chronic lymphocytic leukemia, hospitalized for treatment of hemolytic anemia. The LPN/LVN should expect to implement which action?

Reworded Question: What should you do for a client with anemia?

Strategy: Although the client has leukemia, they are admitted with anemia. You must focus on the anemia.

Needed Info: Lymphocytic leukemia: characterized by proliferation of lymphocytes. S/S: fatigue, weakness, hemolytic anemia, easy bruising, bleeding gums, epistaxis, fever, generalized pain. Diagnostic tests: CBC, bone marrow aspiration, lumbar puncture, x-rays, lymph node biopsy. Treatment: total body irradiation or radiation to spleen, chemotherapy. Nursing responsibilities: low-bacteria diet (no raw fruits or vegetables), institute bleeding precautions (soft toothbrush, don't floss, no injections, no aspirin, pad bed rails, use air mattress, use paper tape), antiemetics, comfort measures. Hemolytic anemia S/S: jaundice, splenomegaly, hepatomegaly, fatigue, weakness. Treatment: O_2, blood transfusions, corticosteroids.

Category: Planning/Physiological Integrity/Physiological Adaptation

(1) Encourage activities with other clients in the day room—does not meet need for rest

(2) Isolate the client from visitors and clients to avoid infection—no information given about white blood cell count; protective isolation for neutrophil count less than 500/mm³

(3) Provide a diet that contains foods that are high in vitamin C—needed for wound healing and resistance to infection; not best choice

(4) Maintain a quiet environment to promote adequate rest—CORRECT: primary problem activity intolerance due to fatigue

69. The answer is 3

The LPN/LVN is caring for a client with cervical cancer. The LPN/LVN notes that the radium implant has become dislodged. Which action should the LPN/LVN take **first**?

Reworded Question: What is the best action when a radium implant becomes dislodged?

Strategy: Think about the outcome of each answer choice.

Needed Info: Limit radioactive exposure: assign client to private room; place "Caution: Radioactive Material" sign on door; wear dosimeter film badge at all times when interacting with client (measures amount of exposure); do not assign pregnant health care worker to client; rotate staff caring for client; organize tasks so limited time is spent in client's room; limit visitors; encourage client to do own care; provide shield in room. Client care: use antiemetics for nausea; consider body image; provide comfort measures; provide good nutrition.

Category: Implementation/Physiological Integrity/
Reduction of Risk Potential

(1) Grasp the implant with a sterile hemostat and carefully reinsert it into the client—the implant should be picked up with long-handled forceps, not a hemostat, and deposited into a lead container in the room, not reinserted into the client

(2) Wrap the implant in a blanket and place it behind a lead shield until reimplantation—the implant should be picked up with long-handled forceps and put into a lead container in the room for disposal

(3) Ensure the implant is picked up with long-handled forceps and placed in a lead container—CORRECT: the priority is to secure the implant to prevent unwanted and dangerous radiation exposure; the implant should be picked up with long-handled forceps and then placed in a lead container; this equipment should be kept in the room of any client receiving this therapy so that it is readily available; institutional guidelines and procedures for managing dislodgement should be followed; radiology is usually involved as soon as dislodgement occurs

(4) Obtain a dosimeter reading on the client and report it to the primary health care provider—need to place implant in lead container

70. The answer is 2

The LPN/LVN comes to the home of a client with cellulitis of the left leg to perform a daily dressing change. The client tells the LPN/LVN that the unlicensed assistive personnel (UAP) changed the dressing earlier that morning. Which action by the LPN/LVN is **best**?

Reworded Question: What is the correct chain of command for reporting a problem?

Strategy: Think about the chain of command.

Category: Implementation/Safe and Effective Care Environment/Coordinated Care

(1) Tell the client that the new dressing looks fine—does not address the problem of the UAP performing the dressing change

(2) Notify the RN supervisor of the situation—CORRECT: correctly follow the chain of command for reporting this problem

(3) Ask the client to describe the dressing change—does not address the problem of the UAP performing the dressing change

(4) Report the UAP to the home care agency—incorrect chain of command; should report problem to next person in direct line of authority in same area

71. The answer is 1

The LPN/LVN is caring for a client with pernicious anemia. The LPN/LVN reinforces teaching about the plan of care. The LPN/LVN should report which statement to the RN?

Reworded Question: What is true about pernicious anemia?

Strategy: Determine the outcome of each answer choice.

Needed Info: Pernicious anemia is caused by failure to absorb vitamin B_{12} because of a deficiency of intrinsic factor from the gastric mucosa. Symptoms: pallor, slight jaundice, glossitis, fatigue, weight loss, paresthesias of hands and feet, disturbances of balance and gait. Treatment: vitamin B_{12} IM monthly.

Category: Evaluation/Physiological Integrity/
Physiological Adaptation

(1) "In order to get better, I will take iron pills."—CORRECT: pernicious anemia is due to vitamin B deficiency, not iron deficiency

(2) "I will attend smoking cessation classes."—no reason to report

(3) "I will learn how to perform IM injections."—many clients instructed how to give monthly IM B_{12} injection

(4) "I will make sure to eat a well-balanced diet."—no reason to report

72. The answer is 2

The LPN/LVN is caring for clients on a general medical/surgical unit of an acute care facility. Four clients have been admitted in the last 20 minutes. Which admission should the LPN/LVN see **first**?

Reworded Question: Who is the priority client?

Strategy: Think ABCs.

Needed Info: Factors to consider: chief complaint; age of client; medical history; potential for life-threatening event.

Category: Planning/Physiological Integrity/Reduction of Risk Potential

(1) A client reporting vomiting and diarrhea—airway issue takes priority

(2) A client with third-degree burns to face—CORRECT: face, neck, chest, or abdominal burns can cause severe edema that restricts the airway; airway issues take priority

(3) A client with a fractured left hip—airway issue takes priority

(4) A client reporting epigastric pain—airway issue takes priority

73. The answer is 4

The LPN/LVN is caring for a client with a diagnosis of chronic bronchitis. The client has audible wheezing, and an oxygen saturation of 85%. Four hours ago, the oxygen saturation was 88%. It is **most** important for the LPN/LVN to take which action?

Reworded Question: What is the best action for a client with COPD?

Strategy: Determine the outcome of each answer choice.

Needed Info: Chronic bronchitis: predisposing factors include smoking, chronic infections, environmental pollution. Teaching reinforcement includes breathing exercises; stop smoking; avoid hot and cold air or allergens; instructions regarding medications; avoid crowds or close contact with persons who have colds or influenza; adequate rest and nutrition; oral hygiene;

influenza vaccines; observe sputum for indications of infection.

Category: Implementation/Physiological Integrity/Pharmacological Therapies

(1) Give beclomethasone, 2 puffs via metered-dose inhaler—administer brochodilator first to open passageways

(2) Auscultate the client's bilateral breath sounds—situation does not require further data collection

(3) Increase oxygen flow rate to 4L/minute via mask—increasing the client's blood oxygen level may cause respiratory depression

(4) Administer albuterol, 2 puffs via metered-dose inhaler—CORRECT: a brochodilator, such as albuterol relaxes bronchial smooth muscles and increases airflow to the lungs.

74. The answer is 4

The LPN/LVN is caring for a client hospitalized for observation following a fall. The client states, "My friend fell last year, and no one thought anything was wrong. She died 2 days later!" Which response by the LPN/LVN is **best**?

Reworded Question: What is the most therapeutic response?

Strategy: Remember therapeutic communication.

Needed Info: Therapeutic communication: using silence (allows client time to think and reflect; conveys acceptance; allows client to take lead in conversation); using general leads or broad openings (encourages client to talk, indicates interest in client); clarification (encourages description of feelings and details of particular experience; makes sure LPN/LVN understands client); reflecting (paraphrases what client says; reflects what client says, especially feelings conveyed).

Category: Implementation/Psychosocial Integrity

(1) "This happens to quite a few people."—nontherapeutic; doesn't address client's concerns

(2) "We are monitoring you, so you'll be okay."—
nontherapeutic; "don't worry" response

(3) "Don't you think I'm taking good care of you?"—
nontherapeutic; focus is on the LPN/LVN

(4) "You're concerned that it might happen to you?"—
CORRECT: reflects client's feelings

75. The answer is 2

The LPN/LVN is caring for clients on the pediatric unit. A client with second- and third-degree burns on the right thigh is being admitted. The LPN/LVN should expect the new client to be placed with which roommate?

Reworded Question: Who is the appropriate roommate for a client with burns?

Strategy: Think about the transmission of diseases.

Needed Info: Burns: increase the risk for infection; contact precautions to prevent spread of pathogens transmitted by direct contact or contact with items in the client's environment, such organisms as *Clostridium difficile* and methicillin-resistant *Staphyococcus aureus*; airborne and contact precautions required until chickenpox lesions become dry and crusted.

Category: Implementation/Physiological Integrity/Physiological Adaptation

(1) A client with chickenpox—infectious disease requires airborne and contact precautions

(2) A client with asthma—CORRECT: lowest risk of cross-contamination because client is not infectious

(3) A client who developed acute diarrhea after antibiotic—requires contact precautions because the client may have *Clostridium difficile* diarrhea

(4) A client with methicillin-resistant *Staphylococcus aureus*—resistant organism requires contact precautions

76. The answer is 2

The LPN/LVN is performing chest physiotherapy on a client with chronic airflow limitations (CAL). Which action should the nurse take **first**?

Reworded Question: What should the LPN/LVN do prior to beginning chest physiotherapy?

Strategy: Determine whether to collect data or implement.

Needed Info: Postural drainage: uses gravity to facilitate removal of bronchial secretions; client is placed in a variety of positions to facilitate drainage into larger airways; secretions may be removed by coughing or suctioning. Percussion and vibration: augments the effect of gravity during postural drainage; percussion: rhythmic striking of chest wall with cupped hands over areas where secretions are retained; vibration: hand and arm muscles of person doing vibration are tensed, and a vibrating pressure is applied to chest as client exhales.

Category: Data Collection/Physiological Integrity/Reduction of Risk Potential

(1) Perform chest physiotherapy prior to meals—prevents nausea, vomiting, aspiration

(2) Auscultate breath sounds before the procedure—CORRECT: helps identify areas of the lung that require drainage; auscultate breath sounds after the procedure to determine effectiveness

(3) Administer bronchodilators after the procedure—given before chest physiotherapy to dilate the bronchioles and to liquify secretions

(4) Percuss each lobe prior to asking the client to cough—may cause fractures of the ribs; percussion helps loosen thick secretions

77. The answer is 2

In which situation would it be **most** appropriate for the LPN/LVN to wear a gown and gloves?

Reworded Question: Which of these clients poses the greatest risk for spreading disease, requiring the use of gloves and a gown?

Strategy: Note how microorganisms are most frequently spread.

Needed Info: Spread of microorganisms: contact directly with a source of infection, contact with surfaces contaminated with microorganisms, some airborne diseases, includes all bodily waste and fluids except sweat. Standard precautions: Centers for Disease Control and Prevention (CDC) recommends barrier techniques to prevent spread of microorganisms; common barriers include gloves, masks, goggles, and gowns; choose appropriate barrier for the situation.

Category: Implementation/Safe and Effective Care Environment/Safety and Infection Control

(1) Administering oral medications to a client with with human immunodeficiency virus disease—there is no contact with blood or other potentially infectious body fluids

(2) Assisting in the care of a motor vehicle accident victim who continues to bleed—CORRECT: blood from this client may contact the LPN/LVN's skin when performing care or gathering data; gloves protect hands and gowns protect the skin from exposure to blood and body fluids

(3) Bathing a client with an abdominal wound infection—gloves provide adequate protection

(4) Changing the linen of a client with sickle-cell anemia—if bed is soiled, gloves should provide adequate protection; linen should not be in contact with the LPN/LVN's uniform

78. The answer is 2

A client is receiving 1,000 mL of 5% dextrose in half normal saline solution IV to infuse over 8 hours. The IV administration set tubing delivers 15 drops per milliliter. The LPN/LVN should expect the flow rate to be how many drops per minute?

Reworded Question: What is the correct IV flow rate?

Strategy: Use the correct formula and be careful not to make math errors.

Needed Info: Formula: total volume × drip factor divided by the total time in minutes.

Category: Planning/Physiological Integrity/Pharmacological Therapies

(1) 15—incorrect

(2) 31—CORRECT: $(1{,}000 \times 15)$ divided by (8×60)

(3) 45—incorrect

(4) 60—incorrect

79. The answer is 3

A client is admitted to the hospital reporting seizures and a high fever. A positron emission tomography (PET) brain scan is prescribed. Before the PET brain scan, the client asks the LPN/LVN what position is necessary for the test. Which statement by the LPN/LVN is **most** accurate?

Reworded Question: What is the proper position for a PET brain scan?

Strategy: Visualize the procedure.

Needed Info: PET brain scan: measures amount of uptake by the brain of radioactive isotopes. Damaged tissue absorbs more than normal tissue. Nursing care before: withhold medicationss (antihypertensives, vasoconstrictors, vasodilators for 24 hours). Test is painless. After test, force fluids to promote excretion of isotopes. Urine doesn't need special handling.

Category: Implementation/Physiological Integrity/Reduction of Risk Potential

(1) "You will be in a side-lying position, with the foot of the bed elevated."—incorrect

(2) "You will be in a semi-upright sitting position, with your knees flexed."—incorrect

(3) "You will be lying on your back with a small pillow under your head."—CORRECT

(4) "You will be flat on your back, with your feet higher than your head"—incorrect

80. The answer is 3

A client is to receive 3,000 mL of normal saline solution IV to infuse over 24 hours. The IV administration set delivers 15 drops per milliliter. The LPN/LVN would expect the flow rate to be how many drops of fluid per minute?

Reworded Question: What should the IV flow rate be?

Strategy: Use the formula and avoid making math errors.

Needed Info: Total volume × the drop factor divided by the total time in minutes

Category: Planning/Physiological Integrity/Pharmacological Therapies

(1) 21—inaccurate

(2) 28—inaccurate

(3) 31—CORRECT: (3,000 × 15) divided by (24 × 60)

(4) 42—inaccurate

81. The answer is 4

The LPN/LVN is caring for a client diagnosed with asthma. The primary health care provider prescribes neostigmine IM. Which action by the LPN/LVN is **most** appropriate?

Reworded Question: Can neostigmine be administered to a client with asthma?

Strategy: "*Most* appropriate" indicates that discrimination is required to answer the question.

Needed Info: Neostigmine: parasympathomimetic used to treat myasthenia gravis and as an antidote for nondepolarizing neuromuscular blocking agents; potentiates the action of morphine; side effects include nausea, vomiting, abdominal cramps, respiratory depression, bronchoconstriction, hypotension, and bradycardia; nursing considerations include monitor vital signs frequently, have atropine injection available, take with milk.

Category: Evaluation/Physiological Integrity/Reduction of Risk Potential

(1) Administer the medication, as prescribed—causes bronchoconstriction; notify the primary health care provider

(2) Obtain the client's blood pressure and pulse—data collection; neostigmine causes hypotension and bradycardia; important to monitor vital signs, but priority is to notify the supervising RN or primary health care provider because medication can precipitate an acute exacerbation of asthma

(3) Ask pharmacist if the medication can be given orally—medication used cautiously for clients with asthma

(4) Notify the primary health care provider—CORRECT: cholinergics can cause bronchoconstriction in asthmatic clients; may precipitate an acute exacerbation of asthma

82. The answer is 4

The LPN/LVN is caring for a client with a history of Addison disease who has received steroid therapy for several years. The LPN/LVN would expect the client to exhibit which change in appearance?

Reworded Question: What changes are seen in a client after taking steroids long-term?

Strategy: All the options in an answer choice must be correct for the option to be right.

Needed Info: Medications: cortisone and hydrocortisone usually given in divided doses: 2/3 in morning and 1/3 in late afternoon with food to decrease GI irritation. Reinforce teaching to report S/S of excessive drug therapy (rapid weight gain, round face, fluid retention).

Category: Data Collection/Physiological Integrity/Physiological Adaptation

(1) Buffalo hump, girdle-obesity, gaunt facial appearance—buffalo hump and girdle-obesity true with long-term steroid use; gaunt face seen with lack of steroids

(2) Skin tanning, mucous membrane discoloration, weight loss—tanning and weight loss seen with lack of steroids; mucous membrane discoloration not seen

(3) Emaciation, nervousness, breast engorgement, hirsutism—nothing to do with steroids; hirsutism: excessive growth of hair

(4) Truncal obesity, purple striations on the skin, moon face—CORRECT: effects of excess glucocorticoids

83. The answer is 1

The LPN/LVN is caring for a client with a history of pancreatic cancer who appears jaundiced. The LPN/LVN should give the **highest** priority to which need?

Reworded Question: What is the highest priority for a client with pancreatic cancer?

Strategy: Remember Maslow.

Needed Info: Medical treatment: high-calorie, bland, low-fat diet; small, frequent meals; avoid alcohol; anticholinergics; antineoplastic chemotherapy

Category: Planning/Physiological Integrity/Reduction of Risk Potential

(1) Nutrition—CORRECT: profound weight loss and anorexia occur with pancreatic cancer

(2) Self-image—a client who appears jaundiced may be concerned about personal appearance, but physiological needs take priority

(3) Skin integrity—jaundice causes dry skin and pruritis; scratching can lead to skin breakdown

(4) Urinary elimination—obstructive process caused by pancreatic cancer darkens urine; kidney function is not affected

84. The answer is 4

The client diagnosed with anorexia nervosa is admitted to the hospital. Which statement by the client requires immediate follow-up by the LPN/LVN?

Reworded Question: Which problem has the highest priority for this client?

Strategy: Remember Maslow's hierarchy of needs.

Needed Info: Anorexia nervosa: a disorder characterized by restrictive eating resulting in emaciation, disturbance in body image, and an intense fear of being obese. Physical needs must be met first to maintain the client in stable condition. Adequate fluid and electrolyte balance are difficult to maintain.

Category: Planning/Psychosocial Integrity

(1) "My gums bled this morning."—vitamin deficiencies may cause bleeding gums, but not the highest priority

(2) "I'm getting fatter every day."—body image disturbance occurs in clients diagnosed with anorexia nervosa, but such psychosocial needs do not take priority

(3) "Nobody likes me, I'm so ugly."—chronic low self-esteem commonly occurs with anorexia nervosa; this psychosocial need does not take priority

(4) "I'm feel dizzy and weak today."—CORRECT: fluid volume deficit takes highest priority; dehydration, a common occurrence with anorexia nervosa, could lead to irreversible kidney damage and vital sign instability

85. The answer is 4

A client is admitted to the hospital for treatment of *Pneumocystis jiroveci* pneumonia and Kaposi's sarcoma. The client informs the LPN/LVN about a personal decision to become an organ donor. Which response by the LPN/LVN is **best**?

Reworded Question: Can this client be an organ donor?

Strategy: Think about each answer choice.

Needed Info: Criteria for organ and tissue donation: no history of significant disease process in organ or tissue to be donated; no untreated sepsis; brain death of donor; no history of extracranial malignancy; relative hemodynamic stability; blood group compatibility; newborn donors must be full-term (more than 200 g); only absolute restriction to organ donation is documented case of human immunodeficiency virus (HIV) disease. Family members can give consent. Nurse can discuss organ donation with other death-related topics (funeral home to be used, autopsy request).

Category: Implementation/Physiological Integrity/Physiological Adaptation

(1) "What does your family think about your decision?"—client has the right to make the decision

(2) "You will help many people by donating your organs."—clients with documented HIV disease are prohibited from donating organs

(3) "Would you like to speak to the organ donor coordinator?"—passes responsibility for the discussion to the organ donor coordinator

(4) "Your illness prevents you from becoming an organ donor."—CORRECT: clients with documented HIV disease are prohibited from donating organs

86. The answer is 3

The LPN/LVN is caring for a client 2 days after a pancreatectomy for cancer of the pancreas. The LPN/LVN observes minimal drainage from the nasogastric (NG) tube. It is **most** important for the LPN/LVN to take which action?

Reworded Question: What is the best action when an NG tube is not draining?

Strategy: Determine whether it is appropriate to collect data or implement.

Needed Info: Insertion of NG sump: measure distance from tip of nose to earlobe, plus distance from earlobe to bottom of xyphoid process. Mark distance on tube with tape and lubricate end of tube. Insert tube through nose to stomach. Offer sips of water and advance tube gently; bend head forward. Observe for respiratory distress. Secure with hypoallergenic tape or securement device. Verify tube position initially and before feeding. Aspirate for gastric contents and check appearance and pH.

Category: Data Collection/Physiological Integrity/Basic Care and Comfort

(1) Notify primary health care provider—should collect data first

(2) Monitor vital signs every 15 minutes—does not address lack of drainage

(3) Check the NG tube for kinking—CORRECT: collect data prior to implementing; maintain tubing in a dependent position to promote drainage

(4) Replace the NG tube immediately—collect data before implementing

87. See explanation for answers

Potential Condition	
Aspiration.	✓

CORRECT OPTION: The LPN/LVN is most concerned that the client could **aspirate** due to dysphagia. The client has been placed on a pureed diet, but due to weakness or damage to the cranial nerves, which control the pharynx and larynx, the client is at high risk of aspirating when trying to swallow.

INCORRECT OPTIONS: There is a risk of malnutrition for a client having difficulty swallowing. However, the greater concern is that the client will aspirate while attempting to swallow. The client may need to receive supplemental nutrition in the initial period after a stroke until swallowing ability improves. Clients are also at high risk of developing depression following a stroke due to the many physical changes and challenges they face. Clients with dysphagia may also become dehydrated due to poor ability to spontaneously hydrate or issues with swallowing liquids. Neither depression nor dehydration are the most concerning potential conditions for this client.

Actions to Take	
Place the client upright in a chair to feed.	✓
Encourage the client to tuck the chin when swallowing.	✓

CORRECT OPTIONS: To decrease the risk of aspiration for the client with dysphagia, the LPN/LVN will **ensure the client is sitting up as high as possible, preferably in a chair**. The client should be instructed to **tuck the chin when swallowing** to help close the glottis and propel the food into the esophagus. Stroking the throat may also help with this.

INCORRECT OPTIONS: The LPN/LVN will not encourage the use of straws to drink fluids. The client has little control of a thin liquid when using a straw and may inhale the fluid into the lungs when sucking on the straw. The client can continue to have fluids but may need to add a thickener to them to assist with swallowing. The client will need to concentrate on eating and drinking. Distractions should be kept to a minimum. Food and fluids should be set up on the client's left for better visualization, and the client should be encouraged to use the unaffected side to hold any eating utensils.

Parameters to Monitor	
Lung sounds.	✓
Temperature.	✓

CORRECT OPTIONS: To determine whether the client is aspirating, the LPN/LVN will monitor the client's **lung sounds** and **temperature**. Gagging and choking are more obvious signs the client is aspirating. Gurgling, noisy respirations indicate liquid has entered the upper airway. The development of adventitious lung sounds indicates the client may have developed aspiration pneumonia. A fever of $100.4°F$ ($38°C$) or greater may develop within 2 hours of aspiration.

INCORRECT OPTIONS: Heart rate may elevate or the client may grimace or appear anxious when choking or in distress. However, clients may silently aspirate, with no outward indications of distress. A change in the level of consciousness would not be a consistent indicator of aspiration. Loss of consciousness with choking is an airway emergency.

88. The answer is 3

The LPN/LVN is planning to administer furosemide 20 mg PO to a client diagnosed with chronic kidney disease. The client asks the LPN/LVN the reason for receiving this medication. Which response by the LPN/LVN is **best**?

Reworded Question: Why is furosemide given to a client diagnosed with stage?

Strategy: Think about the action of furosemide.

Needed Info: Chronic kidney disease is progressive, irreversible kidney damage that can be caused by hypertension, diabetes mellitus, lupus erythematosus, or chronic glomerulonephritis; symptoms include anemia, acidosis, azotemia, fluid retention, and urinary output alterations; nursing care includes monitoring potassium levels, daily weight, intake and output, dietary teaching about regulating protein intake, fluid intake to balance fluid losses, and some restrictions of sodium and potassium.

Category: Implementation/Physiological Integrity/Reduction of Risk Potential

(1) "To increase the blood flow to your kidney."—Furosemide is a loop diuretic that inhibits sodium and chloride reabsorption at the proximal and distal tubules and the ascending loop of Henle

(2) "To decrease your circulating blood volume."—Furosemide used to treat fluid overload due to chronic kidney disease

(3) "To increase excretion of sodium and water."—CORRECT: nursing considerations when administering furosemide include monitoring blood pressure, measuring intake and output, monitoring potassium levels; don't give at hour of sleep

(4) "To decrease the workload on your heart."—correcting the fluid overload will decrease the workload on the heart, but the primary reason furosemide is given to clients diagnosed with chronic kidney disease is to augment the kidney's functioning

89. The answer is 3

The LPN/LVN is reinforcing discharge teaching for a client with chronic pancreatitis. Which statement by the client indicates that further teaching is necessary?

Reworded Question: What is an incorrect statement about pancreatitis?

Strategy: This is a negative question; you are looking for incorrect information.

Needed Info: Plan/implementation: nothing by mouth (NPO), gastric decompression. Medications: antacids, analgesics, antibiotics, anticholinergics. Maintain fluid/electrolyte balance. Monitor for signs of infection. Cough and deep-breathe; semi-Fowler position. Monitor for shock and hyperglycemia. Treatment of exocrine insufficiency: medications containing amylase, lipase, trypsin to aid digestion. Long-term: avoid alcohol; low-fat, bland diet; small, frequent meals. Monitor S/S of diabetes mellitus.

Category: Evaluation/Physiological Integrity/Reduction of Risk Potential

(1) "I do not have to restrict physical activity."—no specific restrictions on activity

(2) "I should take pancrelipase before meals."—pancreatic enzyme replacement should be taken before or with meals

(3) "I will eat three large meals every day."—CORRECT: small, frequent meals are most beneficial with chronic pancreatitis

(4) "I must not drink any alcoholic beverages."—chronic pancreatitis requires complete abstinence from alcohol

90. The answer is 3

After a laparoscopic cholecystectomy, the client reports abdominal pain and bloating. Which response by the LPN/LVN is **best**?

Reworded Question: What is the best intervention for a client reporting free air pain?

Strategy: "*Best*" indicates there may be more than one response that appears correct.

Needed Info: Cholecystectomy: removal of gallbladder. T-tube inserted to ensure drainage of bile from common bile duct until edema diminishes. Check amount of drainage (usually 500–1,000 mL/day, decreases as fluid begins to drain into duodenum). Protect skin around incision from bile drainage irritation (use zinc oxide or water-soluble lubricant). Keep drainage bag at same level as gallbladder. Maintain client in semi-Fowler position after T-tube removal; observe dressing for bile; notify primary health care provider for significant drainage. Evaluate pain to check for other problems. Monitor for signs of potassium and sodium loss; flattened or inverted T-waves on electrocardiogram; muscle weakness; abdominal distension; headache; apathy; nausea or vomiting; jaundice.

Category: Implementation/Physiological Integrity/Physiological Adaptation

(1) "Increase intake of fresh fruits and vegetables"—no indication of constipation

(2) "I'll give you the prescribed pain medication."—laparoscopic procedure requires less pain medication than open cholecystectomy

(3) "Why don't you take a walk down the hallway?"—CORRECT: carbon dioxide insufflated during laparoscopic surgery causes pain; ambulation increases absorption and decreases pain

(4) "You may need an indwelling urinary catheter."—carbon dioxide insufflated during laparoscopic surgery causes pain; an indwelling urinary catheter does not relieve associated pain

91. See explanation for answers

The LPN/LVN identifies client findings that are consistent with **anemia**, a decrease in the normal concentration of erythrocytes (RBCs) that transport oxygen. The client is exhibiting fatigue, dyspnea with exertion, pale skin, and increased radial pulses; these manifestations are consistent with the body's response to tissue hypoxia from decreased RBCs. Anemia can occur in clients receiving chemotherapy due to the myelosuppressive effects on bone marrow function. Fatigue can occur as a response to decreased oxygen in the tissues. INCORRECT OPTIONS: Leukopenia is a decrease in the overall white blood cell count, including granulocytes, monocytes, and lymphocytes. Pancytopenia occurs when all components of the complete blood count (i.e., white blood cells, red blood cells, platelets) are decreased. The client findings do not indicate leukopenia or pancytopenia.

Alternating activities with rest also allows for oxygen consumption that is needed for vital functions. INCORRECT OPTIONS: Providing examples of foods high in potassium is important when serum potassium levels are decreased; potassium concentration is not affected by the quality or quantity of RBCs. The client should engage in regular activity, but rest often. Complete bedrest is not necessary and may result in issues related to immobility.

The LPN/LVN anticipates that due to a low hemoglobin and hematocrit, the client may need **supplemental oxygen**. Cardiopulmonary symptoms of anemia may require oxygen therapy to maintain cardiac output and stabilize the client, especially if underlying cardiac disease is present. INCORRECT OPTIONS: Meticulous skin care and oral hygiene are appropriate for clients with weakened immune systems when protection from skin irritation and potential opportunistic infection from the client's normal flora is needed. Pernicious anemia is the most common type of cobalamin deficiency (vitamin B_{12}) that occurs in absence of intrinsic factor that is needed for absorption of vitamin B_{12}.

As anemia becomes more severe, an increase in cardiopulmonary symptoms can occur due to insufficient tissue perfusion. Signs and symptoms include **heart palpitations**, shortness of breath at rest, tachycardia, and chest pain. INCORRECT OPTIONS: The cause of the client's anemia is most likely due to the myelosuppressive effects of chemotherapy. Bleeding from mucosa surfaces (e.g., nose, gums) may occur when a reduction of platelets is present. An increased oral temperature may be a sign of infection in immunocompromised clients.

92. The answer is 3

The nursing team consists of an RN, an unlicensed assistive personnel (UAP), and an LPN/LVN. The PN/LVN would expect to be assigned to which client?

Reworded Question: What is a correct client assignment for an LPN/LVN?

Strategy: Think about each answer.

Needed Info: LPN/LVNs care for stable clients with predictable outcomes. Unlicensed assistive personnel (UAPs) perform standard, unchanging procedures.

Category: Implementation/Safe and Effective Care Environment/Coordinated Care

(1) A client scheduled for an MRI of the brain—requires assessment and teaching; should be cared for by RN

(2) An unconscious client who requires a bed bath—bed bath for an unconscious client can be assigned to the UAP

(3) A client in balanced suspension traction—CORRECT: LPN/LVN must care for client; collect data on client airway, adequate respirations, and circulatory status

(4) A client with diabetes who needs help bathing—UAP can assist with bath

93. The answer is 125

The primary health care provider orders 1 L dextrose 5% in half normal saline solution IV to infuse over 8 hours. The drip factor stated on the IV administration set tubing is 15 gtt/mL. How many milliliters should the LPN/LVN expect to be infused every hour?

Reworded Question: How much fluid needs to infuse every hour to infuse 1,000 mL in 8 hours?

Strategy: Think about the question being asked. Note that there is unnecessary information provided.

Needed Info: One liter is equal to 1,000 milliliters. Dividing the total amount of fluids to infuse by the number of hours in which the infusion should be completed equals hourly fluid amounts.

Category: Planning/Physiological Integrity/Pharmacological Therapies

1 liter = 1,000 mL; 1,000 mL/8 hours = 125 mL/hour

The correct answer is 125.

94. The answer is 1, 3, 4, and 5

CORRECT OPTIONS: Clients receiving diuretics are at risk for hypovolemia and fluid volume deficit. Orthostatic hypotension occurs if the client has a drop of 20 mmHg in the systolic BP or a drop of 10 mmHg in diastolic BP within two to five minutes of standing. **Encouraging PO fluids** may be necessary to prevent dehydration and minimize these adverse effects of fluid volume deficit. For the client in heart failure, close attention to intake and output is important as well. **Ongoing monitoring of BP and HR** is necessary to treat and ensure resolution of symptoms. Loop diuretics, such as furosemide, commonly cause electrolyte imbalances, most notably hypokalemia. **Obtaining electrolyte levels** is an ongoing intervention and crucial to monitor. **Changing positions slowly** can help limit the intensity of orthostatic hypotension and may be something the client should continue for the duration of medication therapy.

INCORRECT OPTIONS: Clients taking loop diuretics are encouraged to increase, not limit, potassium intake. Daily, not weekly, weights are necessary to monitor fluid balance. The client with heart failure will not increase sodium intake, which can cause fluid retention and exacerbate heart failure symptoms.

95. The answer is 1

A client underwent vagotomy with antrectomy for treatment of a duodenal ulcer. Postoperatively, the client develops dumping syndrome. Which statement by the client indicates to the LPN/LVN that further dietary teaching is necessary?

Reworded Question: What is contraindicated for the client with dumping syndrome?

Strategy: Be careful! You are looking for incorrect information.

Needed Info: Antrectomy: surgery to reduce acid-secreting portions of stomach. Delays or eliminates gastric phase of digestion. Dumping syndrome occurs in clients after a gastric resection. It occurs after eating and is related to the stomach's reduced capacity. Undigested food is dumped into the jejunum resulting in distention, cramping, pain, diarrhea 15–30 minutes after eating. Subsides in 6–12 months. S/S 5–30 minutes after eating: vertigo, tachycardia, syncope, diarrhea, nausea. Treatment: sedatives, antispasmodics, high-protein, high-fat, low-carbohydrate, dry diet. Eat in semirecumbent position, lying down after eating.

Category: Evaluation/Physiological Integrity/ Reduction of Risk Potential

(1) "I should eat bread with each meal."—CORRECT: incorrect information; should decrease intake of carbohydrates

(2) "I should eat smaller meals more frequently."—true; 5 to 6 small meals

(3) "I should lie down right after eating."—true; delays gastric emptying time

(4) "I should avoid drinking fluids with my meals."— true; no fluids 1 hour before, with, or 2 hours after meal

96. The answer is 3

The LPN/LVN reinforces discharge teaching with a client with emphysema. Which statement by the client indicates that teaching was successful?

Reworded Question: What is true about emphysema?

Strategy: Determine the outcome of each answer choice.

Needed Info: Emphysema: chronic progressive respiratory disease caused by destruction of alveolar walls. Complications: acute respiratory infections, heart failure or cor pulmonale, cardiac dysrhythmias. Symptoms: cough, dyspnea, wheezing, barrel chest, use of accessory muscles to breathe. Treatment: bronchodilators, corticosteroids, cromolyn sodium, oxygen, diaphragmatic and pursed-lip breathing maneuvers, energy conservation, diet therapy.

Category: Evaluation/Physiological Integrity/Physiological Adaptation

(1) "Cold weather should help my breathing problems."—can exacerbate breathing problems by causing bronchospasms

(2) "I'll eat three balanced meals daily but limit my fluid intake."—small, frequent meals should be consumed to increase caloric intake, limit shortness of breath caused by eating; fluids should not be limited because hydration liquefies secretions

(3) "I'll limit my outside activity when pollution levels are high."—CORRECT: pollution acts as irritant by causing bronchospasms

(4) "Intensive exercise should help me regain strength."—intensive exercise is not tolerated; a conditioning program can help conserve and increase pulmonary ventilation

97. The answer is 3

The LPN/LVN is hearing a client call for help. The LPN/LVN enters the room and finds a client in bilateral wrist restraints with a cool, pale right hand and no palpable radial pulse. Which would be the most appropriate action for the LPN/LVN to take **first**?

Reworded Question: What is the priority response to this situation?

Strategy: Think ABCs and about the risk restraints pose to circulation.

Needed Info: Loss of circulation: loss of all or part of a limb can occur in as little as 15 minutes when blood flow is absent.

Category: Planning/Safe and Effective Care Environment/Safety and Infection Control

(1) Leave to find the client's nurse—this delays the immediate intervention required to protect the hand

(2) Massage the client's wrist and hand—does not address the cause of the impaired hand circulation, delays intervention

(3) Remove the right wrist restraint—CORRECT: provides the most immediate and effective way to help return circulation to the wrist and hand; the LPN/LVN can call for help and turn on the client's call light for further assistance and assessment

(4) Reposition the client to reduce pressure—does not address the cause of the impaired hand circulation, delays intervention

98. The answer is 4

The LPN/LVN is reinforcing discharge teaching for a client with a new colostomy. The LPN/LVN knows teaching was successful when the client chooses which menu option?

Reworded Question: What is the appropriate diet for a client with a colostomy?

Strategy: Recall the type of diet required and then select the menu that is appropriate.

Needed Info: Diet: a low-residue diet for 4–6 weeks postoperatively, avoiding gas-forming, odor-producing, or excessively laxative or constipating foods.

Category: Evaluation/Physiological Integrity/Reduction of Risk Potential

(1) Sausage, sauerkraut, baked potato, and fresh fruit—sausage and sauerkraut are gas-producing and should be avoided with a new colostomy

(2) Cheese omelet with bran muffin and fresh pineapple—bran muffin and fresh fruit are high-fiber (residue)

(3) Pork chop, mashed potatoes, turnips, and salad—turnips are odor-causing and salad is high-residue

(4) Baked chicken, boiled potato, cooked carrots, and yogurt—CORRECT: provides balanced nutrition, high protein, low residue, low fat, and nonirritating foods

99. The answer is 2

The LPN/LVN is implementing the protocol for teaching a new mother how to breastfeed her newborn. The LPN/LVN knows that teaching has been successful if the client makes which statement?

Reworded Question: What indicates that a newborn is receiving adequate nutrition when breastfeeding?

Strategy: Think about each statement. Is it true?

Needed Info: Breastfeeding is recommended for first 6–12 months of life; human milk is considered ideal food. Colostrum is secreted at first; clear and colorless; contains protective antibodies; high in protein and minerals. Milk is secreted after 2–4 days; milky white appearance; contains more fat and lactose than colostrum.

Category: Evaluation/Health Promotion and Maintenance

(1) "My baby's weight should equal the birthweight in 5 to 7 days."—breastfeeding infants should surpass birthweight in 10–14 days

(2) "My baby should have at least 6 to 8 wet diapers per day."—CORRECT: indicates newborn adequately hydrated and therefore, ingesting adequate nutrition

(3) "My baby will sleep at least 6 hours between feedings."—newborns feed approximately every 2 to 3 hours during the day and every 4 hours at night

(4) "My baby will feed for about 10 minutes per feeding."—should feed for approximately 15–20 minutes per breast

100. The answer is 2

A client is admitted to the telemetry unit for evaluation of reported chest pain. Eight hours after admission, the client's cardiac monitor shows ventricular fibrillation. The primary health care provider defibrillates the client. The LPN/LVN understands that the purpose of defibrillation is to do which these?

Reworded Question: Why is a client defibrillated?

Strategy: Think about each answer choice.

Needed Info: Defibrillation: delivers an electrical current to the heart that depolarizes myocardial cells. When the cells repolarize, the sino-atrial (SA) node commonly recaptures its role as the heart's pacemaker.

Category: Implementation/Physiological Integrity/Physiological Adaptation

(1) Increase cardiac contractility, preload, and cardiac output—inaccurate

(2) Depolarize cells allowing SA node to recapture pacing node—CORRECT: electrical current delivered to the heart depolarizes myocardioal cells allowing the SA node to recapture its pacing role

(3) Reduce the degree of cardiac ischemia and acidosis—inaccurate

(4) Provide electrical energy for depleted myocardial cells—inaccurate

101. The answer is 3

The LPN/LVN is caring for a client who suddenly reports chest pains. The LPN/LVN knows that which symptom would be **most** characteristic of an acute myocardial infarction (MI)?

Reworded Question: What type of pain is characteristic in an MI?

Strategy: Think about the cause of each type of pain.

Needed Info: MI signs and symptoms: chest pain radiating to neck, jaw, shoulder, back, or left arm; unrelieved by nitroglycerin. Also fever, apprehension, dizziness, diaphoresis, palpitations, shortness of breath.

Category: Data Collection/Physiological Integrity/Physiological Adaptation

(1) Intermittent, localized epigastric pain—indicates GI disorder

(2) Sharp, localized, unilateral chest pain—symptoms of pneumothorax

(3) Severe substernal pain radiating down the left arm—CORRECT: pain may be crushing; radiate; unrelated to emotion or exercise

(4) Sharp, burning chest pain moving from place to place—may be caused by anxiety

102. The answer is 1

The primary health care provider prescribes packing for a nonhealing open surgical wound. Which is the **first** action by the LPN/LVN?

Reworded Question: Which first step is important prior to packing a wound?

Strategy: Determine what you need to know about the wound and dressing. "*First* action" indicates priority.

Needed Info: Must observe a wound to properly care for the wound and client. Observation allows the nurse to determine what materials are needed, whether another person will be needed to provided assistance, and whether the client will require pain medication prior to the dressing change. Open wounds require sterile technique.

Category: Planning/Safe and Effective Care Environment/Safety and Infection Control

(1) Identify wound size, shape, and depth—CORRECT: it is necessary to observe the wound to adequately prepare for a dressing change and select appropriate dressing materials

(2) Observe for wound drainage or discharge—this is necessary, but not the first step

(3) Plan to set up for clean technique—an open wound requires sterile, not clean, technique

(4) Select the proper dressing material—this is a safe and expected practice, but not the first step

103. The answer is 2

A client returns to the clinic 2 weeks after hospital discharge. The client is taking warfarin sodium 2 mg PO daily. Which statement by the client to the LPN/LVN indicates that further teaching is necessary?

Reworded Question: What is contraindicated for warfarin?

Strategy: Think about what each statement means and how it relates to warfarin.

Needed Info: Warfarin sodium: anticoagulant. Side effects: hemorrhage, fever, rash. Prothrombin time (PT) used to monitor effectiveness; PT usually maintained at 1.5–2 times normal. Antidote: vitamin K (aquamephyton). Nursing responsibilities: check for bleeding gums, bruises, nosebleeds, petechiae, melena, tarry stools, hematuria. Use electric razor, soft toothbrush; provide green leafy vegetables (contain vitamin K).

Category: Evaluation/Physiological Integrity/Pharmacological Therapies

(1) "I take an antihistamine before bedtime."—no contraindication

(2) "I take aspirin whenever I have a headache."—CORRECT: inhibits platelet aggregation increasing the risk for bleeding; avoid use with warfarin

(3) "I put on sunscreen whenever I go outside."—correct behavior

(4) "I take an antacid if my stomach gets upset."—correct information

104. The answer is 3

To enhance the percutaneous absorption of nitroglycerin ointment, it would be **most** important for the LPN/LVN to select which site?

Reworded Question: What is the best site for nitroglycerin ointment?

Strategy: Think about each site.

Needed Info: Nitroglycerin: used in treatment of angina pectoris to reduce ischemia and relieve pain by decreasing myocardial oxygen consumption; dilates veins and arteries. Side effects: throbbing headache, flushing, hypotension, tachycardia. Nursing responsibilities: teach appropriate administration, storage, expected pain relief, side effects. Ointment applied to skin; sites rotated to avoid skin irritation. Prolonged effect up to 24 hours.

Category: Implementation/Physiological Integrity/Pharmacological Therapies

(1) Muscular—not most important

(2) Near the heart—not most important

(3) Non-hairy—CORRECT: skin site free of hair will increase absorption; avoid distal part of extremities due to less-than-maximal absorption

(4) Bony prominence—most important is that the site be non-hairy since hair interferes with absorption

105. The answer is 3

When assisting the RN in planning care for a postoperative client, which should be the **first** choice of the LPN/LVN to reduce the client's risk for pooled airway secretions and decreased chest wall expansion?

Reworded Question: What respiratory intervention is the easiest and most cost-effective to implement?

Strategy: Identify standards of care to prevent respiratory complications for all hospitalized clients.

Needed Info: Causes of respiratory complications in the hospital setting: decreased mobility or immobility of acutely ill clients. To prevent potential complications: frequently reposition clients from side to side, get clients out of bed to a chair, assist clients to ambulate.

These actions are cost-effective, easy, and standard practice.

Category: Planning/Physiological Integrity/Basic Care and Comfort

(1) Chest percussion—not necessary for the majority of clients and requires nursing staff or respiratory therapy intervention

(2) Incentive spirometry—not necessary for the majority of clients, adds cost to care and requires a piece of equipment issued to the client

(3) Position changes—CORRECT: can be encouraged and accomplished easily for all clients without any additional expense for equipment or staff

(4) Postural drainage—not necessary for the majority of clients and requires nursing staff or respiratory therapy intervention

106. The answer is 2

Which action by the LPN/LVN would be **most** helpful in preventing injury to elderly clients in a health care facility?

Reworded Question: What is the most frequent cause of injury for the elderly in a health care facility?

Strategy: Think about the primary injury category for the elderly.

Needed Info: Statistically, falls are the most frequent cause of injury for the hospitalized or institutionalized elderly adult. Must protect clients/residents from falls.

Category: Planning/Safe and Effective Care Environment/Safety and Infection Control

(1) Closely monitor the temperature of hot oral fluids—necessary, but not the most frequent cause of injury

(2) Keep unnecessary furniture out of the way—CORRECT: falls are the most common cause of injury, and maintaining an uncluttered environment can help prevent falls

(3) Maintain the safe function of all electrical equipment—necessary, but not the most frequent cause of injury

(4) Use safety protection caps on all medications—necessary, but bottles of medication should not be accessible to clients

107. The answer is 4

Which statement by a client during a group therapy session requires immediate follow-up by the LPN/LVN?

Reworded Question: Which statement indicates the possibility of impending danger?

Strategy: Think about which statement would make you question the client's intentions.

Needed Info: In *Tarasoff v. The Regents of the University of California* (1976), the court established a duty to warn of threats of harm to others. Failure to warn, coupled with subsequent injury to the threatened person, exposes the mental health professional to civil damages for malpractice. Based on this and other rulings in many states, the mental health caregiver must take responsibility to warn society of potential danger.

Category: Implementation/Psychosocial Integrity

(1) "I know I'm a chronically compulsive liar, but I can't help it."—this statement is revealing, but does not indicate impending threat

(2) "I don't ever want to go home; I feel safer here."—this statement is a response to anxiety or fear, but does not indicate immediate danger

(3) "I don't really care if I ever see my girlfriend again."—this statement does not imply a threat or impending violence

(4) "I'll make sure that doctor is sorry for what he said."—CORRECT: under the Tarasoff Act, a threatened person, including health professionals, must be warned about threats or potential threats to personal safety

108. The answer is 3

A female client visits the clinic reporting right calf tenderness and pain. It would be **most** important for the LPN/LVN to ask which question?

Reworded Question: What is a predisposing factor to developing deep vein thrombosis (DVT)?

Strategy: Determine why you would ask each question.

Needed Info: Thrombophlebitis (phlebitis, phlebothrombosis, or DVT): clot formation in a vein secondary to inflammation of vein or partial vein obstruction. Risk factors: history of varicose veins, hypercoagulation, cardiovascular disease, pregnancy, oral contraceptives, immobility, recent surgery, or injury.

Category: Data Collection/Physiological Integrity/ Pharmacological Therapies

(1) "Do you exercise excessively?"—excessive exercise could cause shin splints

(2) "Have you had any recent fractures?"—not relevant to client's reported symptoms

(3) "What type of birth control do you use?"—CORRECT: increased risk of DVT with oral contraceptives

(4) "Are you under a lot of stress?"—should be concerned about possibility of DVT

109. The answer is 1

Which should be the LPN/LVN's **first** priority in providing care for a client who has end-stage ovarian cancer and has been weakened by chemotherapy?

Reworded Question: What is the most important information needed regarding this client?

Strategy: Think about basic needs of every client. Remember Maslow's hierarchy of needs.

Needed Info: Maslow's hierarchy of basic human needs: physiological needs must be met before higher-level needs of safety and security, love and belonging, self-esteem, and self-actualization. Untreated pain affects all other physiological needs: oxygenation, food and fluid intake, elimination, ability to rest and sleep, comfort, and activity level.

Category: Planning/Physiological Integrity/Basic Care and Comfort

(1) Collect data to see if client has pain—CORRECT: collecting data to see if the client has pain enables the LPN/LVN to plan for the client's pain management needs

(2) Determine if the client is hungry or thirsty— important physiological needs that are difficult to meet for a client in pain

(3) Explore the client's feelings about dying—important psychological safety and security need that is difficult to meet for a client in pain

(4) Observe the client's self-care abilities—important safety and security need that is difficult to meet for a client in pain

110. The answer is 2

The LPN/LVN in the postpartum unit is caring for a client who delivered her first child the previous day. The LPN/LVN notes multiple varicosities on the client's lower extremities. Which action should the LPN/LVN perform?

Reworded Question: What is the best way to prevent thrombophlebitis?

Strategy: Think about what causes thrombophlebitis.

Needed Info: high-risk of developing thrombophlebitis during pregnancy and immediate postpartum period. Thrombophlebitis: inflammation of vein associated with formation of a thrombus or blood clot. Other risk factors: prolonged immobility, use of oral contraceptives, sepsis, smoking, dehydration, and heart failure. S/S: pain in the calf, localized edema of one extremity, positive Homans sign (pain in calf when foot is dorsiflexed). Treatment: bed rest and elevation of extremity, anticoagulant (heparin).

Category: Planning/Health Promotion and Maintenance

(1) Teach the client to rest in bed when the baby sleeps—not preventive; bed rest can cause thrombophlebitis

(2) Encourage early and frequent ambulation—CORRECT: facilitates emptying of blood vessels in lower extremities

(3) Apply warm soaks for 20 minutes every 4 hours—not a preventive measure but an intervention used to treat; must be ordered by primary health care provider

(4) Perform passive range-of-motion (ROM) exercises 3 times daily—early ambulation more effective; passive ROM retains joint function, maintains circulation; passive exercises: no assistance from client

111. The answer is 2

The LPN/LVN is caring for a client who sustained a left femur fracture in a bicycle accident. A cast is applied. The nurse knows that which exercise would be **most** beneficial for this client?

Reworded Question: What exercise is best for a client in a cast?

Strategy: Picture the client as described. Imagine client performing each type of exercise. Also think about the key words "*Most* beneficial."

Needed Info: Fracture: break in continuity of bone. Complications: hemorrhage (bone vascular), shock, fat embolism (long bones), sepsis, peripheral nerve damage, delayed union, nonunion. Treatment: reduction (closed or open), immobilization (cast, traction, splints, internal and external fixation). Cast allows early mobility. Nursing responsibilities: teach isometric exercises.

Category: Planning/Physiological Integrity/Reduction of Risk Potential

(1) Passive exercise of the affected limb—nurse moves extremity; unable to perform with cast in place

(2) Quadriceps setting of the affected limb—CORRECT: isometric exercise: contraction of muscle without movement of joint; maintains strength in the affected limb

(3) Active range-of-motion exercises of the unaffected limb—not best, doesn't strengthen affected limb

(4) Passive exercise of the upper extremities—need strengthening exercises, not passive exercises

112. See explanation for answers

In preparation for a dressing change, the LPN/LVN puts on sterile gloves. Where should the LPN/LVN initially grip the first sterile glove?

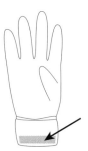

Reworded Question: What is the correct procedure for applying sterile gloves?

Strategy: Remember what part of the glove must remain sterile.

Needed Info: Absolutely necessary for the first glove of the pair to be donned in the proper fashion. Grasp the top end of the folded cuff without touching any part of the rest of the sterile glove to avoid contamination from nonsterile hands.

Category: Implementation/Safe and Effective Care Environment/Safety and Infection Control

113. The answer is 2

A client is being discharged from the hospital following a right total hip arthroplasty. The LPN/LVN reinforces discharge teaching. Which statement by the client would indicate that teaching was successful?

Reworded Question: What should a client do after a total hip arthroplasty?

Strategy: Determine which movements bring the right hip toward the median plane of the body (adduction).

Needed Info: Adduction: movement toward the median plane or midline of the body. Adduction precautions implemented to prevent hip dislocation: legs may not be crossed at knees or ankles, knees must be separated (most often with a special pillow). No hip flexion beyond 90 degrees.

Category: Planning/Physiological Integrity/Basic Care and Comfort

(1) "I can bend over to pick up something on the floor."—this describes flexion, not adduction. It is not allowed for total hip arthroplasty clients

(2) "I should not cross my ankles when sitting in a chair."—CORRECT: even though the client is only crossing the legs at the ankles, the leg is adducted

(3) "I need to lie on my stomach when sleeping in bed."—the prone position does not necessarily adduct the hip

(4) "I should spread my knees apart to put on my shoes."—this movement abducts the hip

114. The answer is 725

The LPN/LVN is caring for a client with continuous bladder irrigation. At 7 A.M., the LPN/LVN notes 4,200 mL of normal saline solution left in the irrigation bags. During the next shift (7 A.M. to 3 P.M.), the LPN/LVN hangs another 3,000 mL and empties a total of 5,625 mL from the urine drainage bag. At 3 P.M., there are 2,300 mL of irrigant left hanging. What is the actual urine output for the client from 7 A.M. to 3 P.M.?

Reworded Question: After subtracting the irrigant, what is the client's urinary output?

Strategy: Calculate irrigant used and subtract it from total fluid output to determine urinary output.

Needed Info: Accurate measurement of urinary output is critical. Subtract the irrigant used from the total fluid output to determine the urinary output.

Category: Implementation/Physiological Integrity/Basic Care and Comfort

The irrigant infused was 4,200 mL left at the beginning of the shift + 3,000 mL added − 2,300 mL remaining at the end of the shift = 4,900 mL infused as irrigant. Total output from the catheter bag was 5,625 mL − 4,900 mL of irrigant infused = 725 mL of urine as output.

The correct answer is 725.

115. The answer is 3

A client with a history of type 1 diabetes mellitus is admitted to the unit reporting nausea, vomiting, and abdominal pain. The client reduced the insulin dose four days ago when influenza symptoms prevented eating. The LPN/LVN observes poor skin turgor, dry mucous membranes, and fruity breath odor. The LPN/LVN should be alert for which problem?

Reworded Question: What do these symptoms indicate?

Strategy: Think about each answer choice.

Needed Info: Diabetes mellitus: disorder of carbohydrate metabolism: insufficient insulin to meet metabolic needs. Type 1 diabetes mellitus: insulin dependent, prone to diabetic ketoacidosis. Type 2 diabetes mellitus: controlled by diet and oral antidiabetic agents, not prone to ketosis. In ketoacidosis, the body becomes dehydrated from osmotic diuresis. The fruity breath odor develops from acetone, a component of ketone bodies. Rate and depth of respiration increase (Kussmaul) in attempt to blow off excess carbonic acid. Hyperosmolar nonketotic syndrome (HHNS)—lacks ketonuria.

Category: Planning/Physiological Integrity/Reduction of Risk Potential

(1) Rebound hypoglycemia—cause: too much insulin after a period of hyperglycemia; blood glucose level falls below 60 mg/dL (3.3 mmol/L); S/S: tachycardia, perspiration, confusion, lethargy, numb lips, anxiety, hunger

(2) Viral gastrointestinal illness—may produce similar symptoms, not best answer based on client history

(3) Diabetic ketoacidosis—CORRECT: cause: insufficient insulin; S/S: polyuria, polydipsia, nausea, vomiting, dry mucous membranes, weight loss, abdominal pain, hypotension, shock, coma

(4) Hyperglycemic hyperosmolar nonketotic coma—extreme hyperglycemia (800–2,000 mg/dL [44.4–111 mmol/L]) with absence of acidosis; some insulin production, don't mobilize fats for energy or form ketones; usually with type 2 diabetes; cause:

infections, stress, medications (steroids, thiazide diuretics), total parenteral nutrition; S/S: polyphagia, polyuria, polydipsia, glycosuria, dehydration, abdominal discomfort, hyperpyrexia, changes in level of consciousness (LOC), hypotension, shock; treatment: fluid and electrolyte replacement, insulin given IV

116. The answer is 1

The LPN/LVN is caring for a group of clients. The nurse knows that it is **most** important for which client to receive scheduled medications on time?

Reworded Question: Which medication, if given late, might cause harm to the client?

Strategy: Think about each answer.

Needed Info: Myasthenia gravis is deficiency of acetylcholine at myoneural junction; symptoms include muscular weakness produced by repeated movements that soon disappears following rest, diplopia, ptosis, impaired speech, and dysphagia.

Category: Planning/Physiological Integrity/Pharmacological Therapies

(1) A client diagnosed with myasthenia gravis receiving pyridostigmine bromide—CORRECT: Pyrostigmine bromide is a cholinesterase inhibitor, which increases acetylcholine concentration at the neuromuscular junction; early administration can precipitate a cholinergic crisis; late administration can precipitate myasthenic crisis

(2) A client diagnosed with bipolar disorder receiving lithium carbonate—Lithium carbonate is a mood stabilizer; targeted blood level = 1–1.5 mEq/L (1–1.5 mmol/L)

(3) A client diagnosed with tuberculosis receiving isonicotinic acid hydrazide—Isonicotinic acid hydrazide (INH) is given in a single daily dose; side effects include hepatitis, peripheral neuritis, rash, and fever

(4) A client diagnosed with Parkinson disease receiving levodopa—Levodopa is thought to restore dopamine levels in extrapyramidal centers; sudden withdrawal can cause parkinsonian crisis; priority is to administer pyrostigmine bromide

117. The answer is 1, 2, 3, 4, 6, 7, and 8

CORRECT OPTIONS: **Rupture of amniotic membranes for > 24 hours prior to delivery** removes the fetus's inherent protection barrier from the vaginal flora and any other infectious organisms. **Recurrent digital cervical assessments accompanying the prolonged labor** are additional opportunities for bacteria to ascend into the uterus when amniotic membranes are ruptured. The laboring client demonstrates symptoms of such an infection (e.g., chorioamnionitis) by having an **elevated temperature** and **foul-smelling amniotic fluid**. A maternal infection can impact the fetus and result in lower Apgar scores. The impact of an **elevated maternal blood pressure** over the course of the pregnancy and at time of delivery can impact the newborn negatively. **Late decelerations and meconium staining of the amniotic fluid** indicate the presence of a placental challenge. The **uncertain gestational age** of this fetus points to concerns regarding lung fetal maturity, despite current large estimated fetal weight and maternal history of uncomplicated delivery of previous large-for-gestational age babies.

INCORRECT OPTION: A maternal history of large for gestational age infants is not a risk factor for poor fetal outcomes or complications.

118. The answer is 3

An school-age client is admitted to the hospital for evaluation for a kidney transplant. The LPN/LVN learns that the client received hemodialysis for 3 years due to stage 5 kidney disease. The LPN/LVN knows that the illness can interfere with this client's achievement of which stage of personality development?

Reworded Question: What developmental stage is altered in a client due to this chronic disease?

Strategy: Picture the person described in the question. Think about this client's activities and interests. This helps eliminate incorrect answer choices. A school-age client may be thinking about homework, or doing chores at home.

Needed Info: Eric Erikson developed a theory of the stages of personality development that progressed in predictable stages from birth to death. Other stages: autonomy versus shame and doubt (task of 1–3 yrs); initiative versus guilt (task of 3–6 yrs).

Category: Planning/Health Promotion and Maintenance

(1) Intimacy—young adult: 20–40 yrs; achieving sexual and loving relationship with another; alternative: isolation

(2) Trust—infancy; results from consistent care by a loving caretaker; teaches that basic needs will be met; alternative: mistrust

(3) Industry—CORRECT: 6–12 yrs; aspires to be the best; learns social skills, how to finish tasks; sensitive about school expectations; may be impaired due to absences from school, growth retardation, and emotional difficulties

(4) Identity—adolescence; peer groups important; used to define identity, establish body image, form new relationships; alternative: role diffusion

119. The answer is 2, 3, 5, and 6

The LPN/LVN notes that a client has an unsteady gait. The LPN/LVN should take which action? **(Select all that apply.)**

Reworded Question: What safety measures are appropriate for a client who is unsteady on their feet?

Strategy: Identify nonrestrictive safety measures.

Needed Info: Safety measures to help prevent falls include: rubber-soled (nonskid) shoes, removal of obstacles and clutter, a method of summoning the help of the nursing staff, assistance when out of bed, adequate lighting, safety bars and hand rails, and adaptive equipment including walkers and raised toilet seats as appropriate.

Category: Implementation/Safe and Effective Care Environment/Safety and Infection Control

(1) Apply a chest or vest restraint at night—restrictive and false imprisonment without a primary health care provider's orders

(2) Help the client put on nonskid shoes for walking—CORRECT: a choice that decreases fall risk without restricting the client

(3) Keep the call light within the client's reach—CORRECT: not restrictive and addresses the client's need to call for assistance when getting out of bed

(4) Lower the bed and raise all four side rails—lowering the bed is appropriate, but raising all the side rails only increases the height from which a client may fall while climbing over the side rails

(5) Provide adequate lighting in room and bathroom—CORRECT: allows client to assess an unfamiliar hospital environment

(6) Remove obstacles and room clutter—CORRECT: provides clear access to room and bathroom

120. The answer is 2

Haloperidol 5 mg PO tid is prescribed for a client with schizophrenia. Two days later, the client reports "tight jaws and a stiff neck." What does the LPN/LVN recognize these complaints to be?

Reworded Question: Why does the client taking haloperidol have these symptoms?

Strategy: Think about each answer choice.

Needed Info: Haloperidol, antipsychotic agent used to treat psychotic disorders. High incidence of extrapyramidal reactions: pseudoparkinsonism (rigidity and tremors), akathisia (motor restlessness), dystonia (involuntary jerking, of muscles, acute muscular rigidity and cramping), tardive dyskinesia (abnormal movements of lips, jaws, tongue). Schizophrenia: retreat from reality, flat affect, suspiciousness, hallucinations, delusions, loose associations, psychomotor retardation or hyperactivity, regression. Nursing responsibilities: maintain safety, meet physical needs, decrease sensory stimuli. Treatment: antipsychotic medications, individual therapy.

Category: Evaluation/Physiological Integrity/ Pharmacological Therapies

(1) Common side effects of antipsychotic medications that will diminish over time—gets worse, untreated, life-threatening
(2) Early symptoms of extrapyramidal reactions to the medication—CORRECT: dystonic reaction, airway may become obstructed
(3) Psychosomatic symptoms resulting from a delusional system—not accurate
(4) Permanent side effects associated with haloperidol therapy—reversible when treated with IV diphenhydramine hydrochloride

121. The answer is 4

A client is receiving a continuous gastric tube feeding at 100 mL per hour. The LPN/LVN checks for gastric residual volume and finds 90 mL in the client's stomach. Which action should the LPN/LVN take?

Reworded Question: What are the standards and procedures for gastric residual volume from a gastric tube feeding?

Strategy: Think about electrolyte balance and gastric emptying.

Needed Info: Standard procedures for clients receiving continuous tube feedings: gastric residual volume and tube placement checked every 4 hours, position clients with head of bed elevated at least 30 degrees. To promote normal function: gastric residual volume with associated gastric enzymes and hydrochloric acid should be returned to the stomach when gastric residual volume measures under 150 mL, feeding should be stopped if the gastric residual volume is over 50% of the volume fed over the last 1 hour.

Category: Physiological Integrity/Basic Care and Comfort/Analysis

(1) Discard the gastric residual volume and continue the tube feeding—gastric residual volume under 150 mL should be returned to the stomach to maintain electrolyte balance; the feeding should be stopped because the gastric residual volume exceeds 50% of the volume fed over 1 hour
(2) Discard the gastric residual volume and stop the tube feeding—return the gastric residual volume and stop the feeding
(3) Return the gastric residual volume and continue the tube feeding—return the gastric residual volume and stop the feeding
(4) Return the gastric residual volume and stop the tube feeding—CORRECT: residuals less than 150 mL should be returned to the stomach to maintain electrolyte balance; the feeding should be stopped because the gastric residual volume exceeds 50% of the volume fed over 1 hour

122. The answer is 4

The LPN/LVN opens several sterile gauze dressings on the client's over-the-bed table. The LPN/LVN knows that taking which action will contaminate the sterile dressings?

Reworded Question: What is incorrect sterile technique?

Strategy: List the basic principles of sterile technique.

Needed Info: To maintain sterility of sterile objects: may only touch other sterile objects, must remain in the LPN/LVN's view, must be above the LPN/LVN's waist, cannot be exposed to air for prolonged periods, must be located inside the 1-inch (2.5 cm) border of a sterile field or within the dressing packaging borders, sterile fluids must not contact a nonsterile object when fluids flow with gravity. The client's over-the-bed table is not sterile.

Category: Evaluation/Safe and Effective Care Environment/Safety and Infection Control

(1) Does not allow the dressings prolonged exposure to the air—a principle of sterile technique

(2) Keeps sterile dressings inside border of the sterile packaging—a principle of sterile technique

(3) Positions top of the over-the-bed table at or above waist level—a principle of sterile technique

(4) Pours sterile saline onto the opened sterile dressing on table —CORRECT: capillary action and gravity lead to contamination of the sterile object because of contact between the nonsterile over-the-bed table and the once-sterile fluid

123. The answer is 1

The LPN/LVN is caring for a client in labor. The primary health care provider palpates a firm, round form in the uterine fundus, small parts on the client's right side, and a long, smooth, curved section on the left side. Based on these findings, where should the LPN/LVN anticipate auscultating the fetal heart tones?

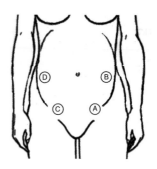

Reworded Question: If a fetus is LOA, where should the nurse listen for the fetal heart tone?

Strategy: Examine the diagram carefully. Know the client's right from left.

Needed Info: Fetal reference point: Vertex presentation—dependent upon degree of flexion of fetal head on chest; full flexion/occiput (O), full extension chin (M), moderate extension (military) brow (B). Breech presentation-sacrum (S). Shoulder presentation-scapula (SC). Maternal pelvis is designated per her right/left and anterior/posterior. Position = relationship of fetal reference point to mother's pelvis; expressed as standard 3—letter abbreviation: left occiput anterior (LOA) (most common), left occiput posterior (LOP), right occiput anterior (ROA), right occiput posterior (ROP), left occiput transverse (LOT), right occiput transverse (ROT).

Category: Planning/Health Promotion and Maintenance

(1) A—CORRECT: point of maximum intensity for fetal heart tones with fetus in LOA position

(2) B—PMI location for fetus in LOP position

(3) C—PMI location for fetus in ROA position

(4) D—PMI location for fetus in ROP position

124. The answer is 4

When completing data collection of an immobilized client, the LPN/LVN knows that edema is commonly observed in which location?

Reworded Question: Where does dependent edema occur in an immobile client? What position is the immobilized client usually in?

Strategy: Identify where dependent edema is likely to settle due to gravity in a client supine.

Needed Info: Immobile clients: most often horizontal in bed, gravity would cause fluid pooling at the most dependent place, namely, the sacrum. Mobile clients: fluids pool in dependent areas such as their feet and ankles.

Category: Data Collection/Physiological Integrity/Basic Care and Comfort

(1) Abdomen—not a likely place for dependent edema

(2) Feet and ankles—a primary place for edema in a client who is sitting up or out of bed walking

(3) Fingers and wrists—not a likely place to initially find dependent edema

(4) Sacrum—CORRECT: gravity causes dependent edema to develop at the sacrum in immobile clients

125. The answer is 1

A client is preparing to take her 1-day-old infant home from the hospital. The LPN/LVN discusses the test for phenylketonuria (PKU) with the client. The LPN/LVN's reinforcement of teaching should be based on an understanding that the test is **most** reliable in which circumstance?

Reworded Question: When is the PKU test most reliable?

Strategy: Focus on the key words in the question. Think about what you know about the PKU test.

Needed Info: PKU: genetic disorder caused by a deficiency in liver enzyme phenylalanine hydroxylase. Body can't metabolize essential amino acid phenylalanine, allows phenyl acids to accumulate in the blood. If not recognized, resultant high levels of phenyl ketone in the brain cause intellectual disability. Guthrie test: screening for PKU. Treatment: dietary restriction of foods containing phenylalanine. Blood levels of phenylalanine monitored to evaluate the effectiveness of the dietary restrictions.

Category: Implementation/Health Promotion and Maintenance

(1) After a source of protein has been ingested—CORRECT: recommended to be performed before newborns leave hospital; if initial blood sample is obtained within first 24 hours, recommended to be repeated at 3 weeks

(2) After the meconium has been excreted—no relationship; dark-green, tarry stool passed within first 48 hours of birth

(3) After the danger of hyperbilirubinemia has passed—no relationship; excessive accumulation of bilirubin in blood; S/S: jaundice (yellow discoloration of skin); common finding in newborn; not cause for concern

(4) After the effects of delivery have subsided—no relationship

126. See explanation for answers

Potential Condition	
Heart failure.	☑

CORRECT OPTION: The client is displaying symptoms of atrial fibrillation which include rapid, irregular heart rate and feelings of a "racing" heartbeat. The client is now having additional symptoms such as shortness of breath, peripheral edema, JVD, diminished pulses, and decreased capillary refill. These findings are consistent with **heart failure**, which is often caused by pre-existing cardiac conditions.

INCORRECT OPTIONS: The client is having some shortness of breath, but is not having other classic symptoms of myocardial infarction (MI) such as chest pain or pressure, jaw pain, indigestion, clammy skin, or diaphoresis. Pulmonary embolism causes sharp pain with shortness of breath, but does not cause peripheral edema. Pneumonia would not cause symptoms of decreased perfusion, and the client with pneumonia would likely have adventitious lung sounds.

Actions to Take	
Obtain manual blood pressure.	☑
Prepare for echocardiogram.	☑

CORRECT OPTIONS: The client has a history of atrial fibrillation with RVR, which places stress on the heart. Obtaining and recording accurate baseline findings on cardiovascular function, such as **blood pressure**, is very important as it appears the client's condition has changed. An **echocardiogram** is a diagnostic test that will give detailed insight about the heart chambers and function, including the left ventricular ejection fraction (LVEF).

INCORRECT OPTIONS: Incentive spirometry (ICS) is a tool used to help prevent atelectasis, most notably in post-operative clients. At this time, it would not be indicated to have the client use ICS. Obtaining a client's temperature can give insight to infection or inflammation, neither of which is suspected in the client. Urine output is a measure of kidney perfusion and function and it will be important to monitor intake and output. Placing an indwelling urinary catheter is not necessary and would increase the client's risk for infection.

Findings to Report	
Abdominal girth.	✓
Daily weights.	✓

CORRECT OPTIONS: It is crucial to monitor progression of heart failure. Fluid overload seen with heart failure is often noted with ascites, which would increase the client's **abdominal girth**. Fluid balance, preload, and afterload are major factors to monitor in the client with heart failure. One of the primary assessments that is done with clients who have heart failure is monitoring **daily weights** (and notifying the health care provider of an increase).

INCORRECT OPTIONS: Oral temperature will not fluctuate or change in response to heart failure. Blood loss is not expected in clients with heart failure so is not something the LPN/LVN would make sure to report. Serum troponin is crucial to obtain in clients reporting symptoms of an MI but does not change in response to heart failure, alone.

127. The answer is 3

The LPN/LVN is caring for an Rh-negative client who has delivered an Rh-positive child. The client states, "The doctor told me about RhoGAM, but I'm still a little confused." Which response by the LPN/LVN is **most** appropriate?

Reworded Question: What is RhoGAM and why is it used?

Strategy: Remember what you know about RhoGAM.

Needed Info: RhoGAM: given to unsensitized Rh-negative (RH–) mother after delivery or abortion of an Rh-positive (Rh+) infant or fetus to prevent development of sensitization. Rh⁻ mother produces antibodies in response to the Rh+ RBCs of fetus. If occurs during pregnancy, fetus is affected. If occurs during delivery, later pregnancies may be affected. An indirect Coombs' test is performed on the mother during pregnancy, and a direct Coombs' test is done on cord blood after delivery. If both are negative and the neonate is Rh+, the mother is given RhoGAM to prevent sensitization. RhoGAM is usually given to unsensitized mothers within 72 hrs of delivery, but may be effective when given 3–4 weeks after delivery. To be effective, RhoGAM must be given after the first delivery and repeated after each subsequent delivery. RhoGAM is ineffective against Rh+ antibodies that are already present in the maternal circulation. The administration of RhoGAM at 26–28 weeks' gestation is also recommended.

Category: Implementation/Health Promotion and Maintenance

(1) "RhoGAM is given to your child to prevent the development of antibodies."—not given to neonate

(2) "RhoGAM is given to your child to supply the necessary antibodies."—not given to neonate

(3) "RhoGAM is given to you to prevent the formation of antibodies."—CORRECT: prevents maternal circulation from developing antibodies

(4) "RhoGAM is given to you to encourage the production of antibodies."—not accurate; given to discourage antibody production

128. The answer is 2

A client is hospitalized with a diagnosis of bipolar disorder. While in the client activities room on the psychiatric unit, the client flirts with other clients and disrupts unit activities. Which approach would be **most** appropriate for the LPN/LVN to take at this time?

Reworded Question: How should you deal with a client with bipolar disorder who is disruptive?

Strategy: Determine the outcome of each answer. Is it desirable?

Needed Info: Nursing responsibilities: accompany client to room when hyperactivity escalates, set limits, remain nonjudgmental.

Category: Planning/Psychosocial Integrity

(1) Set limits on the behavior and remind the client of the rules—too confrontational

(2) Distract the client and escort the client back to the room—CORRECT: clients are easily distracted; nonthreatening action

(3) Instruct the other clients to ignore this client's behavior—does not ensure safety

(4) Inform client of negative behavior and return client to room—too confrontational; may agitate

129. See explanation for answers

CORRECT OPTION: The client is most likely experiencing **orthostatic (i.e., postural) hypotension** (OH). Common medications that cause OH are diuretics, antihypertensive medications, and opioids. INCORRECT OPTIONS: The client was previously stable and is not exhibiting signs of a myocardial infarction, such as chest, jaw, or arm pain. While being pale, diaphoretic, and lightheaded can be associated with hypoglycemia, the client just ate breakfast and has no history of diabetes or use of hypoglycemic medication.

CORRECT OPTION: The LPN/LVN should **measure the client's vital signs** immediately, checking the blood pressure as well as the pulse rate. Hypotension could also be due to bradycardia. INCORRECT OPTIONS: The LPN/LVN needs to check the client's vital signs to determine what the issue could be before taking actions, like giving the client juice or applying oxygen.

CORRECT OPTION: **OH can occur when a client is taking multiple medications that can cause hypotension** as both a desired effect and an adverse effect. The client is taking multiple medications that can cause hypotension, and the client took all of the medications at one time. In addition, the client has other risk factors for OH, including advanced age and prolonged immobility. INCORRECT OPTIONS: The most likely issue is that the client is experiencing additive effects of several medications taken, not that the client is having a complication from surgery or is volume depleted.

CORRECT OPTION: **The LPN/LVN should speak with the RN about adjusting the client's medication regimen so that the client is at less risk for experiencing medication-induced hypotension.** INCORRECT OPTIONS: The client is just beginning to increase PO intake; it is not advisable to push oral fluids. The LPN/LVN cannot withhold or discontinue medications without clear parameters or orders from the physician.

130. The answer is 1

A client is brought to the emergency department bleeding profusely from a stab wound in the left chest area. Vital signs include: blood pressure 80/50 mmHg, pulse 110 beats/minute, and respiratory rate 28 breaths/minute. The LPN/LVN should expect which potential problem?

Reworded Question: What type of shock is described?

Strategy: Form a mental image of the person described.

Needed Info: Symptoms of hypovolemic shock: tachycardia, reduced output, irritability. Treatment: oxygen therapy, IV fluids to restore volume, adrenaline, hydralazine. Nursing responsibilities: check airway, vital signs, insert IV catheter, check arterial blood gas results, central venous pressure measurements, insert indwelling urinary catheter, hourly intake and output, position flat with legs elevated, keep warm.

Category: Planning/Physiological Integrity/Physiological Adaptation

(1) Hypovolemic shock—CORRECT: loss of circulating volume

(2) Cardiogenic shock—decrease in cardiac output; causes include heart failure, MI, cardiac dysfunction

(3) Neurogenic shock—increase in vascular bed; caused by spinal anesthesia, spinal cord injury

(4) Septic shock—decreased cardiac output, hypotension; may be caused by gram-negative or gram-positive bacteria

131. See explanation for answers

Potential Condition	
Asthma attack.	✓

CORRECT OPTION: Most clients with asthma have a history of allergic rhinitis and may have chronic sinus problems. Triggers for an **asthma attack** include allergies; this client has a history of allergies and was outside when the symptoms started. The client was also running around, and exercise can trigger an asthma attack.

INCORRECT OPTIONS: The client is not displaying the classic symptoms of an anaphylactic reaction, aside from shortness of breath. Pericarditis is inflammation of the pericardial sac and usually presents with chest pain and a friction rub that is able to be auscultated. A URI does not necessarily cause severe shortness of breath or wheezing, but often results in nasal congestion, coughing and upper airway secretions.

Medications to Administer	
Albuterol nebulizer.	✓
Beclomethasone nebulizer.	✓

CORRECT OPTIONS: Medication management for an asthma attack must be timely and efficient. Inhaled bronchodilators and oral corticosteroids are the mainstays of treatment for mild to moderate asthma attacks. **Albuterol**, a short-acting beta$_2$ agonist (SABA), is considered a rescue inhaler and has an immediate onset of action. Administering albuterol, followed by an inhaled corticosteroid, such as **beclomethasone**, is beneficial in dilating the bronchioles and decreasing inflammation.

INCORRECT OPTIONS: IM epinephrine is the medication of choice for an anaphylactic reaction but not an asthma attack. It binds to receptors within the sympathetic nervous system but is not specific to the lungs. Metoprolol is a cardioselective beta-blocker, which would not benefit this client. Acetylcysteine is a mucolytic, when given as a nebulizer, but the client is not exhibiting issues with respiratory secretions.

Parameters to Monitor	
Peak expiratory flow rate (PEFR).	☑
Pulse oximetry.	☑

CORRECT OPTIONS: During an acute attack, **PEFR measurements** can be used to help identify the severity of an asthma attack, guide in providing the most appropriate treatment, or monitor the severity of disease. Oxygen levels should be continuously monitored with **pulse oximetry**.

INCORRECT OPTIONS: Sputum culture would be helpful to obtain if the client reported secretions or recent URI, which this client did not mention. CRP is an inflammatory marker that could help guide care of a client with pericarditis or an infection. A TEE is a diagnostic test that will give detailed insight about the heart chambers and function by visualizing the heart through the esophagus, instead of outside the chest wall.

132. The answer is 3

A client is admitted to the hospital for surgical repair of a detached retina in the right eye. In implementing the plan of care for this client postoperatively, the LPN/LVN should encourage the client to take which action?

Reworded Question: What should you do after surgery for a detached retina?

Strategy: Picture the client as described.

Needed Info: Detached retina: separation of retina from pigmented epithelium. S/S: curtain falling across field of vision, black spots, flashes of light, sudden onset. Treatment: surgical repair (photocoagulation, electrodiathermy, cryosurgery, scleral buckling). Complications: infection, redetachment, increased intraocular pressure. Nursing responsibilities postoperatively: check eye patch for drainage, position with detached area dependent; no rapid eye movement (reading, sewing); no coughing, vomiting, sneezing.

Category: Planning/Physiological Integrity/Reduction of Risk Potential

(1) Perform self-care activities—activity restrictions depend on location and size of tear

(2) Maintain patches over both eyes—only affected eye covered

(3) Limit movement of both eyes—CORRECT: bed rest with eye patch or shield

(4) Refrain from excessive talking—no restriction

133. The answer is 2

The LPN/LVN is caring for a client who receives a balanced complete formula through an enteral feeding tube. The LPN/LVN knows that the **most** common complication of an enteral tube feeding is which of these?

Reworded Question: What is a common complication of a tube feeding?

Strategy: Think about each answer choice. Focus on the words "*Most* common," which means there may be more than one answer. And in this situation there is: #4 is a complication but is not common.

Needed Info: Enteral tube feedings are used for clients who are unable to tolerate feeding by the oral route but who have a functioning GI tract. May be given by intermittent or continuous infusion. Elevate head of bed 30–45 degrees. Give at room temperature. Check for placement before feeding. Don't hang solution for more than 6 hrs. Flush tubing with 30 mL water every 4 hrs. Change feeding set every 24 hrs. Balanced complete formula contains intact protein.

Category: Evaluation/Physiological Integrity/Basic Care and Comfort

(1) Edema—not frequently seen; if present primary health care provider may change formula to a low-sodium

(2) Diarrhea—CORRECT: formula intolerance or rate intolerance; give slowly; other symptoms of intolerance: nausea, vomiting, aspiration, glycosuria, diaphoresis

(3) Hypokalemia—normal potassium 3.5–5 mEq/L (3.5–5 mmol/L); not commonly seen; common causes: diuretics, diarrhea, GI drainage

(4) Vomiting—can happen with rapid increase in rate; administer slowly

134. The answer is 1

The LPN/LVN is caring for a preschool-age client diagnosed with a fractured pelvis caused by a motor vehicle accident. The LPN/LVN prepares the child for the application of a hip spica cast. It is **most** important for the LPN/LVN to take which action?

Reworded Question: How do you prepare a preschool-age client for the procedure?

Strategy: "*Most* important" indicates that discrimination is required to answer the question.

Needed Info: Hip spica cast immobilizes the hip and knee. Preschool children (age 36 months to 6 years) fear injury, mutilation, and punishment; allow child to play with models of equipment; encourage expression of feelings.

Category: Planning/Health Promotion and Maintenance

(1) Obtain a doll for the client with a hip spica cast in place—CORRECT: preschoolers need to see and play with dolls and equipment; explain procedure in simple terms and explain how it will affect the client

(2) Tell the client that the cast will feel cold when applied—may feel a warm or burning sensation under cast while it dries due to chemical reaction between the plaster and the water

(3) Reassure the client that the cast application is painless—will be placed on special cast table that holds the client's body; turning to apply the cast may be painful

(4) Introduce the client to another client who has a hip spica cast—more important to allow client to play with doll with a hip spica cast; viewing the cast may be frightening

135. The answer is 3

An infant is brought to the pediatrician's office for a well-baby visit. During the examination, congenital subluxation of the left hip is suspected. The LPN/LVN would expect to see which symptom?

Reworded Question: What will you see with congenital hip dislocation?

Strategy: Form a mental image of the deformity.

Needed Info: Subluxation: most common type of congenital hip dislocation. Head of femur remains in contact with acetabulum but is partially displaced. Diagnosed in infant less than 4 weeks old S/S: unlevel gluteal folds, limited abduction of hip, shortened femur affected side, Ortolani sign (click). Treatment: abduction splint, hip spica cast, Bryant traction, open reduction.

Category: Data Collection/Health Promotion and Maintenance

(1) Lengthening of the limb on the affected side—inaccurate

(2) Deformities of the foot and ankle—inaccurate

(3) Asymmetry of the gluteal and thigh folds—CORRECT: restricted movement on affected side

(4) Plantarflexion of the foot—seen with clubfoot

136. The answer is 2

A client comes to the clinic because for suspected pregnancy. Tests confirm pregnancy. The client's last menstrual period began on September 8 and lasted for 6 days. The LPN/LVN calculates which expected date of confinement (EDC) for this client?

Reworded Question: How do you calculate the EDC?

Strategy: Perform the calculation required and check for math errors!

Needed Info: EDC or estimated date of delivery (EDD): calculated according to the Naegele rule (first day of the last normal menstrual period minus 3 months plus 7 days and 1 year). Assumes that every woman has a 28-day cycle and pregnancy occurred on 14th day. Most women deliver within a period extending from 7 days before to 7 days after the EDC.

Category: Implementation/Health Promotion and Maintenance

(1) May 15—too early

(2) June 15—CORRECT: September 8 minus 3 months = June 8 plus 7 days plus one year = June 15 of next year

(3) June 21—EDC is calculated from first, not last day, of last normal menstrual period

(4) July 8—not accurate

137. The answer is 4

After completing data collection, the LPN/LVN observes that a client is exhibiting early symptoms of a dystonic reaction related to the use of an antipsychotic medication. Which action by the LPN/LVN would be **most** appropriate?

Reworded Question: What is the first thing you do for a client with a dystonic reaction?

Strategy: Set priorities. Remember Maslow's hierarchy of needs.

Needed Info: Dystonic reaction: muscle tightness in throat, neck, tongue, mouth, eyes, neck, and back; difficulty talking and swallowing. Treatment: IM or IV diphenhydramine or benztropine.

Category: Implementation/Psychosocial Integrity

(1) Reality-test with the client and assure the client that physical symptoms are not real—real symptoms, not delusions

(2) Teach the client about common side effects of anti-psychotic medications—physical needs highest priority

(3) Explain to the client that there is no treatment that will relieve these symptoms—diphenhydramine used IM or IV

(4) Notify the primary health care provider to obtain a prescription for IM diphenhydramine—CORRECT: emergency situation, can occlude airway

138. The answer is 1

As a client nears death, the client's family member says, "I wish I could do something for her." Which response by the LPN/LVN is **most** appropriate?

Reworded Question: What is the most therapeutic communication for the family member?

Strategy: Think about the member's need to help the client.

Needed Info: End-of-life research: last of the senses of a dying person is believed to be hearing, reports of survivors support the reassurance they felt from the words of the caregivers present. Therapeutic communication: supports inclusion of significant others, supports "hope" or "usefulness" on the part of significant others.

Category: Evaluation/Psychosocial Integrity

(1) "It may be comforting if you talk to her calmly and clearly."—CORRECT: the client may actually hear her family member's communications; the family member is offered something to do that may be helpful to both the client and the family member

(2) "She does not know that you are here, but you can sit here."—the client may be aware that her family member is there, and it is nontherapeutic to exclude the family member from offering comfort

(3) "Unfortunately, there is little that you can do at this point."—it is nontherapeutic to exclude the family member from offering comfort

(4) "Why don't you take a break? It is just a matter of time now."—it is nontherapeutic to exclude the family member from offering comfort

139. The answer is 4

The LPN/LVN is providing care to clients in a long-term care facility. Four meal choices are available to the clients. The LPN/LVN should ensure that a client on a low-cholesterol diet receives which meal?

Reworded Question: What should a client on a low-cholesterol diet eat?

Strategy: Remember which foods are part of a low-cholesterol diet.

Needed Info: Low-cholesterol diet should reduce total fat to 20–25% of total calories and reduce the ingestion of saturated fat. Carbohydrates (especially complex carbohydrates) should be 55–60% of calories. High-cholesterol foods: eggs, dairy products, meat, fish, shellfish, poultry.

Category: Implementation/Physiological Integrity/Basic Care and Comfort

(1) Egg custard and boiled liver—high amounts of cholesterol

(2) Fried chicken and potatoes—avoid fried foods

(3) Hamburger and french fries—avoid fried foods

(4) Grilled flounder and green beans—CORRECT: fish instead of meat; increase vegetables

140. The answer is 465

The LPN/LVN is removing a client's breakfast tray and notes that the client consumed 4 oz of pudding, 4 oz of gelatin, 6 1/2 oz of tea, and 5 oz of apple juice. How many milliliters should the LPN/LVN record for the client's breakfast intake?

Reworded Question: Calculate the client's oral fluid intake in mL.

Strategy: Remember what is considered oral fluid intake.

Needed Info: Oral fluid intake: any liquid or food in more solid form that melts at room temperature.

Category: Data Collection/Physiological Integrity/ Basic Care and Comfort

The calculation is 4 oz gelatin + 6½ oz of tea + 5 oz of apple juice = 15½ oz × 30 mL = 465 mL. Pudding does not melt at room temperature, so is not considered to be a liquid and therefore it is not included in the calculation.

The correct answer is 465.

141. The answer is 4

A client comes to the clinic at 32 weeks' gestation. A diagnosis of pregnancy-induced hypertension (PIH) is made. The LPN/LVN is reinforcing teaching performed by the RN. Which statement by the client indicates that further teaching is required?

Reworded Question: What is not accurate about the care of a client with PIH?

Strategy: This is a negative question. Look for incorrect information.

Needed Info: PIH, preeclampsia, toxemia: development of hypertension (increase 30 mmHg systolic or 15 mmHg diastolic) with proteinuria and/or edema (dependent or facial) after 20 weeks' gestation. Risk factors: parity

(first-time mothers), age (younger than 20 or older than 35), geographic location (southern or western United States), multifetal gestation, hydatidiform mole, hypertension, and diabetes. Prevention: early prenatal care, identify high-risk clients, recognize S/S early; bed rest lying on L side, daily weights. Treatment: urine checks for proteinuria; diet (increased protein and decreased Na+). Can develop into eclampsia (convulsions or coma).

Category: Evaluation/Health Promotion and Maintenance

(1) "Lying in bed on my left side is likely to increase my urinary output."—true; bed rest promotes good perfusion of blood to uterus; decreases blood pressure and promotes diuresis

(2) "If the bed rest works, I may lose a pound or two in the next few days."—true; causes diuresis; results in reduction of retained fluids; instruct to monitor weight daily and notify primary health care provider if notices abrupt increase even after resting in bed for 12 hours

(3) "I should be sure to maintain a diet that has a good amount of protein."—true; replaces protein lost in urine; increases plasma colloid osmotic pressure; avoid salty foods; avoid alcohol; drink 8 glasses of water daily; eat foods high in roughage

(4) "I will have to keep my room darkened and not watch much television."—CORRECT: incorrect info, not necessary; diversional activities helpful

142. The answer is 4

The LPN/LVN is collecting data about a client's fluid balance. Which finding **most** accurately indicates to the LPN/LVN that the client has retained fluid during the previous 24 hours?

Reworded Question: How can the LPN/LVN most accurately determine fluid retention?

Strategy: Look at the most conclusive means of determining fluid retention.

Needed Info: Means of evaluating fluid retention: recording fluid intake and output; determining areas of edema especially the sacrum, feet, and ankles; listening for wet lung sounds; and measuring short-term weight gain. Weight gain: most objective and accurate. Weight gain of 2.2 lb (1 kg) is equivalent to 1 L of fluid.

Category: Data Collection/Physiological Integrity/Basic Care and Comfort

(1) Edema is found in both ankles—unable to consistently quantify this form of data

(2) Fluid intake is equal to fluid output—this is normal but does not account for insensible fluid loss through the skin and lungs

(3) Intake of fluid exceeds output by 200 mL—provides information, but does not eliminate the possibility of error recording all intake and output

(4) Weight gain of 4 lb (1.8 kg) is noted—CORRECT: identifies fluid retention in a factual, accurate method and is unlikely to represent a gain of actual body substance (muscle or fat) in a 24-hour time frame

143. The answer is 2

The LPN/LVN is caring for a client diagnosed with bipolar disorder. Which behavior by the client indicates that a manic episode is subsiding?

Reworded Question: What indicates normalizing behavior?

Strategy: Think about the behaviors that indicate mania.

Needed Info: Manic clients may tease, talk, and joke excessively, usually cannot sit to eat and may need to carry fluids and food around in order to eat, often try to take a leadership position in an environment, and try to engage others.

Category: Data Collection/Psychosocial Integrity

(1) The client tells several jokes during a group meeting—reflects an elated mood and no real participation in the meeting; manic clients may tease, talk, and joke excessively

(2) The client sits and talks with other clients at mealtimes—CORRECT: manic clients have difficulty socializing because of flight of ideas and

intrusiveness; usually cannot sit to eat and will carry fluids and food around

(3) The client begins to write a book about personal story—manic clients often write voluminously; may help to express feelings, but does not reflect improvement, especially if thoughts are grandiose

(4) The client initiates a unit effort to start a radio station—manic clients often try to take a leadership position in an environment and try to recruit others

144. The answer is 2

A parent brings a child to the pediatrician for treatment of chronic otitis media. The parent asks the LPN/LVN how to prevent the child from getting ear infections. Which response by the LPN/LVN is **best**?

Reworded Question: What will prevent the development of otitis media? What causes otitis media?

Strategy: Think about the causes of otitis media.

Needed Info: Otitis media: frequently follows respiratory infection; reduce occurrence by holding child upright for feedings, encourage gentle nose-blowing, teach modified Valsalva maneuver (pinch nose, close lips and force air up through eustachian tubes), blow up balloons or chew gum, eliminate tobacco smoke or known allergens.

Category: Planning/Health Promotion and Maintenance

(1) "Cover your child's ears during baths"—does not prevent otitis media

(2) "Treat upper respiratory infections quickly"—CORRECT: respiratory fluids are a medium for bacteria; antihistamines used

(3) "Administer nose drops at bedtime"—not preventative

(4) "Isolate your child from other children"—too extreme a measure

145. The answer is 2

A client is calling the suicide prevention hotline to report a personal suicide plan. Which question should the LPN/LVN ask **first**?

Reworded Question: What is most important to know about a client who has threatened suicide?

Strategy: *"First"* indicates priority.

Needed Info: Signs of suicide: symptoms of depression, client gives away possessions, gets finances in order, has a means, makes direct or indirect statements, leaves notes, increase in energy. Predisposing factors: male over age 50, teenagers between 15–19, poor social attachments, clients with previous attempts, clients with auditory hallucinations, overwhelming precipitating events (terminal disease, death or loss of loved one, failure at school, job).

Category: Data Collection/Psychosocial Integrity

(1) "What happened to cause you to want to end your life?"—does not determine immediate need for safety

(2) "Tell me the details of the plan you developed to kill yourself?"—CORRECT: lets you prioritize interventions to assure safety

(3) "When did you start to feel as though you wanted to die?"—does not determine immediate need for safety

(4) "Do you want me to prevent you from killing yourself?"—yes/no question, closed

146. The answer is 2

Prior to the client undergoing a scheduled intravenous pyelogram (IVP), it would be **most** important for the LPN/LVN to ask which question?

Reworded Question: What do you need to know before an IVP?

Strategy: Think about each answer and how it relates to IVP.

Needed Info: IVP: radiopaque dye injected into the body and is filtered through the kidneys and excreted by the urinary tract. Visualizes kidneys, ureters, and bladder. Preparation: NPO midnight, cathartics evening before test. Injection of dye causes flushing of face, nausea, salty taste in mouth.

Category: Data Collection/Physiological Integrity/ Reduction of Risk Potential

(1) "Do you have any difficulty voiding?"—not most important

(2) "Do you have any allergies to shellfish or iodine?"— CORRECT: anaphylactic reaction; itching, hives, wheezing; treatment: antihistamines, oxygen, cardiopulmonary resuscitation, epinephrine, vasopressor

(3) "Do you have a history of constipation?"—not essential information

(4) "Do you have a history of frequent headaches?"— not most important

147. The answer is 3

A client observes the LPN/LVN in the delivery room place drops in her newborn's eyes. The client asks the LPN/LVN why this was done. Which response by the LPN/LVN is **best**?

Reworded Question: Why are eyedrops placed in a newborn's eyes?

Strategy: "*Best*" indicates that discrimination may be required to answer the question.

Needed Info: Prophylactic care of newborns includes administration of vitamin K to prevent hemorrhage; erythromycin and tetracycline are used for prophylactic eye care.

Category: Implementation/Health Promotion and Maintenance

(1) "The drops constrict your baby's pupils to prevent injury."—erythromycin or tetracycline eye drops do not cause myosis

(2) "The drops will remove mucus from your baby's eyes."—does not remove mucus from baby's eyes

(3) "The drops will prevent infections that might cause blindness."—CORRECT: precaution against opthalmia neonatorum (inflammation of the eyes due to gonorrheal or chlamydia infection)

(4) "The drops will prevent neonatal conjunctivitis."—conjunctivitis is inflammation of the conjunctiva

148. The answer is 3

The LPN/LVN is caring for a client admitted for a possible herniated intervertebral disk. The primary health care provider prescribed ibuprofen, propoxyphene hydrochloride, and cyclobenzaprine hydrochloride to be given as needed for pain. Several hours after admission, the client reports increased discomfort. Which action should the LPN/LVN take **first**?

Reworded Question: What should you do first?

Strategy: Set priorities. Collect data before implementing.

Needed Info: Herniated disk: knifelike pain aggravated by sneezing, coughing, straining.

Category: Planning/Physiological Integrity/Pharmacological Therapies

(1) Give the client ibuprofen to promptly manage the pain—implementation; not first step

(2) Ask the primary health care provider which drug to give first—collect data before implementing

(3) Gather more information from the client about the pain—CORRECT: collect data; first step in nursing process

(4) Allow the client some time to rest to see if the pain subsides—implementation; not first step

149. The answer is 4

A client is transferred to a long-term care facility after a stroke. The client has right-sided paralysis and dysphagia. The LPN/LVN observes an unlicensed assistive personnel (UAP) preparing the client to eat lunch. Which situation would require an intervention by the LPN/LVN?

Reworded Question: What option is wrong?

Strategy: This is a negative question. Determine if you are looking for a correct situation or a problematic situation.

Needed Info: Dysphagia: difficulty swallowing. Provide support if necessary for the head, have the client sit upright, feed the client slowly in small amounts, place food on unaffected side of mouth. Maintain upright position for 30–45 minutes after eating. Good oral care after eating.

Category: Evaluation/Physiological Integrity/ Reduction of Risk Potential

(1) The client remains in bed in the high Fowler position—correct positioning, or may sit in chair

(2) The client's head and neck are positioned slightly forward—correct positioning; helps client chew and swallow

(3) The UAP places food in back of the mouth of unaffected side—helps client handle food

(4) The UAP adds tap water to pudding to help the client swallow—CORRECT: requires intervention, usually able to better handle soft or semi-soft foods; difficulty with liquids

150. The answer is 2, 3 and 4

The LPN/LVN is collecting data and a client's blood pressure is 146/92 mmHg with labored respirations at a rate of of 24 breaths/minute. Bloody drainage appears on the client's IV dressing. The client reports pain in the left hip, depression, and hunger. The LPN/LVN identifies which of these as subjective data? **(Select all that apply.)**

Reworded Question: What data have been reported by the client?

Strategy: Look for client-reported data.

Needed Info: Subjective data: client's perceptions. Objective data: information perceptible to the senses (sight, hearing, touch, smell, taste) or measurable data.

Category: Data Collection/Safe and Effective Care Environment/Coordinated Care

(1) Blood pressure—measurable objective data

(2) Depression—CORRECT: subjective client-reported data

(3) Hip pain—CORRECT: subjective client-reported data

(4) Hunger—CORRECT: subjective client-reported data

(5) IV drainage—measurable objective data

(6) Respirations—measurable objective data

PART FIVE

NCLEX-PN® EXAM RESOURCES

SUMMARY OF CRITICAL THINKING PATHS

The 9 charts in this appendix illustrate different paths you must choose from in order to correctly answer NCLEX-PN® exam questions. The stepping stones stand for steps that you must follow in order to find the correct answer for that question type. Use the chart to refresh your memory with respect to the various steps for each type of question. Tear out this page and refer to it to practice using this book's strategies when answering practice NCLEX-PN® exam-style questions.

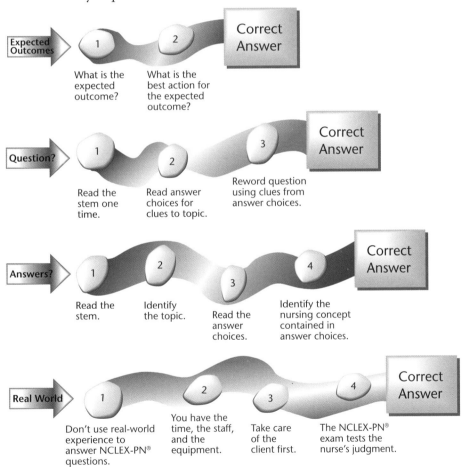

Expected Outcomes
1. What is the expected outcome?
2. What is the best action for the expected outcome?
Correct Answer

Question?
1. Read the stem one time.
2. Read answer choices for clues to topic.
3. Reword question using clues from answer choices.
Correct Answer

Answers?
1. Read the stem.
2. Identify the topic.
3. Read the answer choices.
4. Identify the nursing concept contained in answer choices.
Correct Answer

Real World
1. Don't use real-world experience to answer NCLEX-PN® questions.
2. You have the time, the staff, and the equipment.
3. Take care of the client first.
4. The NCLEX-PN® exam tests the nurse's judgment.
Correct Answer

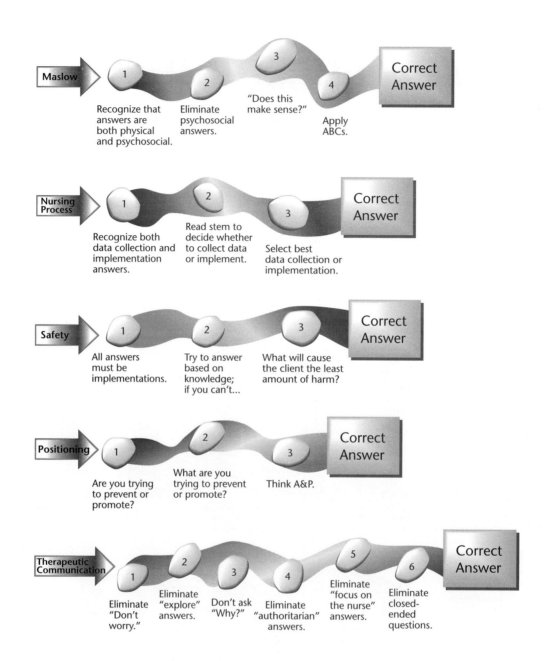

Maslow

1 Recognize that answers are both physical and psychosocial.

2 Eliminate psychosocial answers.

3 "Does this make sense?"

4 Apply ABCs.

Correct Answer

Nursing Process

1 Recognize both data collection and implementation answers.

2 Read stem to decide whether to collect data or implement.

3 Select best data collection or implementation.

Correct Answer

Safety

1 All answers must be implementations.

2 Try to answer based on knowledge; if you can't...

3 What will cause the client the least amount of harm?

Correct Answer

Positioning

1 Are you trying to prevent or promote?

2 What are you trying to prevent or promote?

3 Think A&P.

Correct Answer

Therapeutic Communication

1 Eliminate "Don't worry."

2 Eliminate "explore" answers.

3 Don't ask "Why?"

4 Eliminate "authoritarian" answers.

5 Eliminate "focus on the nurse" answers.

6 Eliminate closed-ended questions.

Correct Answer

NURSING TERMINOLOGY

abduction – movement away from the midline

abraded – scraped

acetonuria – acetone in the urine

adduction – movement toward the midline

afebrile – without fever

albuminuria – albumin in the urine

ambulatory – walking

amenorrhea – absence of menstruation

amnesia – lack of or defective memory

ankylosis – stiff joint

anorexia – lack of appetite

anuria – total suppression of urination

apnea – short periods when breathing has ceased

arthritis – inflammation of joint

asphyxia – suffocation

atrophy – wasting

auscultation, auscultate – to listen for sounds

bradycardia – heart rate lower than 60 beats per minute

Cheyne-Stokes respirations – alternating periods of apnea and hyperventilation

choluria – bile in the urine

conjunctivitis – inflammation of the inner lining of the eyelid (conjunctiva)

copious – large in quantity, abundant

cyanotic – bluish in color due to poor oxygenation

defecation – bowel movement

dental caries – decay of the teeth

dentures – false teeth

diarrhea – excessive or frequent defecation and passage of liquid, unformed feces

diplopia – double vision

distended – appears swollen

diuresis – large amount of urine voided

dorsal recumbent – lying on back, knees flexed and apart

dysmenorrhea – painful menstruation

dyspnea – shortness of breath

dysrhythmia, arrhythmia – abnormal heartbeat

dysuria – painful urination

edematous – puffy, swollen

emaciated – thin, underweight

emetic – agent given to produce vomiting

enuresis – bed-wetting

epistaxis – nosebleed

eructation – belching

erythema – redness

eupnea – normal breathing

excoriation – raw surface

exhibit – an NCLEX question type that includes a client chart or medical record, which becomes visible when the exam candidate clicks an on-screen tab

exophthalmos – abnormal protrusion of eyeball

extension, extend – to straighten

fatigued – tired

feigned – pretended

fetid – foul smelling

fixed – motionless

flaccid – soft, limp, and flabby

flatus, flatulence – expulsion of gas from the digestive tract

flexion – bending

flushed – pink or hot

Fowler position – semierect, knees flexed, head of bed elevated 45–60 degrees

gavage – forced feeding through a tube passed into the stomach

glossy – shiny

glycosuria – glucose in the urine

gustatory – dealing with taste

heliotherapy – using sunlight as a therapeutic agent

hematemesis – blood in vomitus

hematuria – blood in the urine

hemiplegia – paralysis of one side of the body

hemoglobinuria – hemoglobin in the urine

hemoptysis – spitting of blood

horizontal – flat

hydrotherapy – using water as a therapeutic agent

hyperpnea – labored breathing characterized by deep and rapid respirations

hypertonic – concentration greater than body fluids

hypotonic – concentration less than body fluids

infrequent – not often

insomnia – inability to sleep

instillation – pouring into a body cavity

intermittent – starting and stopping, not continuous

intradermal – within or through the skin

intramuscular – within or through the muscle

intraspinal – within or through the spinal canal

intravenous – within or through the vein

involuntary – occurring without conscious control

incontinent – unable to control bladder or bowels

isotonic – having the same tonicity or concentration as body fluids

jackknife position – prone with hips over break in table and feet below level of head

jaundice – abnormal yellowness of the skin or whites of the eyes

knee-chest position – in face-down position resting on knees and chest

kyphosis – humpback, concavity of spine

labored – difficult, requires an effort

lacerated – torn, ragged edged

lateral position – on the side, knees flexed

lithotomy position – on the back, buttocks near edge of table, knees well flexed and separated

lochia – drainage from the vagina after delivery

lordosis – sway-back, convexity of spine

manipulation, manipulate – to handle

menopause – cessation of menstruation

menorrhagia – profuse menstruation

metrorrhagia – variable amount of uterine bleeding at irregular intervals between expected menstrual periods

micturate – to pass urine, urinate

moist – wet

monoplegia – paralysis of one limb

mucopurulent – drainage containing mucus and pus

mydriasis – dilation of pupil

myopia – nearsightedness

myosis – contraction of pupil

nausea – desire to vomit

necrosis – death of tissue

nocturia – frequent voiding at night

obese – overweight

objective – involving verifiable information based on facts and evidence

oliguria – scant urination, less than 400 mL per 24 hours

orthopnea – inability to breathe or difficulty breathing while lying down

palliative – offering temporary relief

pallor – abnormal paleness of the skin

palpation, palpate – to feel with hands or fingers

paraplegia – paralysis of legs

paroxysm – a sudden or violent onset of symptoms (e.g., seizures, atrial fibrillation)

pediculi – lice

pediculosis – lice infestation

percussion, percuss – to strike

persistent – lasting over a long time

petechia – small rupture of blood vessels

photophobia – sensitivity to light

photosensitivity – skin reaction caused by exposure to sunlight

pigmented – containing color

polyuria – excessive voiding of urine

prescription – an order, intervention, remedy, or treatment directed by an authorized health care provider

primary health care provider – a member of the health care team (usually a medical physician, nurse practitioner, etc.) who is licensed and authorized to prescribe for clients

profuse – large in amount

projectile – ejected or projected some distance

pronation – turning downward

prone – on abdomen, face turned to one side

prophylactic – preventative

protruding – extending outward

pruritus – itching

ptosis – drooping eyelid

purulent drainage – drainage containing pus

pyrexia – elevated temperature

pyuria – pus in the urine

radiating – spreading to distant areas

radiotherapy – using x-ray or radium as a therapeutic agent

rales, crackles – abnormal breath sounds

rapid – quick

rhinitis – inflammation of nasal mucosa causing swelling and clear watery discharge

rotation – movement in circular pattern

sanguineous drainage – bloody drainage

scanty – small in amount

semi-Fowler position – semi-erect, head of bed elevated 30–45 degrees

serous drainage – drainage of lymphatic fluid

Sims position – on left side, left arm behind back, left leg slightly flexed, right leg slightly flexed

sprain – wrenching of a joint

stertorous – characterized by snoring

stethoscope – instrument used for auscultation

strabismus – misalignment of visual focus

stuporous – partially unconscious

subcutaneous – under the skin

subjective – involving information that cannot be verified externally (e.g., sensations, opinions, emotions)

sudden onset – started all at once

superficial – on the surface only

supination – turning upward

suppurating – discharging pus

syncope – fainting

syndrome – group of symptoms

tachycardia – fast heartbeat, greater than 100 beats per minute

tenacious – tough and sticky

thready – barely perceptible

tonic tremor – continuous shaking

Trendelenburg position – flat on back with pelvis higher than head, foot of bed elevated 6 inches

urticaria – hives or wheals; eruptions on skin or mucous membranes

vertigo – dizziness

vesicle – fluid-filled blister

visual acuity – sharpness of vision

void – to urinate or pass urine

COMMON MEDICAL ABBREVIATIONS

ABC – airway, breathing, circulation

abd. – abdomen

ABG – arterial blood gas

ABO – system of classifying blood groups

AC – before meals

ACE – angiotensin-converting enzyme

ACS – acute compartment syndrome

ACTH – adrenocorticotrophic hormone

ad lib – freely, as desired

ADH – antidiuretic hormone

ADLs – activities of daily living

AFP – alpha-fetoprotein

AIDS – acquired immunodeficiency syndrome

AKA – above-the-knee amputation

ALL – acute lymphocytic leukemia

ALP – alkaline phosphatase

ALS – amyotrophic lateral sclerosis

ALT – alanine aminotransferase

AMI – antibody-mediated immunity

AML – acute myelogenous leukemia

amt. – amount

ANA – antinuclear antibody

ANS – autonomic nervous system

AP – anteroposterior

A&P – anterior and posterior

APC – atrial premature complexes

aq. – water

ARDS – adult respiratory distress syndrome

ASD – atrial septal defect

ASHD – atherosclerotic heart disease

AST – aspartate aminotransferase

ATP – adenosine triphosphate

AV – atrioventricular

BCG – Bacille Calmette-Guerin

BID – two times a day

BKA – below-the-knee amputation

BLS – basic life support

BMR – basal metabolic rate

BP – blood pressure

BPH – benign prostatic hypertrophy

bpm – beats per minute

BRP – bathroom privileges

BSA – body surface area

BUN – blood urea nitrogen

C – centigrade, Celsius

c̄ – with

Ca – calcium

CA – cancer

CABG – coronary artery bypass graft

CAD – coronary artery disease

CAL – chronic airflow limitations

CAPD – continuous ambulatory peritoneal dialysis

caps – capsules

CBC – complete blood count

CC – chief complaint

CCU – coronary care unit, critical care unit

CDC – Centers for Disease Control and Prevention

CHF – congestive heart failure

CK – creatine kinase

Cl – chloride

CLL – chronic lymphocytic leukemia

cm – centimeter

CMV – cytomegalovirus

CNS – central nervous system

CO – carbon monoxide, cardiac output

CO$_2$ – carbon dioxide

comp – compound

cont – continuous

COPD – chronic obstructive pulmonary disease

CP – cerebral palsy

CPAP – continuous positive airway pressure

CPK – creatine phosphokinase

CPR – cardiopulmonary resuscitation

CRP – C-reactive protein

C&S – culture and sensitivity

CSF – cerebrospinal fluid

CT – computed tomography

CTD – connective tissue disease

CTS – carpal tunnel syndrome

cu – cubic

CVA – cerebrovascular accident or costovertebral angle

CVC – central venous catheter

CVP – central venous pressure

D&C – dilation and curettage

DCBE – double-contrast barium enema

DIC – disseminated intravascular coagulation

DIFF – differential blood count

dil. – dilute

DJD – degenerative joint disease

DKA – diabetic ketoacidosis

dL, dl – deciliter (100 mL)

DM – diabetes mellitus

DNA – deoxyribonucleic acid

DNR – do not resuscitate

DO – doctor of osteopathy

DOE – dyspnea on exertion

DPT – vaccine for diphtheria, pertussis, tetanus

Dr. – doctor

DRE – digital rectal exam

DVT – deep vein thrombosis

D/W – dextrose in water

Dx – diagnosis

ECF – extracellular fluid

ECG, EKG – electrocardiogram

ECT – electroconvulsive therapy

ED – emergency department

EEG – electroencephalogram

EHR – electronic health record

EMD – electromechanical dissociation

EMG – electromyography

ENT – ear, nose, and throat

ERCP – endoscopic retrograde cholangiopancreatography

ESR – erythrocyte sedimentation rate

ESRD – end-stage renal disease

ET – endotracheal tube

F – Fahrenheit

FBD – fibrocystic breast disease

FBS – fasting blood sugar

FDA – U.S. Food and Drug Administration

FFP – fresh frozen plasma

FHR – fetal heart rate

FHT – fetal heart tone

fl – fluid

FOBT – fecal occult blood test

4 × 4 – piece of gauze 4 inches by 4 inches; used for dressings

FSH – follicle-stimulating hormone

ft. – foot, feet (unit of measure)

FUO – fever of undetermined origin

g – gram

GB – gallbladder

GCS – Glasgow Coma Scale

GFR – glomerular filtration rate

GH – growth hormone

GI – gastrointestinal

gr – grain

gtt – drops

GU – genitourinary

GYN – gynecological

h, hrs – hour, hours

Hb, Hgb – hemoglobin

HCG – human chorionic gonadotropin

HCO_3 – bicarbonate

HCP – health care provider

Hct – hematocrit

HD – hemodialysis

HDL – high-density lipoprotein

HF – heart failure

Hg – mercury

HGH – human growth hormone

HHNK – hyperglycemia hyperosmolar nonketotic coma

HIPAA – Health Insurance Portability and Accountability Act

HIV – human immunodeficiency virus

HLA – human leukocyte antigen

H_2O – water

HR – heart rate

HSV – herpes simplex virus

HTN – hypertension

Hx – history

Hz – hertz (cycles/second)

IAPB – intra-aortic balloon pump

IBBP – intermittent positive pressure breathing

IBS – irritable bowel syndrome

ICF – intracellular fluid

ICP – intracranial pressure

ICS – intercostal space

ICU – intensive care unit

I&D – incision and drainage

IgA – immunoglobulin A

IM – intramuscular

I&O – intake and output

IOP – increased intraocular pressure

IPG – impedance plethysmography

IPPB – intermittent positive-pressure breathing

IUD – intrauterine device

IV – intravenous

IVC – intraventricular catheter

IVP – intravenous pyelogram or intravenous pyelography

JRA – juvenile rheumatoid arthritis

K^+ – potassium

kcal – kilocalorie (food calorie)

kg – kilogram

KO, KVO – keep vein open

KS – Kaposi's sarcoma

KUB – kidneys, ureters, bladder

L, l – liter

lab – laboratory

lb – pound

LBBB – left bundle branch block

LDH – lactate dehydrogenase

LDL – low-density lipoprotein

LE – lupus erythematosus

LH – luteinizing hormone

liq – liquid

LLQ – left lower quadrant

LOC – level of consciousness

LP – lumbar puncture

LPN – licensed practical nurse

Ⓛⓣ, Ⓛ – left

LTC – long-term care

LUQ – left upper quadrant

LV – left ventricle

LVN – licensed vocational nurse

m – minum, meter, micron

MAOI – monoamine oxidase inhibitor

MAST – military antishock trousers

mcg – microgram

MCH – mean corpuscular hemoglobin

MCV – mean corpuscular volume

MD – muscular dystrophy, medical doctor

MDI – metered dose inhaler

mEq – milliequivalent

mg – milligram

Mg – magnesium

MG – myasthenia gravis

MI – myocardial infarction

mL, ml – milliliter

mm – millimeter

MMR – vaccine for measles, mumps, rubella

MRI – magnetic resonance imaging

MS – multiple sclerosis

N – nitrogen, normal (strength of solution)

Na^+ – sodium

NaCl – sodium chloride

NANDA – North American Nursing Diagnosis Association

NG – nasogastric

NGT – nasogastric tube

NLN – National League for Nursing

NPO – nothing by mouth (nil per os)

NS – normal saline

NSAID – nonsteroidal anti-inflammatory drug

NSNA – National Student Nurses' Association

NST – non-stress test

O_2 – oxygen

OB-GYN – obstetrics and gynecology

OCT – oxytocin challenge test

OOB – out of bed

OPC – outpatient clinic

OR – operating room

OSHA – Occupational Safety and Health Administration

OTC – over-the-counter (drug that can be obtained without a prescription)

oz – ounce

$\bar{p}$ – with

P – pulse, pressure, phosphorus

PA chest – posterior-anterior chest x-ray

PAC – premature atrial complexes

$PaCO_2$ – partial pressure of carbon dioxide in arterial blood

PACU – postanesthesia care unit

PaO_2 – partial pressure of oxygen in arterial blood

PAD – peripheral artery disease

Pap – Papanicolaou smear

PC – after meals

PCA – patient-controlled analgesia

pCO_2 – partial pressure of carbon dioxide

PCP – *Pneumocystis jiroveci* pneumonia (formerly *Pneumocystitis carinii* pneumonia)

PD – peritoneal dialysis

PE – pulmonary embolism

PEEP – positive end-expiratory pressure

PERRLA – pupils equal, round, react to light and accommodation

PET – postural emission tomography

PFT – pulmonary function test

pH – hydrogen ion concentration

PICC – peripherally inserted central catheter

PID – pelvic inflammatory disease

PIPEDA – Personal Information Protection and Electronic Documents Act

PKD – polycystic disease

PKU – phenylketonuria

PMS – premenstrual syndrome

PND – paroxysmal nocturnal dyspnea

PO, po – (per os) by mouth

pO₂ – partial pressure of oxygen

PPD – positive purified protein derivative (of tuberculin)

PPE – personal protective equipment

PPN – partial parenteral nutrition

PRN, prn – as needed, whenever necessary

pro time – prothrombin time

PSA – prostate-specific antigen

psi – pounds per square inch

PSP – phenolsulfonphthalein

PT – physical therapy, prothrombin time

PTCA – percutaneous transluminal coronary angioplasty

PTH – parathyroid hormone

PTSD – post-traumatic stress disorder

PTT – partial thromboplastin time

PUD – peptic ulcer disease

PVC – premature ventricular contraction

q – every

QA – quality assurance

QID – four times a day

qs – quantity sufficient

R – rectal temperature, respirations, roentgen

RA – rheumatoid arthritis

RAI – radioactive iodine

RAIU – radioactive iodine uptake

RAS – reticular activating system

RBBB – right bundle branch block

RBC – red blood cell or red blood count

RCA – right coronary artery

RDA – recommended dietary allowance

RF – rheumatic fever, rheumatoid factor

Rh – antigen on blood cell indicated by + or –

RIND – reversible ischemic neurologic deficit

RLQ – right lower quadrant

RN – registered nurse

RNA – ribonucleic acid

R/O, r/o – rule out, to exclude

ROM – range of motion (of joint)

RR – respiratory rate

(Rt), (R) – right

RUQ – right upper quadrant

Rx – prescription

s̄ – without

S., Sig. – (Signa) to write on label

SA – sinoatrial node

SaO₂ – systemic arterial oxygen saturation (%)

sat sol – saturated solution

SBE – subacute bacterial endocarditis

SDA – same-day admission

SDS – same-day surgery

S/E – side effects

sed rate – sedimentation rate

SI – International System of Units

SIADH – syndrome of inappropriate antidiuretic hormone

SIDS – sudden infant death syndrome

SL – sublingual

SLE – systemic lupus erythematosus

SMBG – self-monitoring blood glucose

SMR – submucous resection

SNF – skilled nursing facility

SOB – shortness of breath

sol – solution

sp gr – specific gravity

spec. – specimen

SpO₂ – oxygen saturation

SS – soapsuds

S/S, s/s – signs and symptoms

SSKI – saturated solution of potassium iodide

stat – immediately

STD – sexually transmitted disease

subcut – subcutaneous

sx – symptoms

Syr. – syrup

T – thoracic (followed by the number designating specific thoracic vertebra)

T, temp – temperature

T&A – tonsillectomy and adenoidectomy

tabs – tablets

TB – tuberculosis

T&C – type and crossmatch

TED – antiembolitic stockings

TENS – transcutaneous electrical nerve stimulation

TIA – transient ischemic attack

TIBC – total iron binding capacity

TID – three times a day

tinct, tr. – tincture

TLC – total lymphocyte count

TMJ – temporomandibular joint

TPA, t-pa – tissue plasminogen activator

TPN – total parenteral nutrition

TPR – temperature, pulse, respiration

TQM – total quality management

TSE – testicular self-examination

TSH – thyroid-stimulating hormone

tsp. – teaspoon

TSS – toxic shock syndrome

TURP – transurethral prostatectomy

UA – urinalysis

UAP – unlicensed assistive personnel

um – unit of measurement

ung – ointment

URI – upper respiratory tract infection

UTI – urinary tract infection

VAD – venous access device

VDRL – Venereal Disease Research Laboratory (test for syphilis)

VF, Vfib – ventricular fibrillation

VPC – ventricular premature complexes

VS, vs – vital signs

VSD – ventricular septal defect

VT – ventricular tachycardia

WBC – white blood cell or white blood count

WHO – World Health Organization

WNL – within normal limits

wt – weight

INDEX